DISTINGUISHED MEN AND WOMEN OF SCIENCE,
MEDICINE AND THE ARTS

LEEWAY

REACHING BEYOND EXPECTATIONS

DR. K. J. LEE'S JOURNEY FROM THE HIDEOUTS OF PENANG TO HARVARD AND BEYOND

DISTINGUISHED MEN AND WOMEN OF SCIENCE, MEDICINE AND THE ARTS

Additional books and e-books in this series can be found on Nova's website under the Series tab.

DISTINGUISHED MEN AND WOMEN OF SCIENCE,
MEDICINE AND THE ARTS

LEEWAY

REACHING BEYOND EXPECTATIONS

DR. K. J. LEE'S JOURNEY FROM THE HIDEOUTS OF PENANG TO HARVARD AND BEYOND

K. J. LEE

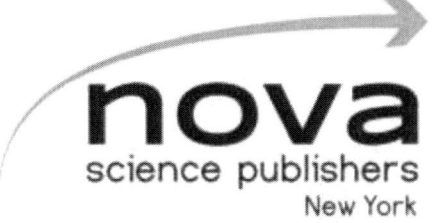

Book front cover designed by Olivia Jang Lee

Copyright © 2020 by Nova Science Publishers, Inc.

All rights reserved. No part of this book may be reproduced, stored in a retrieval system or transmitted in any form or by any means: electronic, electrostatic, magnetic, tape, mechanical photocopying, recording or otherwise without the written permission of the Publisher.

We have partnered with Copyright Clearance Center to make it easy for you to obtain permissions to reuse content from this publication. Simply navigate to this publication's page on Nova's website and locate the "Get Permission" button below the title description. This button is linked directly to the title's permission page on copyright.com. Alternatively, you can visit copyright.com and search by title, ISBN, or ISSN.

For further questions about using the service on copyright.com, please contact:
Copyright Clearance Center
Phone: +1-(978) 750-8400   Fax: +1-(978) 750-4470   E-mail: info@copyright.com.

NOTICE TO THE READER

The Publisher has taken reasonable care in the preparation of this book, but makes no expressed or implied warranty of any kind and assumes no responsibility for any errors or omissions. No liability is assumed for incidental or consequential damages in connection with or arising out of information contained in this book. The Publisher shall not be liable for any special, consequential, or exemplary damages resulting, in whole or in part, from the readers' use of, or reliance upon, this material. Any parts of this book based on government reports are so indicated and copyright is claimed for those parts to the extent applicable to compilations of such works.

Independent verification should be sought for any data, advice or recommendations contained in this book. In addition, no responsibility is assumed by the Publisher for any injury and/or damage to persons or property arising from any methods, products, instructions, ideas or otherwise contained in this publication.

This publication is designed to provide accurate and authoritative information with regard to the subject matter covered herein. It is sold with the clear understanding that the Publisher is not engaged in rendering legal or any other professional services. If legal or any other expert assistance is required, the services of a competent person should be sought. FROM A DECLARATION OF PARTICIPANTS JOINTLY ADOPTED BY A COMMITTEE OF THE AMERICAN BAR ASSOCIATION AND A COMMITTEE OF PUBLISHERS.

Additional color graphics may be available in the e-book version of this book.

Library of Congress Cataloging-in-Publication Data

ISBN: 978-1-53617-894-4

Published by Nova Science Publishers, Inc. † New York

"Leeway" chronicles the life and times of Professor KJ Lee.

Best-known to generations of ENTs world-wide for his renowned *"K.J.Lee's Essential Otolaryngology; Head and Neck Surgery"* - this memoir focuses on lesser-known aspects of the great man's life.

Born in war-torn Malaya in 1940, his early story is one of danger and hardship, overcome by hard-work, tenacity and loving family support. Aged 17, he sets off by cargo ship to Harvard where he's awarded a full tuition scholarship. In the US through continued hard work, ingenuity, perseverance, charm and 'not taking no for an answer', he succeeds not only in his chosen field of Otolaryngology, but goes on to propose solutions for the US healthcare delivery system and become advisor to successive Presidential administrations.

Because the memoir is narrated by three different writers – Sally Hyun Jung Jee, Clementine Xinyi Li and Coco Kejia Ruan, all from Columbia University, the life story takes on a fable-like quality, brimming with humorous anecdotes, honest accounts of trials and set-backs and tips and advice that benefit us all, whatever our chosen field.

ENTs in particular, will be intrigued to hear the surprising back-story to the publication of the *"K.J.Lee's Essential Otolaryngology"* as well as by the fascinating insights into some of the historical 'Greats' in the US Otolaryngology field.

Most of all, what shines through, is the incredible compassion, positivity and humanity that is the truly special character of KJ Lee himself.

A heart-warming read!

Rosaleen Shine
ENT & Audiology News

An inspirational book!

The two most important take aways from this book was the habit of double-checking and making a "to do" list. I think Ahchu's carefulness and double checking are one of the most important habit in the practice of medicine and life in general. After I have read this book, I wanted to appeal to all young readers to embrace this double, triple checking habit into their lives. I am sure that writing a "to do" list every day and checking it frequently is another great habit. It will prevent me from forgetting something sometimes. I feel that this book is so interesting and easy to read and have many lessons to learn from it. By reading this book, young people like me can enhance the aspiration to reach the success in their life. There is no mountain too tall to climb. Make lemonade out of lemons.

Misheelt Batjargal, MD
Health Policy Consultant

In Dr. K.J. Lee's book one walks beside him in the jungle as he is being raised by his grandmother there. It was safer in the jungle during the early 1940's under the Japanese occupation of Malaya than it would have been in a big city. The journey continues as he applies to college in the United States as one of a very few Malayan students. K.J. Lee never leaves any stone unturned. He became a doctor in America active in medical politics with "consumer" patients as his central focus in a not for profit start-up. His life is a mixture of remarkable problem solving intelligence filtered by a strong compassion. I think this remarkable book will appear as an amazing movie seen as a guide to living well and meaningfully.

Benjamin Zucker
Author of multiple books on gems

Dr. K.J. Lee is a true leader, a giant in the field of medicine and also a great businessman with an attitude of gratitude toward his patients, colleagues, and friends.

By reading his book, we learn about his many contributions, his hard work, his leadership and expertise. Many of us who have been fortunate to know him, know that he always practiced what he is trying to convey in this book to the new generation of professionals. He practiced what he preaches today.

Alfonso Panico
Former Honorary Consul of the Republic of Italy
for the State of Connecticut

Doctor K.J. Lee's memoir, "Leeway" is a must read! With an authentic desire to help others, Dr. Lee has devoted his life to supporting people on their healing path. Woven within the pages of this transformative book, you'll discover the love of God and family, secrets of success, and genuine compassion that are outlined with humor and honesty. I wholeheartedly recommend this book.

Catherine Galasso-Vigorito
Nationally Syndicated Columnist and
Best-Selling Author of
God Will do the Rest and The Open Window

Dr. Lee's memoir is an inspiring tale about a boy with a mind of determination like no other to make his dreams a reality. It is about how a boy with a brilliant mind came from nothing and pushed himself to be a ground-breaking doctor. Even with the success he gained for himself he never forgot where he came from, he never forgot that sense of determination, he recognized failure, he never lost heart, which helped form him into the doctor that does what's best for his patients and those around him. Dr. Lee and his story are a great example to everyone to never forget who you are, to always look out for the best well-being of others, and to never give up.

Elisa Palmieri
Physician Assistant Student

This memoir is dedicated to God, K.J.'s parents, Linda's parents, Linda, Ken, Susan, Lloyd, Chieko, Mark, Jennica, Morgan, Olivia, Mason, Juliet and Elias.

CONTENTS

Foreword — xv
Polly Chester

Preface and Acknowledgments — xvii
K. J. Lee

Introduction — xix
Keyu Liu

Chapter 1   The Lemons of His Life   1
Clementine Xinyi Li

Chapter 2   Don't Take No for an Answer   11
Coco Kejia Ruan

Chapter 3   Father and Son   19
Clementine Xinyi Li

Chapter 4   Departure for a New World   25
Sally Hyun Jung Jee

Chapter 5   The Ferncliff   31
Sally Hyun Jung Jee

Chapter 6   Space Race and the Race of Life   37
Clementine Xinyi Li

Chapter 7	Broken Cars and Broken Dreams, Everyone's Hero *Clementine Xinyi Li*	51
Chapter 8	Surprise after Surprise *Coco Kejia Ruan*	59
Chapter 9	The Trip Where Everything Went Wrong *Clementine Xinyi Li*	63
Chapter 10	Off Guard *Coco Kejia Ruan*	71
Chapter 11	Have I Met You Before? *Coco Kejia Ruan*	77
Chapter 12	'K.J.' Was Coined *Coco Kejia Ruan*	85
Chapter 13	Residency *Sally Hyun Jung Jee*	119
Chapter 14	The Army *Sally Hyun Jung Jee*	129
Chapter 15	K. J. Lee's Essential Otolaryngology *Sally Hyun Jung Jee*	135
Chapter 16	The Man from Timbuktu *Sally Hyun Jung Jee*	143
Chapter 17	The Items He Left Behind *Sally Hyun Jung Jee*	149
Chapter 18	"Dr. Lee, Please Pray before You Operate" *Coco Kejia Ruan*	159
Chapter 19	K. J.'s Cardinal Rules *Coco Kejia Ruan*	167
Chapter 20	It Does Not Have to End This Way *Clementine Xinyi Li*	175

Chapter 21	Appreciate Strengths and Manage Weaknesses *Coco Kejia Ruan*	**181**
Chapter 22	Untangling the Healthcare Web *Clementine Xinyi Li*	**189**
Chapter 23	The Patient Is U Foundation, Inc. *Sally Hyun Jung Jee*	**195**
Chapter 24	Postscript	**209**
Appendix 1.	A Selection of the Lee Family's Christmas Cards (1966-Present) *Cards designed by Linda Lee*	**223**
Appendix 2.	Articles by DoctorLee	**229**
Appendix 3.	Patient Handouts	**333**
Index		**355**

FOREWORD

Polly Chester

K.J. Lee is a world-renowned otolaryngologist and head and neck surgeon. Born in Malaya in 1940, he travelled to Harvard on a scholarship in 1958 and went on to make an indelible contribution to his chosen medical specialty. In this memoir, he shares his incredible story, from his childhood in war-torn Malaya to his personal and professional success in the U.S.A. In his usual spirit of encouraging and supporting the development of junior colleagues, Dr. Lee has chosen to tell his story through three Columbia University writers – Sally Hyun Jung Jee, Clementine Xinyi Li and Coco Kejia Ruan. Their own education and background have enabled them to fully understand and appreciate his story and communicate it to you, the reader, in the words and style of K.J. himself. Leeway is a tale of hard work and perseverance, positivity and forward thinking, love and family, and above all, success against the odds. As K.J. himself says, "When life gives you lemons, always, always make lemonade."

PREFACE AND ACKNOWLEDGMENTS

K. J. Lee

"With God, all things are possible" — Matthew 19:26

"God helps those who help themselves."

I am thankful for and humbled by the story the writers have penned in this 'memoir'. They have chronicled the simple life of an ordinary boy from childhood to near retirement, as well as capturing his concerns and vision for solutions in the US healthcare delivery system. Polly Chester did a great job as Editorial Consultant. Heather Pownall, Publishing Consultant, efficiently managed the publishing process from beginning to end. Jeannie Grenier, my Editorial Assistant for many of my publications over the last 35 years, delivered her usual high-quality work.

I give thanks to our Creator and my parents for their DNA and for my upbringing: nature and nurture. My beloved, devoted wife of 54 years has been my constant companion, best friend and advisor. Our three sons have not only made me proud but have contributed humor, ideas and solutions to my projects. We chat several times a week and I take great pleasure from my relationship with them, our daughters-in-law and our grandchildren. I thank Olivia Jang Lee for designing the front cover of Leeway.

Contributing Authors – Columbia University writers:

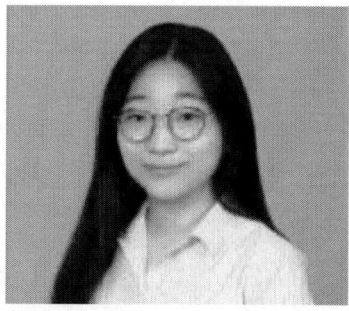

Sally Hyun Jung Jee.

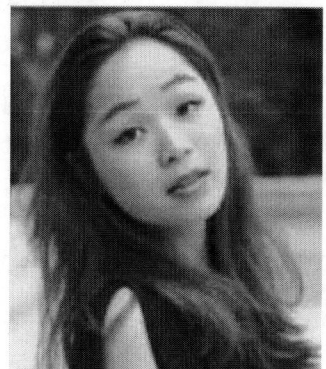

Clementine Xinyi Li.

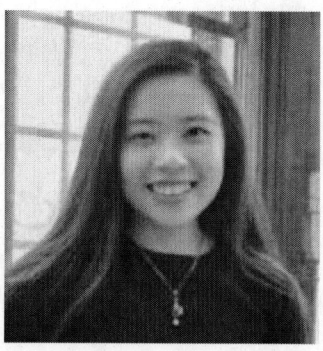

Coco Kejia Ruan.

INTRODUCTION

Keyu Liu

"His achievements can be matched by any ordinary, industrious young person."

Among the various principles and lessons Dr. K.J. Lee carries with him, there is one quite literally close to his heart. In his left blazer pocket is a pen with a ballpoint on one end and a light on the other. Along the side of the pen is a line by Hippocrates, the ancient Greek Father of Medicine who established medicine as a profession around 400 BC: "Cure sometimes, treat often, comfort always." As one of the core objectives behind The Patient Is U Foundation, Inc. (TPIU), co-founded by Dr. Lee, Hippocrates' words encapsulate the essence of medical practice, a standard that Dr. Lee adopts in his own practice during his decades of work as an ENT doctor.

The lives that have been changed under these principles of practice can be weaved into an anthology. Karen has been a patient of K.J. since her late teens in the early 1980s. She suffered from perforated eardrums as a young child, which caused her to have chronic ear and sinus infections. Karen's condition required surgery accompanied by various medical treatments. She came across K.J. when he was practicing at New Haven, and he swiftly delivered his diagnosis and treatment plan. Now in her 60s, Karen shares her gratefulness for the decades of medical care she received from K.J., and her awe at the depth of attention K.J. devoted to her case: "I have never heard of another doctor who does this, but his discharge paper far exceeds the typical format. He printed out specific information on what to expect before and after my surgery, what would be normal, what would not be normal, and what to do when a list of possible symptoms occurred."

The magic underlying effective patient care is simply the ability to feel and understand the pain of those being treated. K.J.'s own childhood could hardly be described as smooth sailing, but rather one that tasted the saltiness of a tumultuous ocean. He contracted malaria and parasitic diseases as an infant and toddler. Having suffered from chronic ear infections, facial paralysis, and undergone the resulting surgery, K.J. knows. He knows that the effects of a physical implication influence not only the body, but the mind. Those aspects of life that are impeded by a health condition trouble the physical and, sometimes more drastically, the social environment one lives in.

If there were one thing that K.J. would wish each of his patients to feel after his diagnosis and treatment, it would be trust. To lay one's own health in the hands of another is an action that takes substantial faith and confidence. K.J. strived to earn this with every patient from the moment he introduced himself with the words, "Nice to meet you, I am Dr. K.J. Lee."

Carol did not feel that trust when she had her ears checked at 28-years-old. Her doctor told her she had undeveloped eardrums and needed surgery. Even now, she can distinctly recall that day and the fear accompanying the uncertainty of her future health. "When my first doctor reappeared, he brought another doctor, who smiled, sat down, and with a reassuring voice said to me, 'Don't worry, I will take care of it.'" For Carol, it was the beginning of a long, trusting friendship with Dr. Lee. The procedure went smoothly. K.J. adeptly took a piece of tissue from the back of Carol's ear (the fascia) to build a new eardrum. Carol, now 73, remembers this encounter more than four decades ago with deep appreciation, not only for the swift procedure that K.J. elegantly performed, but for the kindness, attention, and reassurance he offered which consoled Carol throughout.

Introduction

Upon hearing that Dr. Lee had retired a few years ago, Carol was brought to tears. "All these years, I have regarded Dr. Lee as a brilliant doctor and a true friend. What makes him remarkable is not just his expertise, but that he never loses sight of small acts of kindness. I was sad that a doctor like him had left the field."

Carol need not worry, K.J. would say. He hopes that future generations of medical students, interns, and residents will continue to practice the same level of expertise, and adhere to his code of practice. K.J. Lee's *Essential Otolaryngology-Head and Neck Surgery* welcomed its 12th and 45th anniversary edition in the spring of 2019[1]. The book is well-known as a must-read for prospective ENT doctors taking the Board Exam. The book has witnessed and documented tremendous growth in the field of ENT in the latter half of the last century until now, propelled by many esteemed doctors whose dedication has made ENT-Head and Neck Surgery the renowned field it is today.

At the American Academy of Otolaryngology-Head and Neck Surgery 2017 convention in Chicago, K.J. was awarded the Presidential Citation for the third time. As he looks back on his decades as an ENT doctor, K.J. recognizes the invaluable contributions from numerous dedicated colleagues in the same field. In the 1960s, an ENT doctor was not permitted to perform neck dissection, parotid or thyroid surgery. Dr. Stuart Strong, an esteemed Head and Neck Surgery practitioner, recalls how ENT was viewed as "a field for the dropouts" and that a thyroid tumor was recorded as "a lump in the neck." K.J. also remembers his initial embarrassment when announcing his chosen specialty at the academic year end dinner at St. Luke's Hospital in 1967. He mumbled quickly that he was heading to Harvard for Head and Neck Surgery, with no one at the event even recognizing the name of the specialty which he unknowingly coined. There was no such specialty then, but today the specialty is known as otolaryngology-head and neck surgery worldwide.

Over the past five decades, fields including laryngology, pediatric otolaryngology, plastic surgery and sleep medicine have undergone

---

[1] K.J. Lee, "KJ Lee's Essential Otolaryngology, 12th Edition," eds. Y. Chan, J. C. Goddard, McGraw-Hill Education, 2019.

tremendous growth and integration into the collective specialty of Otolaryngology-Head and Neck Surgery. Dr. Eugene Meyers recounted the "battle of ownership" between the American Society for Head and Neck Surgery, established in 1958 by ENT doctors, and the Society of Head and Neck Surgeons, founded in 1954 by general surgeons[2]. Head and Neck practices were not initially considered as part of the ENT specialty, and it was only through gradual improvements in surgical training that ENT doctors gained the respect of general surgeons. The two associations finally merged as the American Head and Neck Society in 1998.

Breakthroughs such as the development of cochlear implants by Dr. William House, refined stapedectomy by Dr. Howard House, skull base surgeries by Dr. Derald Brackmann and others likewise propelled the growth of Otolaryngology-Head and Neck Surgery. K.J.'s own groundbreaking research papers, 'Results of Tympanoplasty and Mastoidectomy at the Massachusetts Eye and Ear Infirmary'[3] and 'The Sublabial Transseptal Transsphenoidal Approach to the Hypophysis'[4] in 1971 and 1978 likewise contributed to ear and pituitary surgical practices. And the future of the specialty is bright. As Dr. Pablo Stolovitzky remarked, the American Academy of Otolaryngology- Head and Neck Surgery has expanded on an international scale to further spread the worldwide influence of the field of ENT[5].

K.J. feels deeply honored to have witnessed such transformation. Following his retirement, he has continued to update *Essential Otolaryngology* to its current version, while advocating for patients through the TPIU foundation. ENT practitioners attending the Chicago convention paid tribute to K.J.'s contribution to the field. However, when asked if they had any questions, many of them humorously inquired if K.J. had any free

---

[2] K.J. Lee, "KJ Lee's Essential Otolaryngology, 12th Edition," eds. Y. Chan, J. C. Goddard, McGraw-Hill Education, 2019.

[3] K.J. Lee, H. F. Schuknecht, "Results of Tympanoplasty and Mastoidectomy at the Massachusetts Eye and Ear Infirmary," *The Laryngoscope*, vol. 81, no. 4 (1971): 529-543. Available at: https://onlinelibrary.wiley.com/doi/10.1288/00005537-197104000-00004.

[4] K.J. Lee, "The Sublabial Transseptal Transsphenoidal Approach to the Hypophysis," *The Laryngoscope*, vol. 88, no. 7 (S10) (1978).

[5] K.J. Lee, "KJ Lee's Essential Otolaryngology, 12th Edition," eds. Y. Chan, J. C. Goddard, McGraw-Hill Education, 2019.

time from work, and what he did during that spare time. While mostly known for his extraordinary work ethic among fellow ENT doctors, K.J.'s life as an international student in the 1950s, his family background, and the personal experiences that made him the man he is today remained an untold story, until now.

This book is a tale of K.J., not only as an ENT doctor, but first as a Malaysian student, then a medical student, a husband, a father, and above all, as someone who wishes to cure, to contribute to a healthier world, and to turn his experiences into stories and lessons that may be shared with future generations. This is the memoir of an ordinary, hard-working boy who has always been guided by principles of common sense. His success can be achieved by any ordinary, industrious young person. At a New Haven Medical Economic Development event in the summer of 2017, my family and I were fascinated to hear about K.J.'s wish to transform his experiences into a biographical work. I was able to introduce him to three of my peers who shared my passion to turn this project into reality, Clementine Li, Coco Ruan, and Sally Jee. Through the work of these dedicated writers, whose tireless interviews, drafting and editing have resulted in the book as it prints today, the life story of Dr. K.J. Lee reveals itself at last.

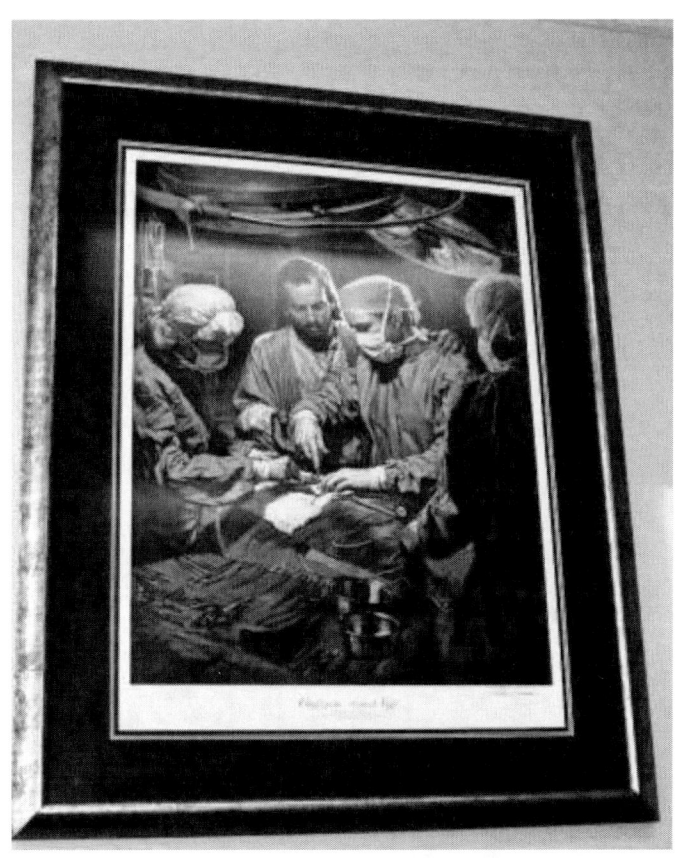

Image 1. *Chief of the Medical Staff* by Nathan Greene, which K.J. first saw a version of in the Aventis Hospital, Penang Malaya, 1954. A print hangs in his office. (Chapter 18).

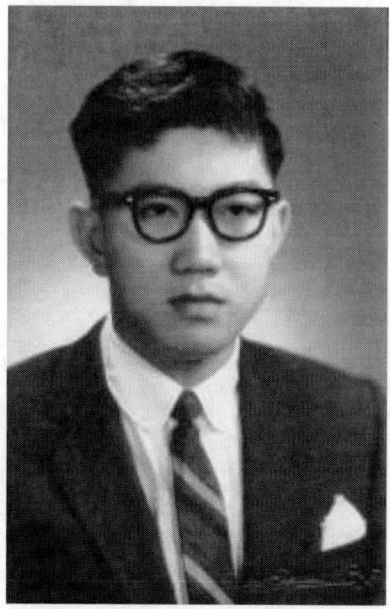

Image 2. K.J. Lee pictured in the Harvard freshman yearbook, 1958. (Chapter 6).

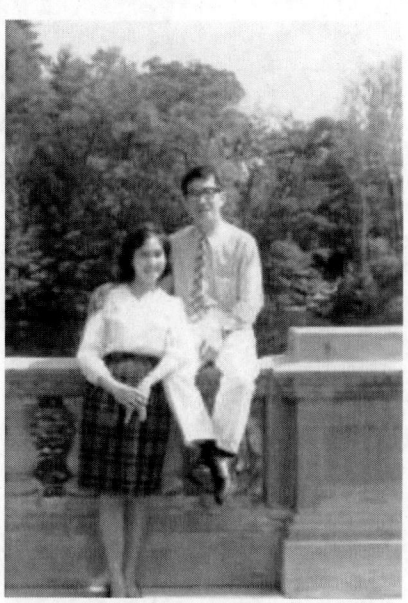

Image 3. Courting Linda at Cloisters, New York, Spring 1966.

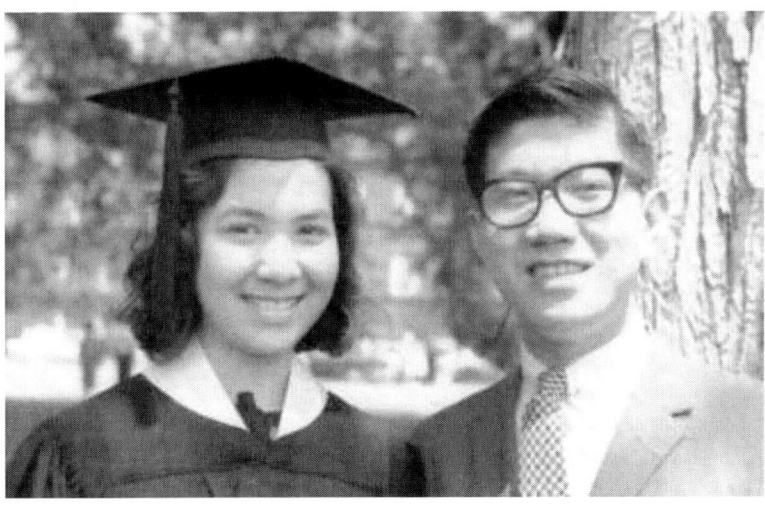

Image 4. Linda's graduation at Vassar, June 1966.

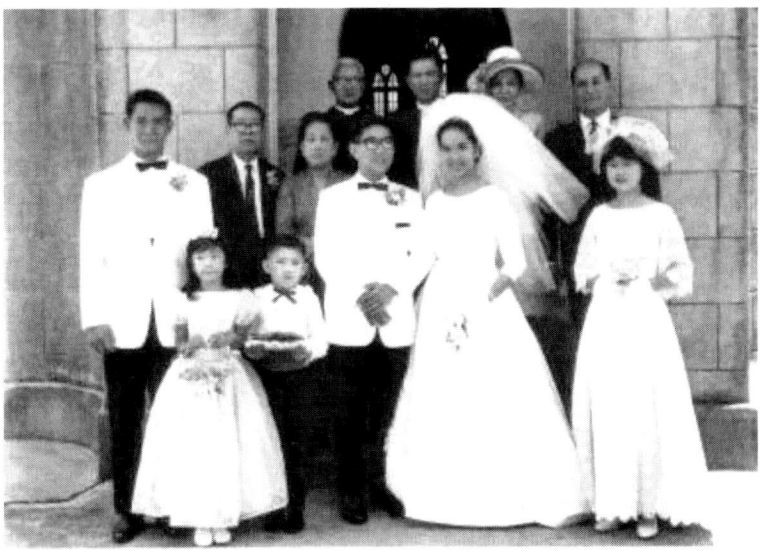

Image 5. K.J. Lee and Linda's wedding, 20 August 1966. The wedding party pictured in front of Madras Lane Methodist Church, Penang, Malaysia.

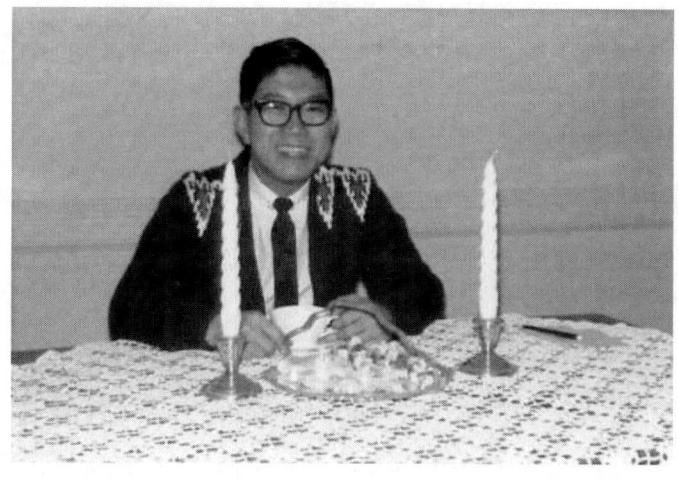

Image 6. K.J. in 1966 wearing the first sweater Linda knitted for him, and he still wears it now!

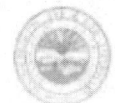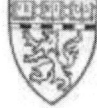

Image 7. K.J. Lee's Harvard Medical School residency graduation diploma from 1970. (Chapter 13).

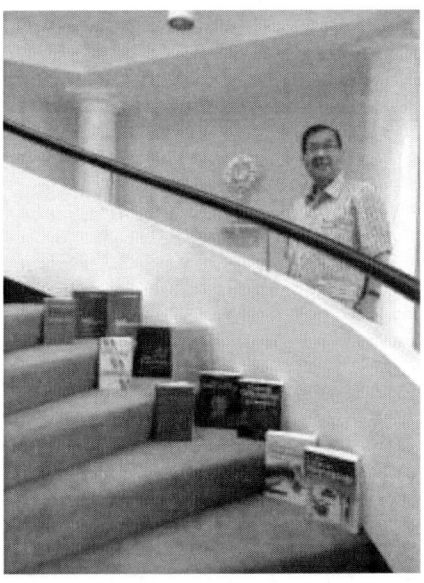

Image 8. K.J. pictured with all the editions published to date of *Essential Otolaryngology-Head & Neck Surgery*. (Chapter 15).

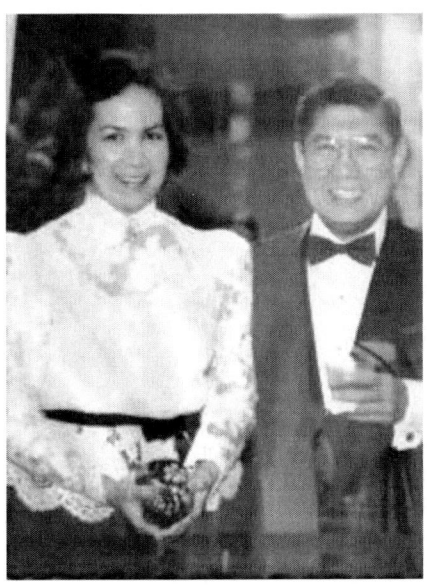

Image 9. K.J. and Linda pictured at the Hospital of St. Raphael gala dinner in the eighties.

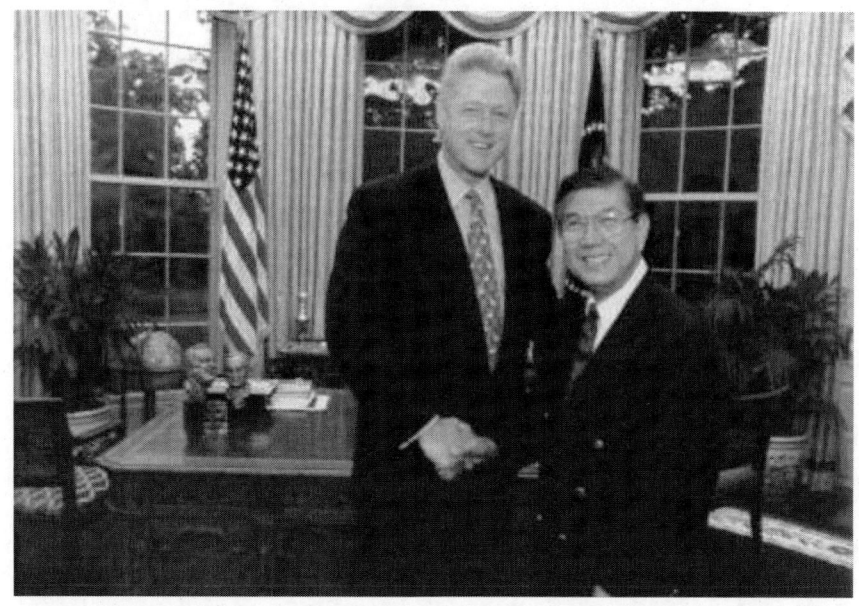

Image 10. K.J. and Bill Clinton in the oval office in 2001. (Chapter 22).

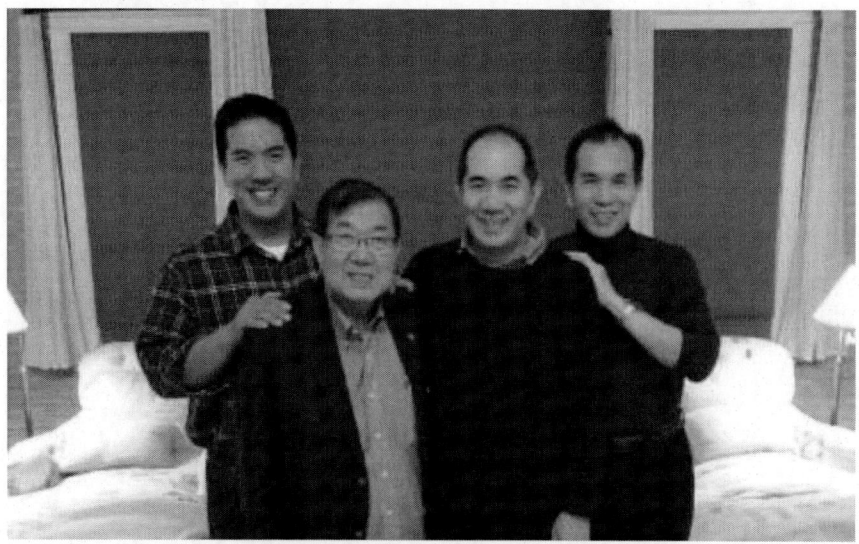

Image 11. K.J. and his sons in Ken's country home, 2017.

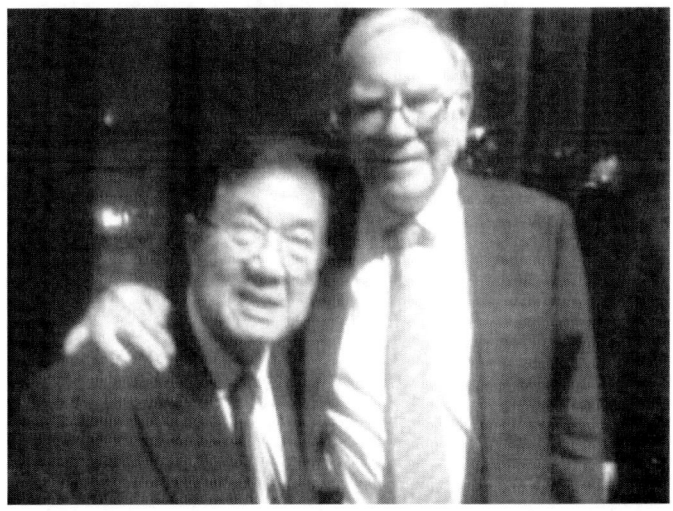

Image 12. K.J. with Warren Buffet, 2011.

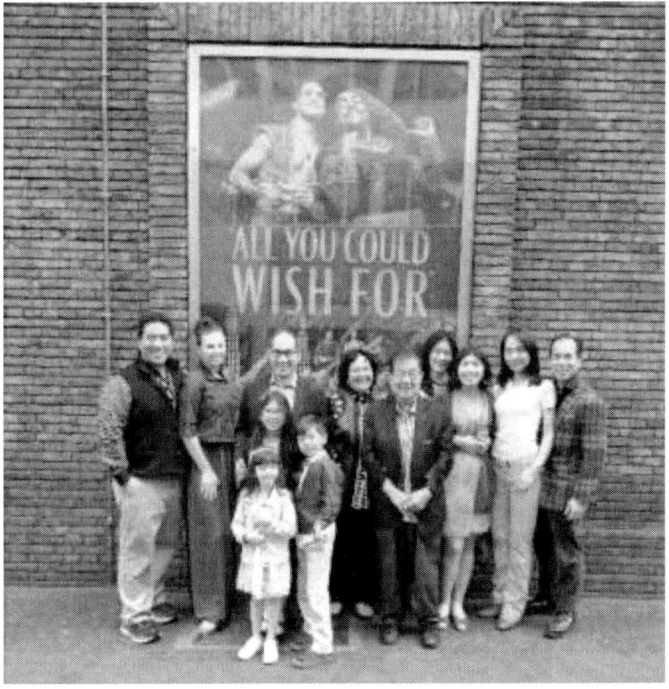

Image 13. Family trip to London, 2018.

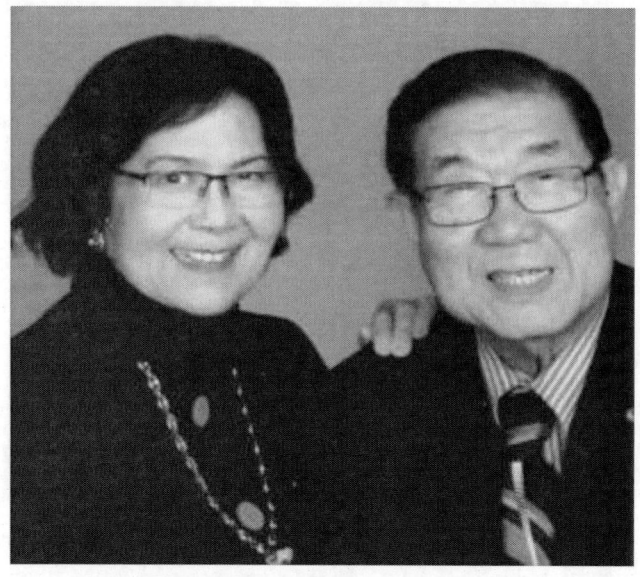

Image 14. Dr. and Mrs. Lee, pictured in the 2018 handbook of their Church.

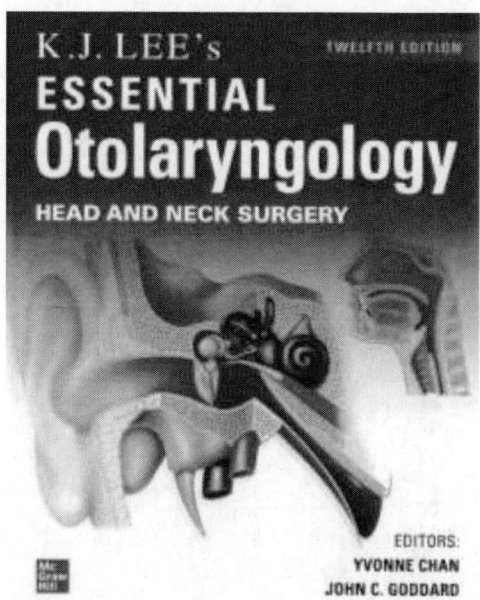

Image 15. K.J. Lee's *Essential Otolaryngology*, widely considered to be one of the most widely-read texts in the field around the world. (Chapter 15).

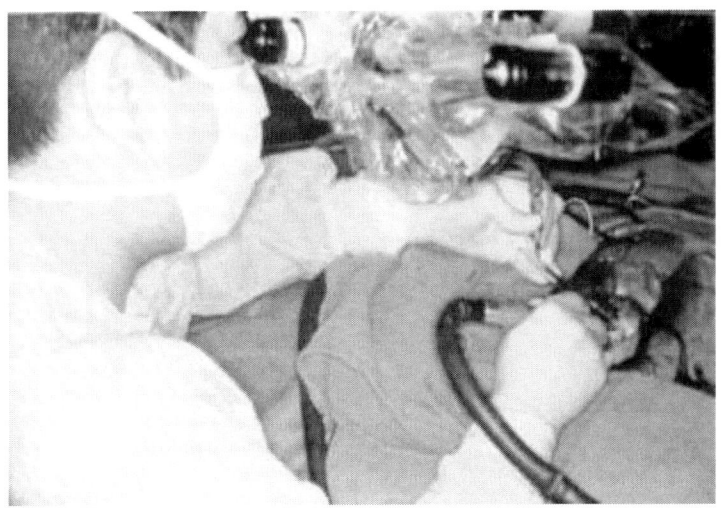

Image 16. K.J. performing an operation in 1973.

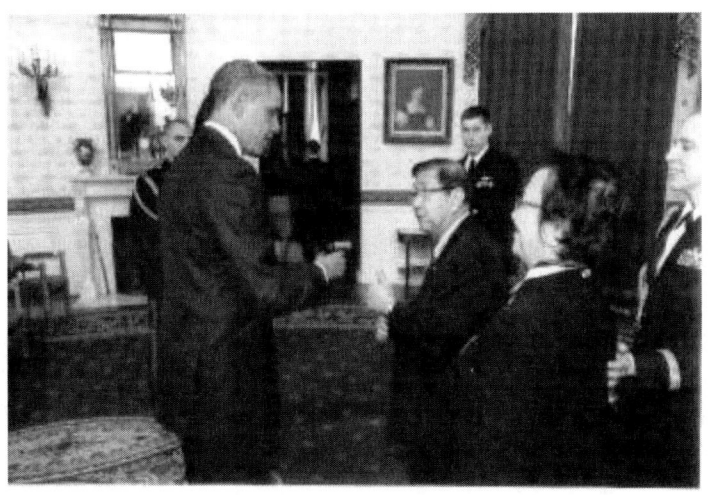

Image 17. K.J. and Linda at the White House, 2010.

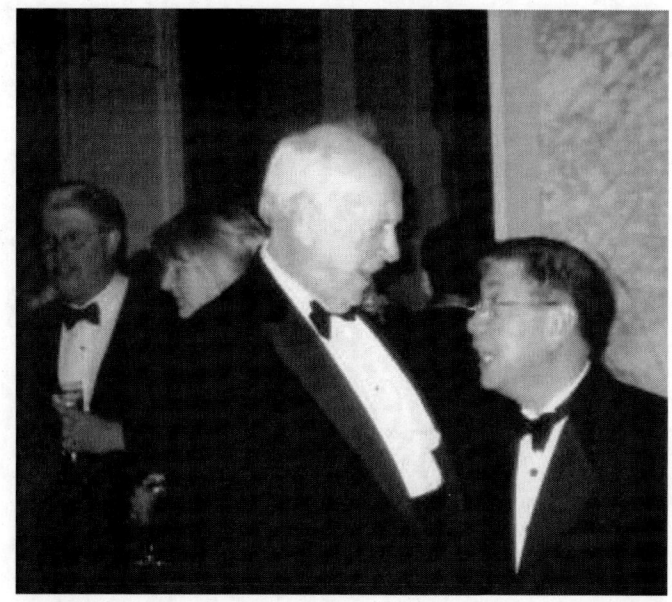

Image 18. K.J. and Professor Watson, who discovered DNA.

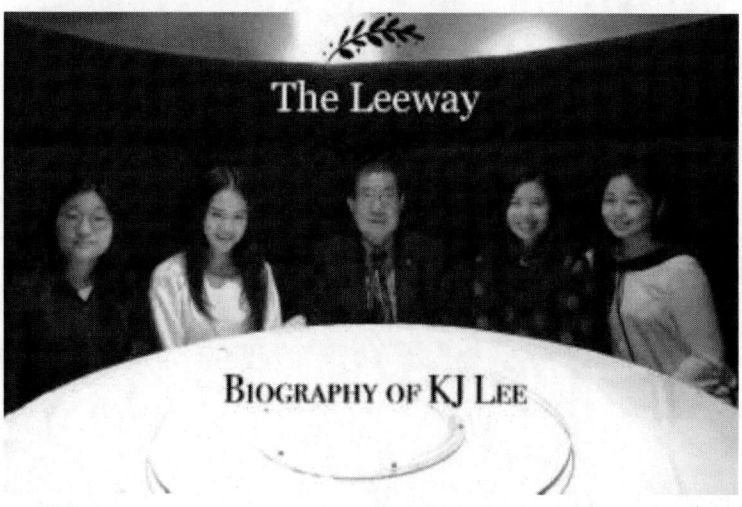

Image 19. The authors of Leeway with Dr. Lee. [L-R] Sally Hyun Jung Lee, Keyu Liu, K.J. Lee, Coco Kejia Ruan and Clementine Xinyi Li.

Chapter 1

THE LEMONS OF HIS LIFE

Clementine Xinyi Li

"Make lemonade out of lemons."

We've all heard the saying, "when life gives you lemons…" It's one that K.J. Lee, known in his younger days as Ahchu, repeats often with a keen-witted, confident smile, as someone who knows how to deal with whatever challenges life presents.

A lemon can be defining. Sucking on the sour juice hurts your teeth and acidifies your dreams, until your subsequent life is merely an extended, latent bitterness. Or, you may throw that lemon back in life's face and grow another fruit of choice. Maybe you are fortunate enough to not have been given lemons at all. None of this was true for Ahchu. In his world it had never been about the bitterness of certain life experiences. It was about redefining and learning from those experiences. This is a story about a man given more than his fair share of lemons who invented his own brand of lemonade.

Ahchu arrived in this world in 1940, a pivotal point in the history of the 20th Century. You might say his timing was bad. In 1939 Nazi Germany's territorial ambitions in Poland finally ignited Europe into war. In 1941 America also entered into one of the deadliest conflicts in human history. In the Lee family's corner of the world, a year after Ahchu's birth and mere hours before the bombing of Pearl Harbor, the Japanese arrived in Kota Bahru, British Malaya.[6] Within two months, the Imperial Army and their *kyokujitsu-ki*— Rising Sun Flags— had saturated the entirety of Malaya, coloring the land with the redness of their flags and the blood of local anti-Japanese sympathizers. Thus, Ahchu first encountered the world and its people at their worst.

It was a grand setting for a tumultuous childhood. War ravaged the country, entering the doors of each ordinary household. In the Lee family's case, the war split them in half: the parents remaining in their city-center bicycle repair shop, while the three young children fled with their grandmother to the tropical jungle of Southeast Asia, hiding from the Japanese soldiers.

Deep in the jungle and the safety of their woody tropical shelters, Ahchu's grandmother needed to exploit all her wit and resourcefulness to

---

[6] "The history of British involvement in Malaya goes back to 1786, when the East India Company established a trading post on Penang Island. Sir Stamford Raffles founded a British settlement on the island of Singapore in 1819 and by 1830 the British Straits Settlements also included Malacca. From the 1870s the sultans of the small Malay states began accepting British 'advisers', who were effectively rulers. In 1896 a federation of Negri Sembilan, Perak, Selangor and Pahang was established with its capital at Kuala Lumpur. Heavy immigration from China and India was encouraged to supply labor for British rubber plantations and tin mines.

Invading from the north, the Japanese rapidly overran Malaya and took Singapore in 1942. After the war, in 1948, a Federation of Malaya was created under British protection, but British and Commonwealth troops had to put down a Communist insurrection, which lasted into the early 1950s. It was by now agreed that Malayan independence was the answer to the Communist claim that they were fighting to free the Malayan people from the British yoke. An election in 1955 was won hands-down by the United Malay National Organisation (UMNO) by running Malay candidates in Malay-dominated areas, Chinese candidates in Chinese areas and Indian candidates in Indian ones. The UMNO's leader Tunku Abdul Rahman became prime minister when the independent Federation of Malaya came into being in 1957...

The federation was renamed Malaysia in 1963, when besides Singapore and all the Malay states it also included two areas in North Borneo – Sarawak and Sabah. Singapore opted out and went its own way in 1965."

Richard Cavendish, "Malayan Independence," *History Today*, vol. 57, no. 8 (2007): available at https://www.historytoday.com/archive/malayan-independence#comment-0 [last accessed 31 March 2019].

invent such games that would distract the children from missing their parents, or asking too many questions about the ongoing, bloody war. Ahchu remembers, "There wasn't much to do in the jungles and we hardly had enough for food, let alone toys. My grandmother, to keep me entertained and distracted from the fact that there was a war going on, would play the game of the rice merchant with my sisters and I."

Young Ahchu played the merchant, while his grandmother and two older sisters acted as his 'customers' from different villages. The little rice merchant would mount his makeshift horse— a pillow between his legs— and happily ride from village to village trading his goods. "Lady, lady, would you like a *katie* of rice?" he politely inquired (*katie* was the Malayan unit of measure). "Oh, maybe not today, Whan Chu. I don't want a *katie* of rice today," his grandmother answered. Whan Chu meant 'sweet potato'. Superstition had it that if the evil gods knew there was a male child in the family, they might come and take him away. To fool the gods, parents would create a nickname for their son, *Ah Too* (pig), *Ah Kow* (dog) or *Whan Chu* (sweet potato). Whan Chu was shortened to Ahchu. His official name is Keat Jin Lee, or following the Chinese rule of putting the family name first: Lee Keat Jin.

"Are you sure? I have my last three sacks left, if you want to buy them, I'll give you half price! Or I could always come back tomorrow." In this way, Ahchu would visit each of his three customers, until everyone received their desired amount of rice at a reasonable price. Then, the little merchant would go 'home', with sacks 'emptied' of rice and 'filled' with coins, having made everyone happy through compromises and deal-making. Ahchu's definition of a good deal seems to have found its roots in this game: where all parties could proclaim victory, and at the same time believe they could have done better. Ahchu credits his grandmother and his two elder sisters for this early training in business.

That plot of Malayan jungle fostered the very beginnings of Ahchu's talent for negotiation and business, which grew and flourished during the course of his life. As an adult, his goods of choice changed from imaginary rice to modest real estate, start-up software companies and consulting firms, and his pool of customers expanded from his immediate family to buyers all over the globe. His early learning was not confined to the time he spent hiding in the jungle during the Japanese occupation. During his teens, his father brought him along to business meetings. His mother also had good business instincts and a strong moral compass, despite her lack of education, formal or otherwise.

That little rice merchant would one day (thanks to modern technology) simultaneously sit at four separate negotiating tables in four different time zones. These meetings overflowed with numbers, facts and interests at stake— but Ahchu did not even need to use notes. With his nimble mind he was more than able to keep track of the immense flow of information, and make swift, accurate decisions. Working alone and moving between different sets of negotiators while they considered his terms, Ahchu would remain as cool as a cucumber, showing no signs of stress or fatigue. He would only express frustration when he felt another party was behaving irrationally, although even this may have seemed like part of his negotiation strategy,

Ahchu's family was not one to give into circumstance. He and his siblings were the champions of the most exciting game of their childhood, affectionately known as 'inner city sports'. A game that had both a functional and an entertainment factor. Old Malayan houses at this time were typically infested with pests, most notably food stealing, pipe-chewing rats the size of small cats, with menacing little red eyes and an all-encompassing hunger. In the Lee household, when someone spotted a rat, they would yell "Aha!" Everyone would stop what they were doing, usually studying, and the game of 'inner city sports' would commence. Ahchu and his siblings would hurriedly bar the gates, the windows, every possible escape route for the unfortunate creature, and begin chasing the rat with broomsticks, pans, or whatever was at hand. You might compare them to English dignitaries hunting deer or foxes across open fields with packs of hounds and glistening shotguns. It was the sole source of entertainment during evenings without television or neighborhood children to play with.

From the game of the rice merchant as a young child and the sport of rat hunting as a pre-teen, to the greater, far more complex game of life, Ahchu showed that the most important rules of the game were those that were fair to all parties involved. A war in Malaya didn't stop him from enjoying his childhood, nor from fostering the necessary skills to become a skillful surgeon and entrepreneur. In life, a hectic schedule only pushed him to do more, achieve more, in spite of the constraints of time, geography, and resources.

The three Lee children lived quietly in an invaded country. Beyond the limits of their lives, unimaginable horror was present in Malaya. Ahchu's family was ethnically Chinese, and during this time the Japanese secret police, *Kenpeitai*, took away more than 50,000 lives, in what would be known as the Sook Ching massacre— 'the purging of ethnic Chinese', when the burning racial hatred of countries at war birthed monsters in men's skin. In every city, schools, prisons, and office buildings were converted into detention and execution centers and Chinese Malayans were targeted most of all. Ironically, the imperial armies had launched a propaganda campaign promoting "Asia for the Asiatics" to justify their occupation of Malaya and gain local peoples' trust. These "Asiatic" posters covered every wall, stained with Asian blood.

None of this reached the small sphere inhabited by the Lee children. Their grandmother, in possession of nothing but a lifetime of wisdom and a maternal fierceness, preserved and defended a haven safe from the imperial forces; the inhumanity, the blood-stained flags of another man's war. Cultivating talents useful to her grandchildren in later life, and most importantly cultivating kindness, she raised children of peace in a time of war.

Though a mother's instinct is always to shelter their children from harm, the outside world can never quite be kept at bay. Hard as Ahchu's grandmother tried and successful as she was, there is no denying the era's imprint on all who lived through it. No parents would choose for their children to live in the jungle unless the cities had inspired enough fear in them for their welfare— and Ahchu's life had been under threat.

Of his earliest years, Ahchu says: "I forgot how old I was exactly when everything began. I must have been one or younger when the invasion happened, when they tried to get rid of anti-Japanese people." Jungles were safer than villages, and villages were safer than cities, where the Japanese were brutally massacring those who defied the imperialist regime. Cities and towns took on an atmosphere of paranoia. People were paid to be informants for the Japanese, and this fostered a deep mistrust that turned son against father, wife against husband, neighbor against neighbor. On a typical day of judgement in a Malayan town at this time, three lone figures could be seen standing in the central square, wearing boxes to hide their faces, and temporarily erase their humanity. With only two holes cut out for seeing—two dark, ominous gaps like the muzzle of a double-barreled gun, ready to betray or be betrayed.

One by one, all the men over the age of 14 would walk in a straight line in front of the masked informants. They were met with either silence, meaning they could return to their daily business, or a nod from the informant, in which case they were immediately dragged away for execution. Their lives hung in the balance, and as each man approached, he typically closed his eyes, shutting out the two dark, judging holes and unbearable possibilities.

Executions were carried out using Samurai swords. Historians have argued that this could be attributed to a nostalgia for bushido codes of honor. However, the idea that decapitation could be about honor seems too kind a supposition. Surely the reason was to provoke fear of the horror of cold steel on flesh, and thereby to intimidate and silence onlookers.

If a nod did not happen for any of the men in line, the informants' necks would be under the blade. They were therefore bound to nod at some point, and this certainty poisoned the air they breathed.

It was a sick game of chance, and Ahchu's father was not a gambler—whether it was nature or nurture that meant Ahchu grew up to develop the same trait of cautiousness or touch of paranoia is debatable. On that day this careful man hid his family in a nearby empty building as the fatal procession went on.

"They told a friend to lock the door from the outside so the Japanese would think there was no one inside the building. If it was locked from within, they would know someone was trying to hide inside." Ahchu's parents told him the story, years later. Hidden away in the building locked from the outside, Ahchu's father must have felt the palpable tension, and with a newborn in one arm, his wife in another, it was easy to be reminded of just how much there was to lose. At some point during the day, Ahchu started to cry. For fear of nearby Japanese soldiers hearing, his parents almost suffocated him, choking him into silence. So, before the age of one, he almost died in the protective hands of his own father and mother.

Ironically, this hiding was not really necessary, as Ahchu's father was neither an anti-Japanese sympathizer nor a spy. He was an innocent, humble, small businessman. This over-cautiousness could have backfired. Similarly, in Ahchu's less dramatic business and real estate encounters, this overly cautious trait may have helped or hurt him— it is not easy to tell.

Ahchu had another encounter that could have ended his life at a very young age. Tropical Penang weather brought forth frequent rain showers. Rain showers in the jungle cause pools of stagnant water, a breeding ground for mosquitos. Mosquitos carry malaria. Ahchu contracted this disease causing him to have frequent high fevers and chills and making him delirious. Since medicine was hard to come by during the Second World War, Ahchu almost succumbed to this illness. However, through the grace of God, he was miraculously cured of the disease and has been free of it ever since.

When relating these events Ahchu underplays his own personal involvement and trauma, instead recounting the story as if it were the plot of a favorite play, smiling and even getting somewhat excited at the suspenseful turns. He has a calm, impartial acceptance of why it happened and how it affected his personality. "If you liked me, you'd call me cautious; if you didn't, you'd call me paranoid. It's not that I don't trust people. I trust, and verify that trust, and verify again. I take risks but only measured ones."

Before saying goodnight to his wife, he always asks, "Have you checked the stove in the kitchen? Locked the door? Checked everything?" If the answer is less than satisfactory, he will get up from the warmth of his bed and go downstairs to check for himself. Only after completing this routine is he content to resume his usual four hours' sleep per night, a habit that he has kept for decades.

This over-cautiousness made an excellent quality for his work as a surgeon. A nurse or resident working under Ahchu would possibly get quite annoyed before each major operation. "Did you check the apparatus, the lab tests…? Could you check again?" Then, quietly and without embarrassing them, Ahchu would always check yet again himself. However, these additional run-throughs that take barely five minutes to execute could make all the difference to the wellbeing of his patients. Decades after Ahchu's rigorous 'checks and double checks' routine, he and his wife were lining up to board a plane in Tampa. Suddenly, from behind he heard, "check and double check." It was the voice of a retired nurse who had worked with Ahchu decades before. He was pleased to know that his practice and teaching had made such an impact.

Unbeknown to Ahchu and his parents on the day he cried in that building locked from the outside, it seems he was destined to become a meticulous surgeon. Out of an era of information warfare, Ahchu learned to check his stove before bedtime, be extra responsible for his patients, and give out well-deserved trust in careful quantities.

Experiences of the war in Malaya clearly left an imprint on Ahchu. However, his childhood also involved quieter, every-day household conflicts, which may pale in comparisons of scale, but nevertheless affect a child's malleable mind in equally significant ways. At this point, Ahchu's tale turns to a quarrel between parents, the movie *Bambi*, and a fire that stayed in his mind for the rest of his life.

One day, Ahchu's mother hid him and his sisters in the church minister's house. There, the three children waited for one uncertain, fearful, confused afternoon, unable to understand their mother's actions and desperate for her, or anyone, to return and restore them to the comfort of their home.

Their solemn-faced father eventually found them hours later, but those moments spent in utter cluelessness and fear cut deep: "To this day I don't know why we were hiding, what happened between them." This incident at the minister's house, it turned out, was only a prelude that would build up to the breaking point of long-accumulated marital tension.

Months later, Ahchu's mother left, taking the two daughters with her and leaving Ahchu with his father. It was a sudden, unexpected disappearance, without giving the other family members much time to prepare or cope— or so it seemed at the time to young Ahchu. As he remained in the bicycle repair shop which doubled as the family home, where the once big, bustling family of five was suddenly more than halved in number, his young mind must have found the procession of events frighteningly incomprehensible. "Why were they gone? Are they coming back?"

His father, sympathetic to what he was going through, took Ahchu to see a new cartoon movie in the theater, hoping to lift his spirits. In mid-20th Century Malaya going to the movies was a luxurious affair, and Ahchu would have been considered lucky to have the opportunity of enjoying such a treat. However, all he remembers from that afternoon is a single provocative scene: a blazing fire, consuming the forest around it, devouring the luscious greenery in its path and spitting out charred, formless chunks of black and brown.

"I don't actually remember what movie that was, but I described the fire in the forest to my wife and children, and they told me it must have been *Bambi*." The vagueness of the rest of his memory brought the fire into sharp focus, and that scene must have had a raw, emotional impact rather than forming a conscious memory. The fire on the silver screen mirrored the fire in Ahchu's mind, as his whole world seemed to perish in flames around him, and he knew neither how the fire started, nor how to put it out. A haunting metaphor for his life, his emotions, and his confusions at that point in time, that fire was charred into Ahchu's memory forever.

To this day, Ahchu still has a fear of fire that has never subsided, "When we built our house, I didn't want a fireplace. However, that posed a problem, because if we didn't build one, the house would not look right in New England and we wouldn't be able to sell it in the future." The fireplace that Ahchu reluctantly conceded to has only ever been used once. Apart from an initial test to see how high the flame would light up, and if it vented properly it has never been lit, and slowly gathers dust in the corner, waiting to perhaps one day boost the house's real estate value.

Although Ahchu actively avoids any encounters with fire, there have been times when he has had to confront it. One day the family hosted a cookout, and a Chinese obstetrician friend decided to cook steak on an open flame. Immediately after the cookout, Ahchu sprang into action: "I quickly brought water to douse the remaining smoldering fire, and then took out all the wet charcoal and dumped it in the trash far from the house." Ahchu smiles as he remembers his own nervousness. It was the first and last cookout he hosted at his home.

It is interesting how memory functions, and how we selectively preserve those that resonate most deeply with us. Though there may not be a choice in which memories are preserved, there's a choice in what to do with them. To be able to reflect on how experiences of trauma have affected your personality and brush them off with a sense of humor and a ready smile is characteristic of Ahchu's philosophy in life.

At this point of his narrative, Ahchu says, "I feel like I need to add a good part here. Too many sad stories have been told." So he shares a story of sweetness and joy.

When the British had retaken Malaya and all seemed well again, Ahchu remembers a gathering one afternoon at the church. Ahchu's mother was in charge of serving ice cream: "For every few scoops she gave out, there was a scoop for me, and I was so happy. I felt so privileged and happy." And on this note he ends the first part of his story.

Ice cream on a tropical afternoon compared to years of the physical and psychological trauma of war doesn't seem to balance out on the scale of life, but a child's mind is a wondrous place, with the simplest moments of happiness and the briefest of sorrows. Perhaps that ability to remember those precious scoops of ice cream on a warm Malayan afternoon as vividly as the sword blades of imperialists enables Ahchu to appreciate even the lemons of his life and integrate them into his own philosophy: being kind, careful, and always managing risk.

"When life gives you lemons, always, always make lemonade. Even if you only make half a cup, just remember the cup is never half empty, it is half full." Ahchu appreciates the role models in his family who taught him this lesson in his early, formative years.

Chapter 2

DON'T TAKE NO FOR AN ANSWER

Coco Kejia Ruan

"Be strong and courageous. Do not be afraid or terrified because of them, for the LORD your God goes with you; he will never leave you nor forsake you."
– Deuteronomy 31:6

The peak of Ahchu's high school career was not when he became one of the few Malayan students in the 1950s ever to receive two acceptance letters from Ivy League schools in the U.S.A. It wasn't when he skipped a grade to join the next class in the second half of the academic year, nor was it when his score of eight subjects trumped his classmates' scores of nine subjects combined. Like his classmates, he took nine subjects. The final exam for each subject was given a numerical score, 100 being the highest. Hence a 'perfect' student could get an aggregate score of 900 for the nine subjects. Although he joined the class in the middle of the academic year, the final exam results showed Ahchu was so ahead of his class, his aggregate score for any eight of the nine subjects he took was still higher than the cumulative score for nine subjects achieved by any of his classmates, many of whom went on to be successful doctors, dentists, lawyers and engineers.

Rather, he would remember the day when he waited outside the American Consulate on a July afternoon, hopped on a bicycle and chased after the Consul along the narrow, paved roads of Penang. Back then, he was not the famous ENT doctor, Professor Lee, but the 15-year-old boy, Ahchu, could only dream about medicine, college, and his future, with the steadfast belief that he would not take no for an answer.

When Ahchu was in the ninth grade at the Methodist Boys' School in Penang, Malaya, he came across the names of three universities in the United States— Harvard, Yale, and Columbia. He imprinted the 19 letters of these three words in his mind and grasped onto them as hard as a person trapped in a fire would a firefighter. The situation in Malaya in the 1950s was indeed a tinder box. With the Malayan Communist Party (MCP) and the government in conflict, the entire country was lacking in direction, and the sense of unease and instability permeated the sultry, tropical atmosphere. But this boy had his eyes fixed on the verdant college towns of New England and New York, where summer heat was never a problem.

H, A, R, V, A, R, D. He did not even know where Cambridge, Massachusetts was on the gigantic map of the United States, but he knew he would somehow cross the vast ocean and get there.

Y, A, L, E. He flipped through every book remotely related to U.S. universities but still couldn't find the mailing addresses of their admissions offices, yet he was sure that he would impress them.

C, O, L, U, M, B, I, A. No one at his school had heard of college counselors or SATs. Ahchu had no clue about the qualifications he would need to apply, but he was determined to outperform his competitors overseas to gain acceptance.

He told his parents, "One day in the near future, I will attend two of the three universities and become a professor at the third." This might sound like a line from a corny Hollywood movie about the American dream from a naive and overly confident teenager, but in the context of 1950s Malaya it seemed like complete fantasy. Everybody knew it wouldn't really happen, except him. Ahchu was always studying while his classmates played sports or enjoyed the beaches of Penang Island. Papa and *Ah Mah* (his mother) constantly told him not to work too hard, especially after he was ill, suffering from facial paralysis. Ah Mah never attended a single day of school while Papa, an orphan, attended school for only eight days. Ahchu's kind-hearted Methodist missionary teachers from Tennessee tried to calm his avid passion by recommending smaller universities elsewhere that were easier to get into. Other people could say no to him a thousand times, but Ahchu would nod slightly, take their advice with sincerity, and keep doing things his way.

When all conventional methods failed, he thought the most straightforward way to obtain the addresses of these three universities would be to visit the Consulate of the United States in Malaya. The Consulate staff smiled at the 15-year-old boy and kindly said no to his request. He smiled back but didn't accept the rejection. He would not take no for an answer.

As he walked out of the consulate, Ahchu turned back to stare at the red tiled roof of the typical Malayan building. The star-spangled banner flew in front, the red, white, and blue standing out brightly against the earthy background. "My dream is not ending here," he said to himself. He felt small and trivial in front of the imposing establishment, just as he had done 10 years ago in front of his pre-school teacher. There, he was one of the only two boys at an all-girls school because Papa thought that would better protect him. (The other boy was the son of the headmistress.) At the girls' pre-school, Ahchu knitted socks and needlepointed, perhaps developing the dexterity he would need for a surgical career. The pre-school had a pot of warm boiled water for the children to hydrate themselves in the tropical environment; tap water being considered unhygienic. To this day, whenever Ahchu happens to drink a glass of water that is warm, his mind immediately goes back 75 years to that place and time.

When he transferred to a British school from the Chinese pre-school, his teacher, Mrs. Key proudly announced to the entire class, "Ahchu has only been here for two weeks and he knows the material and the rules better than you all who have been here for months. What's more, he showed up to his first-grade exam even when he had a fever of over 102-degrees. You should all learn from his work ethic! That's the way to be a good student." Ahchu would always remember the warmth that glowed in his heart thanks to her words of praise and encouragement.

Ahchu returned to the Consulate the next day, but he didn't dare enter. The flag wasn't even raised, maybe because of the weather. His legs were heavy, and he felt stuck between his fervent desire for a brilliant future and the uncertainties of the present. His legs weren't new to this tense sensation. They experienced it first in the Second Form year of middle school, when Principle Choo Kheam walked into the classroom in the middle of a lesson and asked Ahchu and two other boys to stand up. The straight-A student Ahchu was worried that he had got into trouble, but instead Principle Choo Kheam announced, "you three boys can skip a grade to Third Form, but that depends on your decision." With only four months left in the school year, Ahchu's mind wavered in uncertainty, "what if I'm not able to keep up after skipping a grade? But if I don't even try to take on the challenge, will I regret it later in life?" Going back home that day, torn and undecided, Ahchu flipped open the Bible to seek help from God, a method he resorted to throughout the years when he felt confused and unsure of himself. The first line that jumped into Ahchu's eyes read, "I, even I, have spoken; yes, I have called him; I have brought him, and he shall make his way prosperous" (*Isaiah 48:15*).

"I have called him; I have brought him, and he shall make his way prosperous," Ahchu mouthed these words repeatedly. His index finger rubbed the two lines of the well-thumbed pages of the Bible. "I have to do my best first, before relying on God's support," he thought. "God helps those who help themselves," is a quote he uses often. Little did he know the life-long implications that these words have for him in his later years. Calmed and satisfied, he simply applied them to the situation at hand and took the Biblical verse to mean that God would watch him prosper in the Third Form. As was God's will, Ahchu went to school the next day confirming his decision to advance a grade. The other two boys selected were also successful, while Ahchu went on to become the top student in the new class. His mentor, Mr. Tio Seng Hee's help was indispensable to his academic success at this time. Impressed by this young boy's ambition and perseverance, Mr. Seng Hee held special review sessions, and 'pre-tests' and 'post-tests' for Ahchu, giving him as much practice and strict instruction as possible. Ahchu was infinitely grateful to Mr. Seng Hee, and when he decided to endow three laboratories in his high school in Malaysia, he named the third one, a chemistry lab, after him. (The first and second labs were named after Ahchu and his wife, and his parents respectively.) Providence sometimes comes in the form of kindness from strangers, and Ahchu learned to appreciate such unexpected kindness with gratitude.

In those moments of solemn contemplation in front of the Consulate, his eyes were fixed on the only moving object— the American flag at the front of the Consul's car, and Ahchu made a discovery. When the Consul was in the car, the flag was raised; otherwise, it was not. Since the secretary at the Consulate would not help him find the address of Columbia, Harvard, and Yale, a wild idea took root in his mind, why not try to meet with the Consul in person? He could be strong and courageous because God had called him! He convinced himself, "I've done this before, just in a different way. God is always with me. This challenge is only a little bigger, but I can do it."

One day after school, Ahchu was waiting outside the Consulate for the Consul to finish work. He stared at the front of the car with the folded flag with intensity. As he eagerly waited for the flag to rise and flutter in the wind, he began an internal dialogue with himself, "Are the stars on the flag symmetrical or asymmetrical? Do all the stripes possess the same width? What does an opened-up flag look like? An eagle, maybe?... Wait! The flag is up!" That meant the Consul was in the car. The red, white, and blue had never seemed so glaring and vivid to Ahchu before, yet he didn't have much time to appreciate the brilliant color palette before he hopped on his old bicycle and chased the Consul's car home. The different colors mixed and became a beam of light shooting straight ahead.

When the car stopped, the Consul rolled down the window, smiling in his light grey seersucker suit. Ahchu didn't know what to say until the Consul broke the silence first, "Here, three Ringgits. I'll buy the newspaper from you. It must have been very tiring for you to sell it in this kind of weather."

It turned out the Consul, Mr. Whitney, thought Ahchu was a newspaper boy. When Ahchu expressed his real intent, he was kind enough to invite him in for tea. By coincidence, Mr. Whitney was an alumnus of Columbia University. When he heard the 15-year-old Malayan boy's plans to study overseas, he gladly provided all the information he had, even putting him in touch with the admissions officers for the three universities. To this day, Ahchu remembers word-for-word the letter that the Harvard Director of Admissions, D.D. Henry, wrote to him in response to his inquiry: "I don't think there is anything that a young man like you, who is far-sighted enough to seek foreign education under meager circumstances and courageous enough to carry out this seemingly impossible task, cannot accomplish in the future. I am afraid that you've looked a little too far ahead as a tenth grader. Finish your last two years of high school well and I'll be delighted to read your application." D.D. Henry and Ahchu continued to exchange letters before he arrived at Harvard, and Mr. Henry was his freshman advisor and mentor throughout his time there. When Ahchu became the president of the American Academy of Otolaryngology — Head & Neck Surgery, he bestowed upon D.D. Henry the prestigious 'Presidential Citation'. Mr. Henry passed away soon after receiving the Citation in person at the national convention in San Diego, attended by thousands of otolaryngology-head and neck surgeons. He was among the influential figures who played a vital role in Achu's early years: Mrs. Key, Mr. Tio, Mr. Choo Kheam and Mr. Whitney are all remembered by him with immense gratitude.

The 1950s were not the ideal time for a Southeast Asian student to apply to Ivy League schools, where the international student population stubbornly remained under five percent and rose only slightly higher after World War II. Even then, as the U.S. became the new world power and its higher education institutions became more respected, most international students were of European heritage. It was uncommon to find an Asian face on campus. It was Ahchu's own hard work and resolute faith that freed him from the usual trajectory of history and the less developed education system in Malaya at that time.

Ahchu was accepted by both Columbia and Harvard in 1958. He eventually chose to attend Harvard with a full tuition scholarship, an incredible achievement at the age of 17. However, Ahchu's elation was fleeting. Rather than glorying in the ephemeral fame associated with the names of the universities, he kept up his habit of hard work. In his memory, his high school career was not defined by those two acceptance letters, but rather by his day-to-day study routines: sitting down at his white marble table, solving a plethora of math and science problems on its surface and then erasing them one by one so that he wouldn't have to spend precious money on paper. Sometimes when he felt inspired, he would sit on the windowsill, memorizing math, physics, and chemistry formulas, and daydreaming of his future in America. You might say he made his way to Harvard on a marble table top with a handful of pencils and erasers.

This is a fitting image of the calm and cautious otolaryngologist that Ahchu would become, but beneath that tranquil surface lies a spirit of untamed resolution with the confidence to say to the world and all its adversities: "I don't take no for an answer!" Yet alongside his ambitions, Ahchu has an unfailingly polite and caring attitude towards those around him. He wants not only to excel, but also to help others achieve new heights. He believes that, "life is better when you are happy, and life is the best when other people are happy because of you."

Live simply, speak kindly, care deeply, love generously. That has been Ahchu's motto from grammar school to the present.

Chapter 3

FATHER AND SON

Clementine Xinyi Li

"The cup is half full and not half empty."

As a red-faced squealing babe, every one of us comes into the world bawling; fragile as a de-shelled egg and more precious than morning dew. Among the first to hold us is the new father, whose gestures may be awkward but always gentle, whose lullabies may be less than melodious but filled with emotion, and who will remain by our side in one way or another, for as long as they live and breathe.

Some say all boys grow up to become their fathers, while girls marry theirs. Be it genetic makeup, the assimilative powers of time, or the human urge for 'legacy' and perpetuity, a portion of the parent is condensed and preserved within the offspring, like the fossilized rocks beneath the landscape, forming the bedrock of the mountains and skyscrapers that rise above it. This is how Ahchu would describe his father— as the founding stones that instilled his habits, taught him his ways, and made him who he is. Their story begins in Papa's small inner-city shop in mid-20th Century Malaya, where as well as fixing bicycles, he bought and sold anything he deemed profitable to put food on the family table, often taking Ahchu along to his business meetings.

Papa, like many others, saw a business opportunity as Malaya proved itself to be a late bloomer in terms of global industrialization. As its keener, more power hungry East Asian neighbors embraced technology and industry, Malaya was slow to let go of its agrarian roots and inched along the path to modernity. As demand grew for a plethora of modern industrial goods produced by neighboring states, men like Papa joined the import/export industry, specializing in buying manufactured goods and machines from other nations and reselling them on the domestic market.

Singer and *Signal* are somewhat similar words. When you utter them, the soft sibilant beginning is swallowed by a guttural incline and released. They look, sound, and feel alike in one's mouth, and this similarity is what Ahchu's father built his living on.

At that time, Singer was one of the best-selling sewing machine brands originating from the United States. Signal, however, was a Japanese sewing machine with similar pronunciation. Papa traded Signal sewing machines, and according to Ahchu's memory, "They were selling like hot cakes. To non-English speakers, Singer and Signal were practically indistinguishable, and they thought they were getting the Singer machines at a fraction of the original price."

It was, more or less, an honest mistake. Papa spoke not a word of English, and in choosing the cheaper import he hit the jackpot. However, his luck turned bad when the Malaya-based general manager of the American brand Singer heard of Papa's flourishing business. If Papa was a billionaire businessman with an army of lawyers able to defend him, it was unlikely that Singer would have taken action against him, but Papa ran a small modest business and had no access to legal counsel. Singer sued.

One day, Papa arrived home with his usually warm and good-spirited face downturned, his brow furrowed into deep lines, so that the rest of the household was immediately worried, "Is there something wrong, Papa?" He looked around at his family members, who were all in need of his support, and gravely pronounced, "Singer is suing us for an astronomical fine that we are definitely unable to pay, and I don't yet know what to do."

Like the rest of the family, Ahchu's oldest sister was naturally distraught on receiving this disturbing news. That Sunday in church she ran into their trusted friend, the Reverend Joe Kennedy, and she couldn't help but tell him of the Singer lawsuit, seeking advice and consolation. Close to the family and a kind, helpful character, the reverend took it upon himself to give aid where he could.

In those days, the expatriate community in Malaya was not nearly as large as it is today. There were very few Americans living in this region, and they were a tight-knit group where everyone knew each other. They all went to the same club and regularly hosted big gatherings for cultural festivals such as Thanksgiving. In this way, although Reverend Kennedy was not among the most prominent and wealthy elite, he was in fact quite good friends with the manufacturing tycoon and general manager of Singer.

The reverend did not only want to help Papa, he wanted to take this opportunity to kill two birds with one stone and help Ahchu's oldest sister as well. Since she had been a little girl, it was common knowledge that the eldest daughter of the Lee family wanted a life as a missionary in the Methodist Church. However, the family was Chinese, strict, and very practical. A life devoted to working as a missionary was not encouraged, as the financial rewards and career prospects were perceived to be minimal. This had been a subject of contention in the household for as long as anyone could remember, and with this in mind, the good Reverend Kennedy visited Papa one day with a proposal, "Look, I know that there is a bit of trouble now regarding matters with Mr. Singer, and I also know that your eldest daughter is eager to join our ranks and become a missionary. Let me make you a deal: if you allow her to join the seminary, I will speak to Mr. Singer and convince him to drop the lawsuit."

Reluctant but at his wit's end, Papa agreed. True to his word, the reverend spoke to Mr. Singer, and the latter agreed to suspend the lawsuit indefinitely with one condition, that Papa could no longer sell Signal sewing machines.

From then on, the family enjoyed a new form of evening entertainment. The entire household, young and old, would sit around the creaky wooden table with one leg shorter than the others, and work on transforming *Signal* machines into '*ignal*' machines under an occasionally blinking, dusky, yellow lamp. The children were best at this task, with their tiny, nimble hands able to precisely scrub off the '*S*' in the logo using dabs of turpentine, without damaging the product and making it unsellable. The adults, with more strength at their disposal, used hammers and hard tools to knock off the '*S*' on the foot pedal, trying not to break it in the process. There were hundreds of Signal machines left in the store house, and this nightly routine became an accepted part of life in Ahchu's household for some time.

In the meantime, the eldest daughter got her wish of attending the seminary. Reverend Kennedy's involvement in obtaining Papa's approval was not publicized, and only they knew the details of the arrangement, so Ahchu's sister never knew that she owed a great debt to the good reverend. Everyone merely interpreted this turn of events as a rare, miraculous moment of generosity and liberalness from the usually stubborn Papa.

The truth lay hidden for many years. Ahchu's sister led a fulfilling career in the seminary, marrying a minister and eventually moving to Atlanta, Georgia where they had three children and live happily to this day. As the children grew up and scattered all over the globe, the family's ties to Reverend Kennedy faded.

Decades later, Ahchu's brother-in-law— the minster his sister married— was retiring from his position in the Chinese church in Georgia. Another minister came to Georgia to replace him, and this female Chinese minister was also named Reverend Kennedy. As the two chatted, they discovered to their amazement that she was the wife of their old friend from Malaya, Reverend Joe Kennedy! Halfway across the globe and almost half a century later, the Kennedys and the Lees were reunited. As the two families re-established their relationship, the old reverend's memory was stirred by this breeze from the past, and he thought of the deal he made all those years ago. He decided to make a call.

Ahchu, now a surgeon and professor, was in Atlanta giving a lecture on ear surgery, and had retired to his hotel room for the night. Close to midnight, as he lay comfortably in his bed, he received a call out of the blue from the 90-year-old Reverend Joe Kennedy. Ahchu was pleasantly surprised by this unexpected reconnection after so many years, and even more startled by what the reverend proceeded to say: "I remember you, the younger child, and I wanted to tell you something before I die. I wanted to tell you a secret that no one else knows."

The reverend explained the deal he and Papa had made all those years ago, and the real reason behind Papa's compromise in agreeing to send his eldest daughter to the seminary. At the end of the call he added, "Whether you tell your sister or not, the choice is yours and only yours. At least now I will have the satisfaction that someone in your family will know God's grace and the truth, and do what you decide is best with it. Goodbye, Ahchu."

Fate is a fascinating thing. It brings people together, and it tears people apart. To this day, Ahchu has never revealed the details of that phone call, and he has yet to decide whether or not to tell. One can't help but wonder how life would have turned out if Reverend Kennedy had not paid that fateful visit decades ago. Would Ahchu's sister have become a minister and met her husband? Would Papa's business have survived the Singer lawsuit? Was this reunion after so long serving some elusive purpose? Perhaps only time will tell.

Chapter 4

DEPARTURE FOR A NEW WORLD

Sally Hyun Jung Jee

"[F]or a transitory enchanted moment man must have held his breath in the presence of this continent, compelled into an aesthetic contemplation he neither understood nor desired, face to face for the last time in history with something commensurate to his capacity for wonder."
– F. Scott Fitzgerald, *The Great Gatsby*

The waves rose, crashing into the sides of the sampan, and fell, gliding to shore. Ahchu looked up at the sky; threatening and heavy with dark clouds — as per usual in tropical Penang — with the possibility of rain. Though he had seen his fair share of cloudy skies, this one, stripped of its sun, made him a little nervous. It was as if the pitch-black sea, with its equally black murmurs, had swallowed the heavens.

Rise and fall, rise and fall. The sea was a creature of its own, and Ahchu's sampan was at its mercy. The small wooden vessel rocked back and forth, responding to every twist and turn of the waves. Now and again, salt water splashed onto Ahchu's face and arms. As the sampan approached the freighter, Ahchu wiped his foggy glasses on his shirt. He could barely make out the name of the ship, inscribed in white letters against the sleek black hull: FERNCLIFF. He stood up to get a better look.

"Whoa there, be careful," the oarsman said. The man had more wrinkles in his face than Ahchu could count, but his arms were like a young man's, their powerfully built muscles shifting underneath the bronzed skin. Letting out a grunt, which seemed more a product of habit than of exertion, he maneuvered the sampan closer to the Ferncliff. As Ahchu stepped out of the sampan and climbed onto the deck of the freighter, a particularly strong wave sent ripples of shock to his feet.

Rise and fall, rise and fall. Trying to avert his gaze from the harbor, where he had said goodbye to his family, Ahchu counted the waves. Rise and fall, rise and fall. He looked out into the open sea, which seemed to have merged with the sky, blurring all natural boundaries. He took a deep breath and braved a smile.

Ahchu had every reason to be excited. He was on his way to Harvard University, his dream school since the ninth grade, when he spotted the word HARVARD in a geography textbook. Just a combination of five different letters of the alphabet, yet the word sounded like a charm. There was another word in the textbook: AMERICA. Ahchu remembered the red and white stripes of the American flag, conspicuous even at a distance as he chased down the Consul's car on his bicycle. He smiled at his own brazenness. "What was I thinking?" But if he could go back in time, he would do it again.

Ahchu recalled the moment he opened the envelope from Harvard with trembling hands. As soon as he saw the word, "Congratulations," on the first page, an electrical sensation had shot through his body. At a time when very few Malayan students went to American colleges, let alone to an Ivy League school with a full tuition scholarship, his acceptance letter meant the world to him. In fact, Ahchu's admission to Harvard was such a rare occurrence that the local press had come to interview him. Dressed up in his only suit, Ahchu posed in front of the reporters. He held in his hands a slide rule, an 'analog computer' used to perform complicated calculations in those days. The expression on his face may have been too grave for someone his age, but it befitted a serious scholar who, as Ahchu told the reporters, was planning to major in nuclear physics.

It was 1957: the year Sputnik was launched and two Chinese nuclear physicists, Tsung-Dao Lee and Chen-Ning Yang, won the Nobel Prize. Physicists believed that nuclear physics would be the discipline to solve all the remaining mysteries in the world, and the public agreed. Ahchu, a young man eager to make his mark on the world, imagined himself becoming the next Asian Nobel Laureate in physics.

But as Ahchu recalled the last night he spent with his family before boarding the ship, his sense of joy receded to shore, and a new wave of emotions came surging. He remembered his argument with his father, who didn't approve of his studying nuclear physics and wanted him to study medicine instead. At that time in Malaya, the discipline you picked depended solely on your grades. If you had top marks, as Ahchu did, you went into medicine. Next was law, followed by engineering. Physics, along with the arts, was at the bottom of the list.

Papa, however, wasn't against nuclear physics simply because of cultural convention. He was a circumspect man, and his memories of World War II were still raw. He had seen Penang invaded by the Japanese Army and placed under Japanese rule. He remembered the atomic bombs dropped on Hiroshima and Nagasaki, and though he was relieved to see the Japanese defeated, the sheer, unimaginable power of a weapon that could decimate entire cities sent a chill down his spine.

Even when the war ended, true peace did not come to Malaya, for the post-war decade was another tumultuous period. There were, of course, pre-existing tensions among different ethnic groups before the war: the Malays found the status quo of British colonial rule unsatisfying, since they felt that Chinese immigrants dominated the economy, while the ethnic Chinese resented the discriminations they faced in Malaya, such as the immigration restrictions of the 1930s.[7] During the Japanese occupation, Malay nationalism grew significantly with the encouragement of Japanese officials, who realized the possibility of the Allied Forces' landing operation on Malaya and hoped to ensure the local population's support of the Japanese

---

[7] C. M. Turnbull, "British Planning for Post-War Malaya," *Journal of Southeast Asian Studies*, vol. 5, no. 2 (1974): 240.

Army.[8] The Malayan Communist Party (MCP), which attracted the support of many ethnic Chinese, had also emerged as a prominent political force during this time. Thus, after the war, tensions peaked when the British abandoned their plan for the Malayan Union— which would grant equal citizenship to the Malay, Chinese, and Indian populations— due to the dissent of the Malays.[9] Soon, a guerilla war erupted between the MCP and the British authorities. On June 18th, 1948, three Europeans and two Asians were killed in the midst of escalating violence, and on June 18th, High Commissioner Edward Gent declared a state of emergency.[10] The Malayan Emergency would last throughout the 1950s, meeting its official end in 1960.

The ongoing social and political unrest convinced Papa, as well as many others of his generation, that the world was still a dangerous place. There could always be another war, and perhaps this one would be even more deadly than the last. Amidst Cold War hostilities, anyone could be caught in the crossfire and become a casualty. So naturally, he worried about his son.

"If you go into nuclear physics, you'll be either a mediocre college professor or someone who invents the next nuclear bomb. Then, the enemies will try to kill you or kidnap you," Papa said, "but no one, not even the enemy soldiers, harms doctors."

Ahchu, taking after his father, was himself a careful young man and fully understood his father's concerns. But Ahchu was only 17. He wanted to pursue a career that he believed would bring amazing new discoveries to the world, along with personal fame and honor, even if it meant taking some risks. However, he hated that the last thing he did before leaving home was argue with his father.

---

[8] Yoichi Itagaki, "Outlines of Japanese Policy in Indonesia and Malaya during the War with Special Reference to Nationalism of Respective Countries," *The Annals of the Hitotsubashi Academy*, vol. 2, no. 2 (1952): 191.
[9] Donna J. Amoroso, "Dangerous Politics and the Malay Nationalist Movement, 1945–47," *South East Asia Research*, vol. 6, no. 3 (1998): 254.
[10] Karl Hack, "The Origins of the Asian Cold War: Malaya 1948," *Journal of Southeast Asian Studies*, vol. 40, no. 3 (2009): 472.

As Ahchu grew accustomed to the rumblings of the sea, his thoughts drifted to his mother's tears, which had streaked the front of her dress like raindrops in Penang's monsoon season. In the 1950s, sending a son to America was like sending him to Mars. A land far, far away, America was a world Ahchu's mother could only imagine, and in her imagination, any number of atrocities could befall her son. There was also the problem of money. Though Ahchu's parents had worked conscientiously their entire lives, keeping a bicycle shop in Penang, they could only just afford his one-way trip to this mysterious country— not in an airplane or a passenger liner but in a freighter that only accepted nine passengers. So Ahchu's mother didn't know if or when Ahchu would be coming home.

Rise and fall, rise and fall. Ahchu inhaled deeply, breathing in the salty air. He knew that his mother, along with his eldest sister, would still be standing where he had left them, trying to catch one last glimpse of the ship before it departed. His breath came out in painful, jagged pieces.

While Ahchu was fighting back tears thinking about her, his mother and sister were hiring a sampan. In the dead of the night, they sailed towards the Ferncliff, anchored a mile away from the harbor. When they reached it, Ahchu's mother told her daughter to knock on the wall of the freighter, hoping against hope that her son would hear. "I might be able to exchange a few words with him before the ship sets sail," she thought. She didn't know what she could say to a son who was leaving for a new world, other than, "I love you so much, take care." But perhaps one last "I love you," could make all the difference, could stay with him like a protective charm and keep him safe. The sister did as instructed, barely hearing her own knock. The sea was, as always, merciless, and the deafening roar of the waves drowned out all other sounds.

"We have to turn back. It's been 15 minutes," the oarsman said. Realizing that Ahchu would never hear them, the two women finally relented. "Ahchu will be okay, mom. Don't worry so much," his sister said, as the two made their way back to the harbor. "I know, it's just…" Their mother's voice trailed off, into the dark, indifferent sea.

Ahchu knows he is fortunate to have such a caring, loving mother who taught him valuable lessons in life: the importance of saving for a rainy day; of never being in debt; of being cautious about lending money to friends or relatives, in case it ruins a relationship. Most significantly she instilled in him the value of respecting those above and, more importantly, below you, a lesson which Ahchu has followed throughout his life.

Chapter 5

THE FERNCLIFF

Sally Hyun Jung Jee

"The real voyage of discovery consists not in seeking new landscapes, but in having new eyes."
– Marcel Proust

Rise and fall, rise and fall. As the Ferncliff glided away from the lights of the harbor, Ahchu looked out into the dark, mysterious ocean ahead of him. He didn't know that his mother and sister had knocked on the ship only a few minutes earlier, hoping to hear from him one last time and that his mother had decided to turn back to the harbor, her heart laden with worry. He couldn't help but think about his family, and homesickness started creeping into the crevices of his heart. Luckily, he didn't have much time to brood.

"Hey, what's your name?" a boy with dark, matted hair asked him. "Ahchu," he answered. The boy tried to pronounce the name as best as he could, and Ahchu smiled at his fervent, yet mostly disastrous, attempts. When Ahchu turned his gaze back to the water, he realized that the ship was already in open sea.

There were eight other passengers on the Ferncliff, all of whom Ahchu would get to know well during his six-week-long journey. The boy with matted hair belonged to a family of four: an American engineer and his wife, along with their two children. The girl was 10 years old, and the boy, who proved to be the mischief-maker of the ship, was 14. Two other Malayan students were on board: a young woman heading to a college in Maine and an older male student going to school somewhere in the Midwest. There was an American woman in her late sixties, with her glasses always perched on the tip of her nose. The last passenger was a missionary teacher who would lead a Bible study session with the three students every morning for the next six weeks. This daily Bible study nurtured Ahchu's Methodist faith and acted as a comforting reminder of home.

The Ferncliff was not a passenger liner but a cargo ship that transported fish to port cities. So naturally, there wasn't much to do. Without swimming pools, shuffleboards, or ping pong tables with which the passengers could amuse themselves, the only source of entertainment was the mischief created by the 14-year-old boy. One of his favorite games was hiding the elderly woman's hearing aid.

"I know you hid my hearing aid again. Tell me where it is or I'll make you regret it!" the woman would yell at the boy, every time her hearing aid went missing. "I don't know what you're talking about, ma'am," the boy would answer, as a devilishly sweet smile spread across his freckled cheeks. The distressed woman would then call for help, and everyone on the ship would go on a scavenger hunt to find where the hearing aid had been hidden this time.

(Another, rather more secret, source of entertainment for Ahchu and the student heading to the Midwest was spying. The girl bound for college in Maine and one of the Ferncliff's young engineers got close to each other, and what started as a series of friendly conversations turned into a passionate fling during the last two weeks of the journey. While the two shared private moments in a quiet corner of the deck, Ahchu and the student looked on from afar).

Partly to keep his homesickness at bay, and partly to prepare for the academic rigor of Harvard, Ahchu kept a regimented schedule on the ship.

Every day, he woke up at 7.30 a.m. and attended Bible study from 8 to 8.30 a.m., before returning to his tiny cabin. From 9 a.m. to 12 p.m., Ahchu would do nothing but study the high school notes he had brought with him from home. He packed more school notes and books than clothes. The only clothing items he carried in abundance were handkerchiefs. It was the custom at that time in Penang to give handkerchiefs as a going away present. His relatives and friends showered him with handkerchiefs. He is still using them as this biography is written, more than half a century later. Of course, there was no library or internet, and since he didn't have any new academic material, he systematically rehearsed all his algebra, chemistry, and physics formulas in his head and reviewed problem sets that he had already solved many times.

"I fear not the man who has practiced 10,000 kicks, but I fear the man who has practiced one kick 10,000 times," Bruce Lee once said. By the time Ahchu reached his destination, he knew his one kick so well that he felt confident even among the brightest minds of the world. Since he didn't take the SATs in Malaya, where such exams were not yet offered, he had to take multiple placement tests at Harvard. Thanks to his tireless practice on the Ferncliff, Ahchu scored highly in all the tests and was allowed to take advanced courses in physics and mathematics.

Despite Ahchu's efforts to make the most of his time on the ship, life on the Ferncliff wasn't always easy. While passing through particularly rough patches of sea, most of the passengers fell ill. When one finally stopped vomiting, others would start, their heads hanging precariously over the safety rail. Luckily, Ahchu never once experienced seasickness throughout the entirety of his voyage. He did however have a serious craving for rice. A Norwegian freighter, the Ferncliff offered only smoked salmon at mealtimes. By the end of the first week, the passengers were so tired of the smell of smoked fish that they longed for anything other than salmon. When they came across one another on the deck, their conversations would inevitably turn to food from home. "I'd kill for a bowl of stir-fried noodles," the student heading to the Midwest would tell Ahchu.

What Ahchu missed the most was, of course, the dishes his mother used to prepare for him, especially home-cooked rice. When the Ferncliff docked at a port for the first time, Ahchu was determined to get himself some Chinese food. Unfortunately, he couldn't find a Chinese restaurant near the port, but he did find an Indian place that served rice. Though the dish was mediocre at best, it was a blessed relief from the smoked salmon that he had been eating for so long. Ahchu tried to savor the food, but the rice melted on his tongue and disappeared all too quickly.

After six weeks on the rough seas, the ship finally arrived at New York harbor. Only four years earlier, in 1954, immigrants who reached the harbor were first processed at Ellis Island. Filing into a three-story brick-and-limestone building, they clutched their passports and other paperwork, trying to keep track of family members in the crowd. Some carried babies and young children in their arms. Upon entering the Registry Room, they underwent a quick medical exam and some preliminary legal questioning. Afterwards, they stood in line for further questions.[11] Ellis Island, having processed more than 12 million immigrants between 1892 and 1954, had closed down by the time Ahchu arrived in New York. He also had a student visa and was not subject to the typical immigration process. He was, however, one of the many young men and women who crossed the ocean to reach the United States. He shared their anticipation of a better future, as well as their anxiety.

At the harbor, Ahchu saw a television for the first time in his life. He couldn't keep his eyes off the moving black-and-white images in an object that resembled a box. While Ahchu was staring at the television screen, someone called his name. "Melvin! Melvin!" Ahchu turned to see a young man with blonde hair. He was the college student who had been sent to Ellis Island to meet Ahchu and take him to Penn Station, where Ahchu would board a train bound for Boston. Ahchu waved at the student, and the student waved back. When the two finally came face to face, they shook hands. "Glad to meet you, Melvin," the student said. "You're quite famous already. We haven't had many students from Malaya, especially ones who get full tuition scholarships."

---

[11] Koman, Rita G. "Ellis Island: The Immigrants' Experience." *OAH Magazine of History* 13, no. 4 (1999): 31-37. http://www.jstor.org/stable/25163308.

(How did the name 'Melvin' fit into Ahchu's life? As Ahchu prepared to leave for Harvard, he thought that having an American name would be useful. His first choice was Kelvin, but his classmates laughed at the name, since Kelvin was an abbreviation for Kelvinator refrigerators sold in Malaya. In the end, Ahchu chose Melvin, which appeared as his official name in the Harvard freshman yearbook. However, he could never get used to the foreign name. During his first semester in college, Ahchu, like many other international students, was seriously homesick and missed everything about his country, even the oppressive Malayan heat and the monsoons. The name Melvin exacerbated his homesickness— Ahchu felt that he had lost all ties to his home country. Besides, he had trouble responding when his classmates called out, "Melvin." "It was not me!" So, after his first month at Harvard, he went to the Registrar and changed his name back to his original, official Chinese name, Keat Jin Lee).

Ahchu and the student started walking towards the train station. It was Labor Day weekend, and soon they were both sweating uncontrollably. "Would you like to get some Coca-Cola before you leave for Boston?" the student asked. Ahchu eagerly agreed. He had been very thirsty for some time. "I'll look for a drug store, then." At the time, American drug stores usually had soda fountains in them. Having lived in Malaya his entire life, Ahchu didn't know this. He also didn't know that 'drug store' was the common name for a pharmacy. Panic-stricken, Ahchu remembered what his father had told him a few days before he left home: "Be careful, Ahchu. In America, they either shoot you or give you drugs." Papa was, it turns out, five decades ahead of his time.

When Ahchu and the student reached the drug store, Ahchu refused to order any drinks. "I'm fine, thanks," he said, "I'm not thirsty anymore." "Are you sure?" the student asked. "Yes," Ahchu answered. Though his throat was parched, he was absolutely sure. Rather than drink a glass of soda infused with questionable chemicals, he would stay thirsty. As the student nonchalantly gulped down his Coca-Cola, Ahchu couldn't help but stare. Envy and anxiety clashed within him: he was dying for a drink, yet he was also scared of what a 'drug store' soda might do to the student. Watching the dark brown liquid dribble from the student's lips, Ahchu felt as if the ground were lurching, as if he were on the ship again. Feeling with full force the seasickness that he never experienced on the Ferncliff, he took a deep breath. "My father was right," Ahchu thought. "I'll have to be extra careful in America."

Papa's own mother died in childbirth while his father died when Papa was eight. He attended less than eight days of school. At 14, he jumped on board a boat sailing from Fukien and worked his passage to Malaya. In exchange for bringing him a basin of water each morning, the ship's book keeper taught him 'the three 'Rs'. He learned so well that he contributed articles to the local press, as well as balancing the books of several businesses. While Ahchu's mother taught him morals and ethics, from his father he learned the value of hard work, organization and perseverance.

Chapter 6

SPACE RACE AND THE RACE OF LIFE

Clementine Xinyi Li

"Every step is a step forward, even if it feels like a step backward. Learn from your mistakes."

October 4th, 1957. A small metal sphere entered into low orbit around Earth. Less than two feet in diameter, with the smooth silver luster of titanium alloy, this seemingly insignificant little ball would catalyze an earthquake in the tumultuous geopolitics of the 20th Century.

Its name was Sputnik. The Soviet Union had launched the first man-made satellite, which successfully completed 1440 orbits around Earth, and America had to suffer the humiliation of coming in second place. Fueled by this defeat, America's national obsession became the idea of entering the vast, enigmatic expanse of space— humankind's ultimate frontier. It permeated not only politics but popular culture, with figures like David Bowie singing "Major Tom to Ground Control…I'm floating in a most peculiar way / and the stars look very different today…"

Thus began the Space Race, an intriguing chapter of the Cold War, where a combination of nationalism and technology resulted in phenomenal progress. Ahchu arrived in America one year after the Sputnik crisis erupted and began his undergraduate education at Harvard University. He was not only a witness to this era of insanity, progress, and sensationalism, but also a participant. He began his very own personal race, a race where the only opponent was his past self. The first goal he set was historically appropriate for this era— to become a nuclear physicist.

Greatly inspired by the two Chinese Nobel Prize laureates in Physics, Yang and Lee, Ahchu was eager to follow in their footsteps. "I was young and top of the class in my high school, the Methodist Boys School in Penang, Malaya. So, when I first came to Harvard, I was a little overconfident, taking all the hardest courses and setting myself impossibly high goals."

Perhaps the most difficult thing about adopting a new culture lies not in the what, but the why. It is not about what different foods you must get used to, languages you must wrap your tongue around, or confusing transportation systems that never take you where you want to go. All these are skills that can be acquired and perfected over time; the real challenge compels you to transform your core values and beliefs and truly think in an entirely different way. Why is this good and the other bad, why must I value this and not that, why do we do anything in life? It is a matter of purpose, and as you plunge into a foreign value system it can easily disorient you into false purpose or, arguably worse, purposelessness. This why is a deeper, more resonant, and more meaningful sort of culture shock, leaving many feeling like a misshapen puzzle piece, knowing that they should belong, need to belong to this great cultural jigsaw that is their new society, but where they cannot fit unless they shave off a few corners and straighten a few curved edges. Multiculturalism is as destructive as it is constructive.

Not every attempt to adapt was fruitful and successful for Ahchu. There is one thing that Ahchu self-proclaims he is not, was never, and will not ever be good at— sports. He had never gone on a single run in his life, had never set foot in a gym, nor did he intend to start. What compelled him to step out of his comfort zone and begin swimming was none other than the tragedy of the great Titanic.

Unfortunately for Ahchu, decades earlier, the son of a Harvard alumnus, Harry Elkins Widener, was aboard the legendary ship, Titanic, and when it sank the poor young man sank with it. His grievous and wealthy mother,

Eleanor Wilkins Widener, subsequently donated the Widener Library to the university with one condition attached: she required every Harvard undergraduate student to pass a swimming test to be eligible for graduation, in order to prevent future young men from succumbing to the same tragedy as her beloved son.

Tragic indeed did Ahchu feel. After inquiring about every other possibility and being firmly told "no" several times, he reluctantly signed up for swimming lessons. His friends were shocked when they saw his lack of ability in the lessons: "Aren't you from Penang, Malaysia? How can you have lived on an island your entire life and still not know how to swim?" It was true. Every single Malaysian probably knew how to swim— except for Ahchu.

Every Monday, Wednesday and Friday at noon, half a dozen freshmen undergraduates gathered in the university's pool stark naked. It was tradition that everyone, including coaches, swam naked in the Harvard pool. (As for the reason, every student had his own suspicions.)

Coach Summers lorded over these practice sessions, and he and Ahchu inspired mutual dread within each other, for entirely different reasons. The coach was baffled and frustrated by Ahchu's inability to float, much less swim freestyle, and watched with disbelief as Ahchu tirelessly failed at the simple movement of turning his head to breathe above water between strokes. Ahchu, sensing this frustration and hating the icy, unyielding brace of the water, also looked on the prospect of his tri-weekly swims with fear and reluctance. The two tormented each other and tried each other's nerves for one painfully long freshman year, until the day of the swimming test finally arrived.

As the pool glistened and gleamed with an ominous glow, Ahchu took a deep breath and refused to give thought to the fact that his excellent grades and his hard work could all be for naught if he couldn't make it across the length of this Olympic-sized pool. He glanced at Coach Summers standing at the side of the starting line, looking down the row of five swimmers who needed to pass the test, and they exchanged one long look.

The coach blew his whistle, "Swimmers ready!" He knelt at the starting line. "Set…Go!" Ahchu jumped into the pool. The water hit him like a solid brick wall and he started paddling ahead in a breaststroke motion, the only style he ever learned. "You better focus. Remember how to breathe!" he thought to himself.

But the water was getting heavier and heavier, and it felt increasingly difficult to lift his head up above the water and draw breath with every single stroke. He thought of how hard he had worked to get to Harvard, to achieve what he did at school. Wouldn't it all be a terrible waste if he was unable to graduate because of one stupid swimming test? Paddling harder and harder, Ahchu still could not ignore the fact that he was sinking further, and it became almost impossible for him to breathe.

At last, K.J. went down about two feet from the finish line. He thought he heard the coach swear quite loudly above the water and yell, "Someone get this boy some help!" As the lifeguards fished him out of the water, he realized with desperation that he would have to continue this torture through his sophomore year and take another test at the end.

He heard the footsteps of Coach Summers and was too ashamed to look up and face the man's eyes. The coach took a hard look at him and sighed, made a few strokes with his pen on the clipboard he was holding and said, "Ahchu, I am going to pass you on paper because I don't want to see you back here next year. Do you understand?" Ahchu almost didn't believe his ears. The fearful Coach Summers was going to let him get away with it that easily? "Just do me a favor. Never go into the water alone. I would feel personally responsible if you drowned because goodness knows you can't actually swim." He could have wept with gratitude and nodded his head with much renewed enthusiasm. The coach gave him a rare smile, patted him on the back and proceeded to direct the next test.

To this day, Ahchu thinks of that as the single most difficult test he ever had to face in his life, even though he went through four years of undergraduate studies in three, followed by another four in medical school. Regretful though unapologetic that he was advancing the Asian student stereotype of that era, Ahchu continued to excel at his studies and despise sports, and this was one part of him that American college culture failed to change. After all, even if every puzzle piece must trim itself to its environment, we must still maintain parts of our old self.

At Harvard classes were numbered based on their level of difficulty. Ahchu did very well when he took Math 1A during the fall semester of his freshman year, so when the spring semester rolled around and it was time to select course difficulty levels again, he decided to run instead of walk.

"Instead of taking Math 1B and Physics 1B, I jumped several orders of magnitude— I decided to take Math 11B and Physics 12C." To put things into perspective, the Math 11A and 11B courses were not intended for the average scientifically-inclined, talented Harvard student; these courses were intended for the geniuses, those with not only natural flair, but for whom equations and definitions came with almost zero effort. Physics 12C, similarly, was for advanced students who had completed Physics 12A and B. Ahchu had not taken any of these prerequisite courses in Physics or Math. Needless to say, a freshman student with little to no prior experience, Ahchu found himself in quite a predicament; there was no way he could keep up.

A graduate student offered to tutor Ahchu, picking him up in his dilapidated car, he drove by to offer Ahchu a ride. In 1958 cars did not have seatbelts, but the student had made and installed a lap and shoulder belt which he handed to Ahchu, insisting that he strap himself in for the ride. Ahchu felt certain that he was the victim of an evil kidnapping attempt. It was only after a few such runs that he became convinced of the older student's friendliness and gratefully accepted the help he offered.

Despite the extra tutoring sessions, Ahchu became increasingly anxious as the semester went on. His performance in class barely improved, and pressure from schoolwork and his own and others' expectations all piled on top of him, like a giant thumb, crushing down on this 18-year-old boy so far away from home. In those days, a Malayan international student could not simply return home if he was stressed or struggling. The first barrier was financial, as intercontinental flights in the 1950s were extravagantly priced, especially for Ahchu's parents. The second was cultural, as custom demanded that a student must return home with a diploma, or not return at all. He could not 'lose face' for himself and his family.

Unable to physically return, he wrote home frequently, making a copy of each letter, and the majority of his contact with his family was written rather than verbal, conducted through the post office, taking over 7-10 days to reach them, rather than verbal communication. There were no cell phones, instant text messages, or emails, so in order to actually talk to his parents, Ahchu had to book a 'trunk call' a week ahead. The call could be connected any time within a 12-hour window, so Ahchu had to skip classes while waiting for the call to go through. It cost more than $20 for a faint, hardly audible three-minute conversation. He could afford only three calls throughout his college years, which worked out as one per year, thanks to Ahchu accelerating his college education and graduating cum laude in three years.

The difficulties of keeping in touch with his family meant that letters were the main form of communication, and to this day, Ahchu keeps the copies of every single letter he sent home during his undergraduate years. These letters dutifully document the warm exchanges between a faraway son and his concerned loving family, "My parents were worried about me back then, afraid that my mental and physical health was seriously at risk from the academic pressure and 'shame' I was facing! They told me, 'Ahchu, you can study whatever you want, you can even major in business if you like, just stay safe and healthy.'"

To the less sophisticated Malayans, the study of business was not a serious discipline and the concept of a business MBA was unheard of in the Lee family. In Malaya, traditionally those with the highest grades went into medicine, followed by law and engineering, whereas disciplines like art and business were at the very bottom of the Malayan academic hierarchy. Ahchu's parents, in this sense, held a more modern, liberal perspective: they just wanted him to be safe and sound.

Encouraged by supportive parents and facing trouble in advanced Math and Physics, Ahchu now reconsidered his chosen career as a nuclear physicist. He remembered a few words of wisdom from his father, "If you are an average nuclear physicist, you will not be world-renowned. If you're a truly good one, you could end up inventing more sophisticated bombs, and enemy countries would send spies to kidnap or assassinate you. Are either of those two things what you want to happen?" At last seeing sense in that logic, Ahchu decided to change his intended major and career to the field of medicine.

There are some moments in life that last forever because their impact lives on far beyond the scope of the present. This moment of doubt and subsequent clarity during Ahchu's freshman year determined the path of his life for decades to come, when he would become a world-renowned otolaryngology-head and neck surgeon, and a professor who would influence this field and the practice of medicine for many future generations

"I believe there has always been a bigger being, God, to help me through life," Ahchu reflects, "I was destined to end up in medicine, and the problems I had in nuclear physics were a subtle way of redirecting me to pursue the right path." Ahchu had finally found his own lane, the one he was meant for and where he would excel in the race of life. He also learned not to take on challenges for which he was not qualified; a lesson that served him well in life.

Ahchu forfeited nuclear physics and any possibility of being personally involved in the Space Race. However, this would be the least of his concerns as an undergraduate, as another race occupied his full attention— the competitive application to medical school.

One day during his senior year, Ahchu was faced with an alarming realization: to get into medical school, not only did he need excellent grades, but equally excellent extracurricular activities. Activities that he did not have because he was studying all the time. Remember, Ahchu completed a four-year undergraduate education in three years and graduated with honors. What was worse was that this realization came a moment too late. Already a senior, Ahchu would have to start at the bottom of any student club he decided to join with no time to work his way into leadership positions, and being at the bottom wasn't going to impress medical school admissions officers enough to give him a place.

With his future on the line, Ahchu wasn't the type to sit and fret; he immediately arranged a meeting with the dean, where he made a bold request. "Sir, I would like you to charter a new student club, the World Cultural Society, and I will serve as the first term president." The dean was somewhat confused and reluctant to grant this request so easily, "What are you going to do with this society that existing clubs do not already do?" Even at this young age, Ahchu knew that a negotiation had to be a win for both parties, and in order for him to get his society chartered, the dean needed to get something in return. What did the dean want? Ahchu asked himself, and quickly came to an answer: funding and scholarships for students.

So he responded, "The Society would promote international understanding, bringing diverse cultures together during our monthly gatherings and in our magazine articles, discussing critical issues such as the apartheid in South Africa or the situation in Southeast Asia. More importantly, we would charge tickets for attendance to these events, in addition to selling advertisement space in our magazine to raise funds: we are going to collect enough to offer a tuition scholarship to an incoming international freshman." Pleased with this answer, the dean chartered the World Culture Society. Ahchu's first step in acquiring a presidency at a student club had succeeded, and now he needed to fulfill his promise to the dean and raise the money for the tuition scholarship.

Ahchu got to work, but where could a college student whose parents weren't exactly Wall Street tycoons get enough money within a few months? It was already late fall of his senior year. When times get desperate, the methods we employ become ever more drastic, and Ahchu came up with a bold, almost reckless idea under intense time pressure.

One afternoon, the ever-resourceful Ahchu stumbled upon a copy of the Boston Symphony booklet where the sponsors' names and addresses were listed— a roll call of wealthy people with the means to donate to Ahchu's society! He immediately made an unlikely connection between this random booklet and his project: he could sell advertising space to the patrons of the Boston Symphony in the World Culture Society program for a cultural event that was suitable for the society's theme and also of interest to this particular target audience.

That weekend, Ahchu and his friend suited up in an attempt to look older than their years, and as professionally credited and convincing as possible, and set out on their wild goose chase. They drove around the city going from door to door based on the addresses in the booklet. This was before the age of email and instant communication, and they were essentially showing up at strangers' homes and asking for money. It was, to be honest, a little rude, and certainly very daring and 'outside of the box'.

Ahchu would politely knock on the doors of these grand, intimidating mansions and inquire, "Would you be interested in purchasing ad space in the magazine of Harvard's prestigious World Culture Society?" Many times, he was simply faced with a door shut in his face: who wanted to deal with such a strange young man holding out an empty palm on a Sunday afternoon? However, Ahchu was not going to let these closed doors end his opportunity to go to a prestigious medical school, and he kept going around town until he had visited every single address listed in the booklet.

To his own amazement, enough of the symphony sponsors purchased advertising space, and they were well on their way towards obtaining enough money for a scholarship. In order to collect the rest of the funds, Ahchu employed similar methods to invite a Neiman Fellow who he had never met to a society meeting to speak about South African apartheid followed by a 'Q&A' session with students. It worked again, and after the ticket fees were counted, Ahchu realized that his promise to the dean was now fulfilled. The World Cultural Society had a fully functional president and a tuition scholarship to bestow, and Ahchu himself had an outstanding extracurricular activity to put on his résumé for medical school. He had turned a deadlock into another win-win scenario and had come out on top in yet another test of himself and his own limits. As well as other medical schools, he was accepted by Columbia University College of Physicians and Surgeons in December of 1960.

Most seniors who had been accepted into medical school took easy courses in the last semester of college. However, Ahchu fell back into his old habit of taking a course far above his level. He took advanced organic chemistry, a course designed for PhD candidates. Not only could he not give any answers in the first quiz, he did not even understand the questions. He panicked and rushed to the Registrar's office. Fortunately, he was just within the deadline for substituting a course. Ahchu realized that he needed more credits to graduate. If he did not graduate, his medical school acceptance would be withdrawn. He had only a few hours to register for a new course.

He needed an easy one where he could catch up in the middle of the semester.

After fruitlessly pacing his dormitory room for hours with furrowed brow, Ahchu had a light bulb moment: many of the varsity athletes talked about taking 'gut courses'— the easiest ones that would ensure minimum workload and high GPA— he just needed to find out what they were. He rushed to the football field, watching the players toss, kick and score, glancing at his watch every now and then to count the minutes before the registrar's office closed. As the athletes in their bulky gear finally exited the field, taking their helmets off and wiping the sweat from their foreheads, Ahchu cautiously approached them and asked, "Hello, I am in a bit of a predicament and would appreciate some advice. What is the easiest possible course I can take this semester?" After exchanging confused, somewhat offended glances, one of the football players finally spoke up, "Try Classics of Russian Literature. No exams in this class and you only need to read 10 Russian novels in English and write a reflection on each of them to pass."

Ahchu was saved. He read the ten novels including War and Peace and Crime and Punishment religiously day and night, finally completing the class with a B. Analyzing books of the literary genre was not Ahchu's strong suit. When questioned about the use of symbolism and motifs in Moby Dick in class, he blurted out, "It's a man going fishing! I really don't see what the fuss is about— is it because it's a particularly large fish?" He was equally poor in music appreciation. In the introductory music class, he could not get past the Gregorian chant, the most basic of rhythms.

Besides competitiveness in academia, an arguably more important form of competition has existed for men and women alike since the dawn of our evolution: the search for a spouse. In Malaya, two generations ago, there was no dating culture. Ahchu recounts, "American high school kids behave differently, but in Malaya in the fifties boys talked to boys and girls talked to girls, there was very minimal intermingling and very few opportunities."

Ahchu fondly recalls the fun days he spent in the Methodist Youth Fellowship, which was divided between the Junior Methodist Youth Fellowship for students under 16 years of age and the Senior Methodist Youth Fellowship was for those aged 16 and older. In July 1956, Ahchu was elected president of the Senior Methodist Youth Fellowship, two months before he turned 16. He was also secretary of the Sunday school. His faith was nurtured during those years. He read the New Testament over and over again. At Harvard his answers to the New Testament course exam were distributed to the class as examples.

In a rare exception to the strict conservative upbringing of an adolescent in Malaya, every Christmas Eve, all the Methodist Youth Fellowship members would go caroling from door to door, girls and boys together. Letters would be sent to all the church members' families, and they would invite the youth members to visit their household and sing. The welcoming families would prepare food and soft drinks, and the crowd would enjoy the music, laughter, and good faith until daylight came. Most importantly, this was a night where the young people could let loose a little and have some fun.

During that last Christmas Ahchu spent in Malaya, a girl was interested in him, and used the caroling night as an opportunity to make her advance. In between caroling, she sat next to Ahchu and talked to him all night. At one point she placed her hand on his, and the two held hands for a while. Ahchu was quite surprised, as this was borderline behavior given the cultural context of that time, and his heart was beating out of pace from this first 'intimate' encounter.

"In the end, I decided not to take it any further. The reason is that I'm attracted to brains more than beauty. Of course, physical beauty is pleasing to the eye, but wisdom and intellectual capacity always came first for me. This girl was not the best student, so I thought it wise not to pursue anything. That was my thinking when I was young, and maybe even now!" Ahchu says with amusement.

In college, even though men and women attended similar classes, their dormitories were separated into Harvard Houses and Radcliffe quads. There would be occasional 'mixers'— dances that accommodated both sexes. In this more liberal environment, the inexperienced young Ahchu's dating life at Harvard was full of unexpected surprises and occasional regrets.

During one mixer, Ahchu and another girl left early and went back to his dorm. The 1960s college dormitories had strict 'parietal hours'. If members of both sexes were inside a dorm room, the door must be left open enough to fit a thick dictionary in the gap. Compliant with these standards, they kept the door open, but at some point during their conversation, the girl suddenly placed Ahchu's hand on her breast.

"I was so scared and felt so unprepared— I didn't know what to do! Harvard is near a beautiful river named the Charles River, so she suggested, 'Why don't we go walk along the Charles River now?' How stupid and naive I was! She wanted to do much more by the Charles River, but I don't think I even managed to summon enough courage to kiss her."

Opportunities like these, unfortunately, did not come often for Ahchu, for faults entirely unrelated to his personality and behavior. There were not many Asians studying at Harvard, and Ahchu's peculiar foreignness made him stand out from the crowd. He was shorter than those around him, and not the best-looking guy on campus, so although many Radcliffe girls would go out with him on dates, this was usually out of sympathy rather than real attraction.

In his senior year, Ahchu's luck turned. He met a freshman Radcliffe girl whose mother was separated from her father and had begun dating a Hawaiian man from San Diego. She was more familiar with and accepting of intercultural relationships. She told Ahchu how her mother's Hawaiian boyfriend got along well with her family and made her mother very happy. The two began dating, and grew close during their brief year together. Ahchu's loneliness at being one of the only international students, so far removed from his home and his culture, was greatly alleviated by her lively presence.

Along came commencement and the end of school. The dormitories slowly emptied out as the students returned home, and the freshmen dorms were no longer in operation— only the seniors' dorms were still open. Being a freshman, Ahchu's girlfriend didn't have a place to stay, and Ahchu could not let her stay in his dorm due to the parietal policies. Therefore, they found a motel friendly to a student's budget, and she stayed there.

"We were talking late into the night. Around midnight, she said I could stay over. We could have gone all the way that night, but instead, I left." There is a strict reason why Ahchu was such a perfect gentleman throughout this relationship. Coming from a conservative family, Ahchu realized that he would want to marry a Chinese girl someday and would need to break up with his American girlfriend at some point in the future. He made this clear to her from the beginning.

"When I tell these stories in medical school, or later on at work, everyone says, 'Ahchu, are you stupid or something? Why didn't you go through with it?' I guess, I was just making the decision I felt was right at the time, and I still respect that decision." Ultimately, none of these 'failed' attempts hindered Ahchu's chances of finding a wife both beautiful and intelligent in the long run. Perhaps this shows another important quality that he possesses— the ability to recognize which competitions do not need to be 'won', and to not hastily sprint in a race of distance and endurance.

In the race of life we compete in many ways. People race against people, nations race against nations, ideologies race against ideologies. We claim our track, kneel in preparation, and set off the minute the referee fires the gun, but too often we are confused as to what we are truly competing for, and who we are actually competing against.

Ahchu has been blessed with rare clarity in this regard, and he always says, "Not everything is a competition, but it is often helpful to maintain a competitive mindset." His true skill lies in distinguishing which competitions matter. He has been fortunate in receiving helpful guidance regarding big decisions in his life, but most importantly, he is blessed with the knowledge that his own uncertainty and limits of capacity are the only enemies in life. He made an enemy of none other.

Chapter 7

BROKEN CARS AND BROKEN DREAMS, EVERYONE'S HERO

Clementine Xinyi Li

"Tell me, Muse, of the man of many ways, who was driven far journeys…"
– Homer, *The Odyssey*

Odysseus the Resourceful lived in pre-historic Ancient Greece, where mythology leads us to believe countless golden, half-immortal heroes walked the earth. The Grecian formula for heroism was simple, a mixture of sculpted muscularity, divine or aristocratic lineage, and a violent battlefield death served as the ultimate testimony to infallible courage. In particular, Odysseus stood out for his extraordinary cleverness and endurance: in a 10-year journey he outwitted man-eating cyclops and shining enchantresses, single-mindedly rejecting all temptation in order to return home to the island of Ithaka.

In the undramatic sobriety of modern age, who are our heroes? There are no more Olympians or kings, no more glory-seeking wars to be won. We have rejected the conformity and patriarchy of the Grecian 'hero' and embraced the 'everyman' as Odysseus. Ahchu is as unlike Odysseus as possible, in possession of no birthright to kingdoms, and no remarkable discus-tossing strength. However, there are striking similarities in the way they constantly rack their brains to devise incredible solutions to tricky situations and succumb to no external force encouraging them to surrender. As Ahchu always says, "Think outside the box."

A painfully practical problem which Ahchu encountered during his student career was the need to raise enough funds to pay for an expensive Ivy League education at Columbia University College of Physicians and Surgeons, in addition to the skyrocketing cost of living in New York. He was successful in overcoming this problem thanks to good fortune, a bit of wit, and President Truman's stringent foreign policy.

In 1949, despite decades of pouring political, military and financial capital into Chiang Kai-Shek's Nationalist Party, America realized its worst 'red scare' when Mao's communist forces triumphed in the Civil War. The incumbent president at this time, Harry S. Truman cut off all diplomatic ties with the newly established People's Republic of China, implementing a comprehensive embargo on the flow of goods, currency, and personnel between the two countries.

Little did Ahchu know, the undercurrents of history were about to wash over him in entirely unexpected ways and at an entirely unexpected moment; that moment came when he happened to be casually skimming the newspaper one morning during his second year at Columbia.

"I stumbled upon a statement by the China Institute explaining that due to the breaking of diplomatic ties with China, it could no longer offer its annual scholarship to a Chinese foreign student attending American medical school. Instead, they offered the scholarship to any student of Chinese descent." Ahchu fit the new criteria perfectly and was now eligible to apply. However, he already had a tuition scholarship, so was he allowed to receive another non-tuition scholarship? Although not explicitly forbidden, it was not exactly common practice either. If he went to the dean and inquired, the dean might say no. Similarly, if he went to the Institute to ascertain this, their answer could come back negative.

A contemplative Ahchu weighed the odds and decided to follow an important principle of negotiation: never worry about too much too soon. As a first-generation student living in the city on his own, a second scholarship covering living expenses would come in handy, so he applied.

The following week he received confirmation that the China Institute were awarding him that year's medical scholarship in recognition of his exemplary grades and academic achievement. Ahchu paid a visit to the dean's office. Standing in front of the formidable hardwood door, he hesitated, and it took him a few moments to muster the courage to tap on the door.

Knock, knock. Ahchu felt fairly confident, but inside his stomach still churned a little. It would be tremendous if this could work out— but if it didn't, it wasn't the end of the world, Ahchu told himself.

As he walked in, he remembered his mother's advice— honesty was the best policy, and he told the dean the whole truth. "I explained how I got the scholarship from the China Institute and the story behind my acceptance. To my delight, the dean said, 'I don't see anything wrong with it, congratulations!'" In the same manner, he notified the China Institute and was congratulated again.

So that fall, Ahchu went to medical school with two scholarships, all above board and with all parties involved aware of the fact. It was quite an Odyssean thing to do: the resourcefulness of never letting an opportunity slip by unnoticed, and the sanguinity to be able to live with the unpredictability of the outcome in the meantime. Ahchu is someone who will take a leap but remain mindful of where he lands, so that he doesn't sprain an ankle in the process.

Despite this fortuitous 'leap' and safe landing, Ahchu knew not to depend on such strokes of luck on a daily basis. Instead he relied on good old-fashioned hard work and making the best possible use of his time. From the moment he entered medical school, Ahchu span himself like a gyroscope, endlessly and rapidly rotating between school work, laboratory hours, and *five* jobs.

His first job was answering the medical school dormitory switch board between midnight and the morning, a few nights a week. His second job was repairing broken 'gas machines' for the anesthesia department. His third job was working as a phlebotomist drawing blood, starting at six o' clock in the morning. His fourth job was collecting fellow classmates' articles of clothing for the laundry company to pick up and redistributing the clean laundry to the students after the company dropped it off. And his fifth job was buying and selling second-hand cars. Looking at this list, it may not be hard to fathom why Ahchu slept only four hours a night; every waking moment he was busy studying or working in one of his many roles.

When Ahchu ran into his old classmate, Tony, decades later, he pulled him aside, and told him with a grin, "I've always wanted to thank you Tony! You're the one that helped put me through med school!" Naturally puzzled Tony asked Ahchu to explain. By this time, they were no longer undistinguished medical students. Tony was head of the Psychiatry Department at a prestigious university and would go on to serve as Dean of the Medical School and then President of the University. Ahchu was also an esteemed professor, well-known in his field around the world, and a surgeon in his own right. "Remember when I got paid picking up student laundry for the laundry company?" Tony nodded, and Ahchu chuckled, "You changed your clothes so frequently, I think at least twice a day, so I got well paid picking up and delivering your clothes!" And the two men, no longer young, had a good laugh over their past laundry. Working five jobs simultaneously and graduating from one of the most rigorous universities in the world are not, as some may think, mutually exclusive. The same spirit of restless resourcefulness underpinned both areas of his life, each supplementing the other by empowering him to achieve success, and at the same time providing respite from each other.

Ahchu channeled his creative, entrepreneurial energies in the classroom as well. First-year medical classes were fast-paced with very heavy workloads. In order to study better, he and a few of his classmates decided to record the lectures on tape. Although not officially against school rules, there was simply no precedent and no explicit allowance for such an idea. Ahchu and his team of daredevils huddled together in his dormitory one night, carefully planning how to sneak the tape recorder into the classroom and working out a rotation for transcribing the recording. The team worked with the cautiousness and skillfulness typical of an espionage mission, and the student spies high-fived each other over their finalized plan. In that era, it was not easy to locate a small tape recorder that could record 60 minutes of a lecture without having to change the tape, and at an affordable price. Ahchu finally located one at a secondhand shop in Times Square and they all chipped in on the cost.

The day soon arrived to set their plan in motion. Ahchu volunteered to be the 'recorder'. He devised a clever way of concealing the machine, threading the wire and microphone through the sleeve of his coat, and sitting in the front row, placing the recorder directly over the amphitheater railing, out of sight of the lecturer. It worked splendidly. The recording was clear and loaded with helpful details. That night the team transcribed it with joy and excitement at the success of their first venture.

One day, a classmate approached Ahchu as he was collecting the recorder after class, "Hey, I just wanted to say I notice what you are doing, coming in every time with that thing." Ahchu froze; being reported to the dean, expelled from school, and returning home to Malaysia in shame quickly and ominously flashed through his mind. He turned to look at the inquirer, an American boy, who said with a half-smile, "I want in."

Their team grew and grew, and copies of their transcriptions were distributed more and more widely, until one day, finally and unavoidably, the dean of students heard of this 'Tape Recorder Gang' and called them to his office. Confronted with the stern face of the dean, they held their breath and decided it was best to look at the ground instead of anything else. Fortunately, the dean smiled, "Don't look too timid! I happen to think you have a good idea. The university will provide you with resources, and in return all first-year students can have a copy of the recordings and transcriptions." After a few years, the daredevil Tape Recorder Gang's audacious plan became the norm, with the majority of lectures being recorded and transcribed to help students study better, and nowadays lectures can probably be found online.

Up to this point, all of Ahchu's extracurricular work and in-class ventures had turned out well, but occasionally he was made to pay the price for his unorthodox approach to life, like any brave soul who steps outside the realm of the norm. It all began when he sold his second-hand 1950s Chevrolet Bel Air convertible to a visiting professor at Harvard for a profit, and subsequently developed this into a business while at medical school. Every weekend, he temporarily transformed from a medical student into an amateur mechanic, working alongside professional mechanics, tinkering with second-hand luxury cars that he could resell for a profit.

"I specialized in broken down Mercedes and Jaguars. My first venture turned out to be lucrative, when I fixed up a Jaguar I bought for about $900 and sold it for $1500. That was a lot by 1960s standards."

Business was going well in Ahchu's rudimentary second-hand car shop, and he soon bought a rusted but dashing model-500S Mercedes. Instead of 'miles', the speedometer registered 'kilometers', and instead of 'gallons' it used 'liters'. It must have been a German car, exposed to salt water while being shipped to America which had caused it to rust considerably. Ahchu worked his magic, removing the rust, repairing its powerful engine and mending its beautiful, beige-colored, genuine leather interior, so that it looked like a brand-new, fashionable luxury car for a dapper young man. Ahchu was very proud of his work, and so when his girlfriend needed to travel from New York to Boston for her medical school interview, he saw an opportunity to impress her and offered to drive her there himself, in his shining, refurbished Mercedes.

It was a road trip of approximately three hours, and the couple set out early in the morning in order to arrive in Boston with plenty of time to spare before the interview. Ahchu was feeling good about himself, going over the speed limit on the empty highway, and pushing the Mercedes to its limits. Fate may have been jealous of Ahchu at that moment, a young doctor driving his gorgeous car, with a beautiful girl by his side. So it decided that somewhere between Poughkeepsie and Boston, it would add a pinch of salt to Ahchu's life. To this day Ahchu does not know what got into him. On a straight stretch of road he floored the gas pedal to see how fast the car could go. The engine suddenly died. Shocked and helpless, the couple struggled to push the car to the side of the highway, from where it was towed to a repair shop in, quite literally, the middle of nowhere. The news went from bad to worse: "They told us that it would take weeks to fix the engine. I had no money, and a medical intern had about five days of holiday in one year. It would be impossible for me to come back and pick up the car later." Ahchu was caught between a rock and a hard place, and worst of all, by that time they were already one hour late for his girlfriend's interview. He needed to do some fast thinking, and being Ahchu, he told the owner of the shop, "Let's make a deal." Ahchu offered to leave the car with him for good and asked the owner how much he was willing to pay for it. The man offered him the pitifully small sum of $50. At this point, Ahchu didn't have many choices. He needed to either accept the $50 and give up the car, or pay the owner hundreds or even thousands of dollars in car repairs, storage, and new parts. It was a no-win situation. So Ahchu tried to strike a slightly better deal: he convinced the owner to trade the car for $50 *plus* a ride to Boston, so his girlfriend could still get to her interview that afternoon. On this occasion it was the best he could achieve with his usually more successful negotiating skills!

However, Murphy's Law was clearly at work that day, as everything that could go wrong did and things got even worse. The university's admissions officers were naturally furious with Ahchu's girlfriend for being so late, and flat-out rejected her application based on old-fashioned misogyny, and for a reason directly related to Ahchu himself.

When she attempted to explain that her long-term boyfriend had driven her to Boston and that they had car trouble during the trip, the admissions officer asked her when she planned to marry to this boyfriend. She told them, truthfully, that it would be sometime soon after graduating from college. "That was why they refused to admit her, stating that all females waste their medical school education by marrying soon after graduation, becoming a wife or a stay-at-home mother and never pursuing medicine again." Ahchu recalled regretfully. Of course, no university admissions office would never be able to get away with such sexism today, but back then, it was sufficient reason for immediate rejection.

So in one day, Ahchu lost his money and his car, and his girlfriend lost her opportunity to go to a prestigious medical school. Ahchu sat in utter misery on the five-hour train journey back to New York. The interstate public transportation infrastructure in the United States was notoriously unsatisfactory, and the train creaked and groaned through the entire journey, drawing a bad day to an appropriately gloomy end. Ahchu ignored the shaky train and the passengers around him— including his girlfriend— and simply stared out the window, never saying a word. Weighing heavily on his heart was the responsibility of failing his girlfriend, and failing his own business, all on the same day!

On that note, Ahchu's brief dabble in second-hand car trading ended. In a rare moment of defeat, fate had played a bad joke and he was forced to live with the consequences. However, he knew that these rare days where everything goes wrong were like sunk costs in economics: there is no way to deal with them other than to move on.

Living on the outside of the proverbial 'box', Ahchu had his share of ups and downs, finding himself gifted with unexpected scholarship surprises, as well as stranded in car repair shops goodness-knows-where. Yet he stayed true to his approach to life for better or worse, remaining outside the box and accepting both the good and the bad as equally valuable in shaping his unique perspective. An outlook that he holds deep in his heart, and that is unchanging regardless of context.

The truest forms of heroism in life do not show themselves in the grand feats of the ancient Greeks, where a spear thrown, a monster slain, or a city conquered would consecrate you with the title of hero, *aristo achaion*. Heroism in our day and age is a constant state— it comes in recognizing defeat but continuing to devote every single iota of passion and zeal to all of life's challenges. Ahchu's humbler version of heroism is the active state of seeking out and exhausting every nook and cranny of possibility.

To be sure, Ahchu is no princely Odysseus, or modern-day megastar. He is one of us, a commoner who works hard, without natural-born Einsteinian genius or phenomenal flair, but with the ability and the grit to 'think outside the box' and drain the giant sponge of life to its very last drop. With this approach, any one of us, indeed any reader of this memoir, can easily excel beyond expectations, and perhaps even beyond Ahchu's remarkable achievements.

Chapter 8

SURPRISE AFTER SURPRISE

Coco Kejia Ruan

"The surprise is that you continue to be surprised."
— Jill A. Davis, *Ask Again Later*

If you see a girl with sleek dark hair walking in the crowds of Times Square, you may think she is just another one of the millions of ordinary Americans rushing to their next destination. But look closer and you notice that she takes baby steps with her toes pointed inward, her head slightly tilted down, and her hands folded in front of her body. Lifting your gaze from her slowly moving feet, you will see her upper body moving in a straight line at a perfect right angle to the ground without the slightest bend or shift, and you can't help asking yourself, "how come she walks this way?" Even in a Western suit, her way of walking is so distinguished that it looks as if she is walking carefully in a kimono. This is Fumiko, one of Ahchu's best female friends from medical school. Her stylistic way of walking embodies reverence, elegance, and femininity and stems from thousands of years of Japanese women sitting on their heels indoors all day long, with their legs neatly bent underneath the fashionable yet restrictive silk garment.

Ahchu had always wanted to marry a Chinese girl according to the traditional values of his family. However, there were very few Asian girls in American higher education at this time, let alone Chinese girls. To his surprise, Ahchu became very close friends with Fumiko, a Japanese American girl. Fumiko attended Vassar College and was a year ahead of Ahchu in medical school. She was not only fun to hang out with, but also warm-heartedly shared her notes with Ahchu and informed him of good elective courses to take and instructors to take them with. With her, Ahchu could work and have fun at the same time. Another of his trademark characteristics is that he does not know how to have fun alone; he feels 'guilty'. Perhaps unfairly, this can make him seem boring to friends and relatives.

The two young people were fond of each other, but bearing their cultural taboos in mind, they never 'dated'. When Fumiko spoke about Ahchu in front of her father to test the water, the staunch Japanese man, who didn't speak English, adamantly decreed, "Sore wa ikemasen. [This is not possible.] You cannot marry this guy because he is Chinese."

In fact, Fumiko's father had arranged for her to marry a tall, handsome Japanese professor. Fumiko's walk was reflective of a highly traditional Japanese family, but her outlook belied her American soul. Having been born and raised in the United States, Fumiko was much more broad-minded than her conventional Japanese father, and she could never be the meek, submissive girl he expected her to be. Shortly after their wedding, Fumiko and her husband had the marriage annulled and she moved to California to continue her medical practice.

When Ahchu saw Fumiko years later, he hardly recognized her. She had taken up motorcycle racing in her new life. When she walked, she still exhibited her characteristic slight, tentative steps, but when she was on her motorbike, these were replaced by the fast, fierce trajectory of her motorcycle with its thundering noise soaring in the air. Her hands, which were usually gently folded in front of her body, now grasped the handlebars tightly, showing pronounced muscles on her arms. This was the real Fumiko that Ahchu had never expected, transcending the borders of cultural heritage and exterior appearances.

By this time, Fumiko had married again. "This time is it a Japanese manga writer that her father wants her to marry? A Japanese doctor in the same field as Fumiko? Or an established and well-off engineer?" Ahchu wondered.

It turned out all his guesses were wrong. Fumiko was now married to a Caucasian named Guido. More importantly, he was a motorcycle racer. Perhaps most intriguing were the circumstances in which they met.

Fumiko, being a motorcycle fanatic herself, attended a motorcycle race in a salt mine in Utah. Guido was racing, and unfortunately, he injured himself badly. Fumiko felt an instant affection for him and took him back to her hospital in a private jet where she doctored and nursed him to full recovery. They married soon after, had a son, and continue to live happily ever after.

You can never judge a person's true character based on how they look, or even by their habits and behavior. If you do, you will be surprised time after time. Who would associate a genteel girl with her traditional Japanese walk, as soft and traceless as the spring rain, with the wild passion of motorcycle racing? Only the heart tells the truth, and it takes great effort to really hear its gradual confession in anyone other than ourselves. It is people like Fumiko and their friendship that make Ahchu's life all the more colorful and meaningful.

Chapter 9

THE TRIP WHERE EVERYTHING WENT WRONG

Clementine Xinyi Li

"Give some leeway, let life happen."

"I have never taken one single vacation without mixing it with work," if asked, Ahchu would so inform you with a hint of pride. Being either in possession of a strong work ethic or what some may call a dire workaholic, Ahchu has never taken a proper holiday in his entire academic and professional career, which collectively spans more than half a century. He approaches fun and recreation the same way he deals with work: with caution, foresight, and strict methodology.

This was how he planned his senior trip after medical school. Senior trip is a beloved tradition, its roots extending to generations of American youths hitting the highways in rented cars, maxing the stereo to full blast, and engaging in raucous, delightfully irresponsible behavior. It is an experience defined by unpredictability, recklessness, and spontaneity— qualities entirely uncharacteristic of Ahchu. This trip involved the unceasingly scrupulous surgeon-to-be in some interesting turns of event, where he would find himself sleeping in cars, handling roadkill, even asking strangers to use their showers. When and how did things go wrong?!

Let us start from the beginning. For medical students in the Sixties, the need to travel the country arose after graduation, as they had to interview for hospital residencies in several different cities. When this situation came about for Ahchu, his friend Jeremy approached him and asked, "Since we have a full month before our internships start, why don't we make a road trip out of it?" They were both single, foreign scholarship students, and neither had seen the American landscape in its full glory. Excited at the prospect of doing so for the first time, the two young men decided to exploit this precious free time (a truly rare happenstance for medical students and residents-to-be), and embark on a precarious adventure.

The first alarm sounded before the trip even began. How would they pay for it? By definition, the primary ingredient of a road trip was a car. Back in the 1960s, the cost of a quality rental car was unaffordable for two first-generation immigrant medical students. Each student had $250 to spend, a moderate if not tight budget for a two-week trip, and renting a car would use up almost half their funds. To avoid this, the resourceful duo put an ad up on a Columbian bulletin board: 'WANTED, ROAD TRIP PARTNERS TO SPLIT COST, SEE AMERICA'.

Soon enough, they received an answer from two Israeli girls. Nina was six-foot-tall and ex-military. Beatrice on the other hand was of average height and build. Though pleased at having found potential partners for their trip, Ahchu was concerned about how appropriate the arrangement was: two boys, two girls, all of them single, alone together on a two-week trip— what would people say? With this in mind, they painstakingly recruited another traveler, a Barnard girl, so that they had five members of the group.

Just as this first crisis was alleviated, the second alarm sounded. Which rental agency would they use? In the 1960s the three main rental car agencies were Hertz, Avis, and Dollar Rent A Car, in order of most to least expensive. Although he was usually thrifty, Ahchu's extreme cautiousness prompted him to select the more well-established company with branches all over the country. He was unusually stubborn regarding such a small matter and countered everyone's suggestion to rent from the cheapest company, so they eventually opted for Hertz with a good insurance plan. Unbeknown to them, the group would be thankful for this choice before long.

On a clear, sunny summer's day, the group of five eager tourists flung their light luggage into the trunk of one rented Chevrolet sedan, and drove through the Columbia University gates to begin their long-awaited trip. The temperature was not too warm, and the sunlight was not too bright, with just the right dose of a cool, morning breeze wafting through the rolled-down windows of their slightly cramped car. It was perfect.

Until it was not. Nina volunteered to be the first driver. As they exited New York City and sped onto the highways, her ex-military instincts kicked in. With both hands gripping the steering wheel and her intense gaze on the road, she pounded the gas pedal as she expertly navigated the vehicle through twists and turns. Enthusiastically, she yelled to the passengers in the backseat, "You wanna see me go from New York to Chicago in under 10 hours? I'll be taking bets now!" The others, struck dumb at each of Nina's crazy turns and quite blanched with fear, murmured something like, "How about no." Nina was too engaged in her driving and brushed them off, "It's fine! I drove trucks in the military. I know what I'm doing!"

Clearly, the Pennsylvania Police Department thought otherwise. A patrol car pulled them over, and two officers got out of the vehicle and began walking towards the car. Everyone started to panic, but Nina glanced at the approaching officers in her rearview mirror and looked back at the rest with a self-assured grin, "Don't worry, I got it."

She fixed her hair, cleared her throat, and rolled down the windows for the two officers, "Something wrong, Mr. Officer?" she asked innocently, tilting her head and flashing her big, charming smile. Ahchu was stunned. Nina spoke impeccable English, but out of her mouth came a string of broken words with a heavy Israeli accent.

"My friends," Nina gestured broadly towards those sitting in the backseat, "from Israel, Malaysia. On trip." She brushed her fingers through her glossy black hair, looking directly at the policemen as her eyes smiled flirtatiously. Smiling too now, they nodded in comprehension and stuck out their thumbs in a gesture of approval. One of them began to say, "Miss, you were going too fast. You see the speed limit on this highway is 65 and you were way over 80..." "What?" Nina's pretty dark eyes widened in false disbelief, "Yes, 80 is too fast!" "Unfortunately, yes. Miss we're gonna need some identification..." Feigning confusion, she shook her head, "Pardon me?" The policeman was going to continue, but his partner gestured slightly towards him to stop, throwing his hands in the air in a 'don't bother' motion. He turned towards Nina and the rest of the group, and spoke slowly and deliberately, "The speed limit is 65 miles per hour. Make sure you don't go over that limit again, can you do that?" The five nodded in unison. "Okay, we're gonna let this one go for now. Have a safe trip, kids."

Waiting until the windows were closed and the police were out of earshot, the group let out a collective, audible exhale. "That was a close one!" Jeremy commented in the back seat. Nina for once did not say a word, but for the rest of the drive she stayed safely within the speed limit.

Travelling from city to city, the group didn't have enough money to stay in hotels, so they made the best of the situation and enjoyed reconnecting with nature— camping. To most, this would entail a well-equipped trailer, sturdy tents with cozy sleeping bags, and roasting marshmallows around a blazing bonfire. To this group, 'camping' meant grabbing a blanket, finding a relatively soft area on a plot of land in the middle of nowhere, and hoping it didn't rain during the night. Being unfamiliar with the country, they were oblivious to the concept of designated camping grounds intended for exactly their situation.

Falling back onto the soft, plush grass every night, looking up at the velvety night sky and gazing at the silver splatter of stars as they drifted off to sleep, they couldn't remember the last time they were surrounded by nature, nor when they had felt this relaxed. Perhaps a 'trip' was just a euphemism for an 'escape', and *where* the unfamiliar destination was mattered less than the fact that there *was* one. Physical displacement provided a context for mental rejuvenation, and something about the absence of bustling city throngs and hectic, competitive work, about being under only a stark dome with no one and nothing else in sight for miles, was philosophically resurrecting.

The group slept in the open-air night after night, with only one exception: Ahchu, who flat-out refused to join them. He explained, "There are wild animals, snakes, insects out there! If you all prefer to stay outside, I'll be perfectly happy in the car by myself." The others thought he was out of his mind, but no matter how good a case they made, they couldn't convince him. Every night, as the group chatted away, and spotted Orion's belt and other patterns in the stars, Ahchu remained safely snuggled on the back seat of the car with all four doors locked and windows up.

Though this return to *tabula rasa* kept the group's soulful needs satiated, physical needs cannot be ignored, and this became painfully obvious when they realized that the last time they had taken a shower had been almost a week ago. Beatrice complained, "I'm jumping into the next river I see. I don't even care about salmonella. I'm practically rotting." Unable to afford hotels, and definitely not about to hop into a stream, Ahchu thought hard: where could they find a clean, usable shower? As they passed a hospital, a stroke of genius hit. Every operating room had showers! They were for the use of nurses and doctors on duty who often needed to stay overnight. Perhaps the two medical students could have an early taste of hospital life on this trip.

The group parked their car and tentatively walked into the hospital's emergency room. Two interns were on their break, snacking and chatting away. Ahchu greeted them and said, "We're medical students who have just graduated, and we're going around the country to interview for our residencies— so I guess we are you, just one year behind! Unfortunately, we can't afford hotels and we really need to take a shower. Could we please quickly use the OR's showers?" In the spirit of commiseration and good will, the interns gladly agreed, and the five wanderers were able to enjoy a heavenly hot shower and running water for the first time in days. As they thanked the interns and exited the hospital, they felt ready to resume their trip.

In this manner, they travelled the country, sleeping under open skies and borrowing others' showers. Things went relatively smoothly until the second week. One morning, the group woke up and found that the car wouldn't start. The gas tank had ruptured, and the liquid inside had been steadily leaking out all night. They were in Iowa, on an almost deserted highway with few other vehicles in sight, and the situation initially seemed quite hopeless.

Luckily, the benefits of Ahchu's insistence on a more expensive rental car agency and a costly insurance plan kicked in: Hertz had a regional agency nearby and quickly came to their aid. A tow truck soon arrived to take their car away to be fixed. With a smirk, Ahchu looked at his friends, "I bet if you got a car from the Dollar Rent A Car, they wouldn't even have an agency here! We'd be stuck!" At the repair station, they discovered that they would need to wait until the leaking fumes dissipated, as the gas tank needed to be sealed using a torch. This meant they would have to leave the car overnight, and since the car was their 'home', where were they going to stay? Exchanging nervous glances, they asked the Hertz staff to take them to the cheapest nearby hotel. There, the five crammed themselves into one $30 room with two double beds and a sofa, and they were grateful for Ahchu's insistence on odd numbers, as it meant they all felt relatively comfortable staying overnight in this arrangement.

The next day, they picked up the car and hit the road again. They were in Nebraska, approaching Wyoming, when disaster struck again. Around 2 a.m., Jeremy, the designated driver, was feeling extremely tired. On the barely-lit highways of the Nebraskan plains, the cramped little car's driver must have lost concentration. He hit a deer. The impact struck them suddenly. The hood flew up against the windshield. The car swerved off the road into a flat meadow. Thankfully, the road was not flanked by a cliff or ravine. Everyone jerked awake and hurried to check for damage. The deer was killed instantly, and their windshield had completely shattered, but luckily remained intact. Most importantly, no one was hurt.

If anyone had been injured, the situation would've been quite different. This was the 1960s, and there were no cell phones, no instant communication, and in the middle of the night no police patrols nor any other highway travelers in sight. Jeremy was obviously distraught, sitting on the ground with his hands folded across his head and refusing to speak. Finally, around four in the morning, they were woken by two troopers arriving to tow their car. It was a great relief to see figures of authority coming to their aid after a dreadfully long night of waiting, but the officers didn't seem interested in talking to them.

"So, what do you think?" One of them gestured towards the dead deer on the road and asked his partner. The group exchanged glances, not sure what the officer was referring to. Ahchu's heart sank: were they going to be held responsible for killing the deer? Was this deer a protected species? Did they have enough money to pay a fine? "I want the legs, and you can have the torso." The other officer answered. Now the group was confused: what were they talking about? Were they going to be punished for killing the deer or not?

"No way! That's where all the good meat is, you can only have two of the legs." The first officer replied, slightly annoyed. They were discussing how to split the meat to take home! The five tourists couldn't help feeling amused— after a whole night of panic and worry and arduous waiting, the two officers were arguing over who got the deer's legs. The group sat on the curb, and quietly listened to their dialogue as they waited for the tow truck. There was something comical about the scene of two patrolmen engaged in discussion with a group of skittish students sitting and watching nearby— an anticlimactic end to a frightful evening.

After the car was towed away, Hertz again sprang to the rescue, "Your insurance plan will cover all the damage, and here is your replacement car at no extra cost!" However, in spite of this good fortune, the group's already tight funds were almost exhausted. On the last day of the trip, all the money they had left was only enough to buy gas and one small bucket of KFC chicken, working out at two pieces per person. The group sat in a circle with the tiny red-and-white colored bucket in the middle, each nibbling their tiny portion, pretending they weren't hungry. As chicken was exchanged from oily finger to oily finger, the group laughed about their bad luck on the two-week trip, and all the fun moments they had shared. To each of them the small pieces of fried chicken tasted absolutely scrumptious. They had made it to Chicago, the Mayo Clinic, the University of Iowa (with its premiere otolaryngology-head and neck residency program), Mount Rushmore, Idaho, Denver, Teton Park, Salt Lake City, and Yellowstone Park.

So that was Ahchu's senior trip. Years later, Jeremy retired from his cardiovascular surgery practice in Boston and moved to Houston. While working as a consultant with M.D. Anderson Cancer Hospital, Ahchu paid him a visit— a long overdue reunion between the two friends. With their families and friends, they sat down to a dinner far more lavish than a single KFC bucket and reminisced about the long-ago trip. They whole-heartedly missed those days when each had barely two pennies to rub together. Ahchu concluded, "Despite everything that happened, it was worth it. However, I would prohibit my children and grandchildren from ever doing the same!"

Chapter 10

OFF GUARD

Coco Kejia Ruan

"Surely what a man does when he is taken off his guard is the best evidence for what sort of man he is."
– C.S. Lewis

Having learned the consequences of lacking extracurricular activities and having to make up for it at the last minute during his college days, Ahchu decided not to make this mistake ever again. Therefore, upon entering medical school, Ahchu took on the responsibilities of the Malaysian Student Association in 1961. Aside from the leadership position, Ahchu genuinely enjoyed connecting with fellow Malaysians and recalling memories long set aside.

When Ahchu was in high school, *To Catch a Thief* was the hit movie of 1955 in Malaya. The attractive retired jewelry burglar, John Robie (Cary Grant), always wore a black turtleneck, whether he was catching the thief, climbing the roof, or on a date with Frances (Grace Kelly). Cary Grant's charisma was boundless, and one day, it seemed that every single Malayan boy spontaneously started wearing black turtlenecks to school. You might think the precocious Ahchu was an exception, but he was not. Wholeheartedly impressed by Cary Grant's swiftness and elegance in his long-sleeve black turtleneck, Ahchu decided to join the fashion trend, which was somewhat unsuited to his surroundings in Penang, where the humidity was constantly above 90% and the temperature over 85°F. In the evenings, he and his buddies would cruise the streets of Penang on their bicycles wearing their turtlenecks, ignoring the sweat that uncontrollably permeated their clothing. What a stupid but fun time!

Another childish act that Ahchu remembered being a part of was the 'competition' to spot Ms. Small, the missionary teacher. Ms. Small was one of the few white women in Penang. With her 5'10" frame she was the exact opposite of 'small', and with her long blonde hair, she managed to stand out wherever she went in Malaya, where few females are taller than 5'4." Although she was not a celebrity by modern standards, she attracted her own young paparazzi in the form of her students. "Hey, breaking news! I spotted Ms. Small in the movie theater yesterday," a student would shout in the classroom. Another would counter with an even greater discovery, "That's nothing. I saw her on a date with a guy the other day, an Australian soldier." The endless gossip surrounding poor, innocent Ms. Small added a bit of flavor to Ahchu's banal school routine. Recalling fond childhood memories such as these gave Ahchu the strength that he needed in more difficult times and similar memories seemed to serve the same role for other Malayan students in America.

"In the good old days back in Malaya, I used to rush to the hawkers in the evening and buy Satay (grilled meat on skewers). There is nothing better than a few satisfactory bites of meat after a long day of studying," one Malaysian student recalled heartily. Another soon followed up, "Me too, although my favorites were Law Bah to eat with a group of friends and Char Keow Teow. I could gobble down the whole plate in no time. You cannot fight with me over this!"

Food was always the main topic of conversation at any gathering of a group of expatriate Malaysian students craving their homeland. New conversations were started, consensus reached, friendships established, misunderstandings resolved, and former bonds rekindled, all through remembering the food of their childhood. Even serious discussions could be sidetracked by the slightest mention of Malayan cuisine. Ahchu liked Malaysian street food as much as any of them, but something else was playing on his mind whilst this ever-expanding daydream of Malaysian food was being built, spoon by spoon, chopstick by chopstick. His mind was clouded by the 'socio-educational-political' situation of Malaysia and the United States: U.S. university degrees were not recognized by the Malaysian government at that time. This meant that having painstakingly earned their university degrees after years of studying, these Malaysian students could not go back to their own country to practice their expertise because they would only be recognized as high school graduates, qualified for less sophisticated jobs.

Ahchu was single-mindedly focused on coming up with a way to resolve this urgent issue, while the conversation surrounding street food went on around him. As hard as he tried to focus, the names of familiar dishes slipped through his fortified wall of concentration; "Nasi Lemak" (rice cooked in coconut milk), "Teh Tarik" (pulled tea), and "Chee Cheong Fun" (rice-noodle rolls) intermingled with his serious planning.

Suddenly, Ahchu had an idea. He had invited the Ambassador of Malaysia to the United States to the Malaysian Student Association's annual meeting, which would be held in Washington, D.C. that year. Walking into the assembly hall filled with nostalgic small talk, the Ambassador understandably thought he had been invited to a casual reception. He was very surprised when Ahchu politely inquired, "Dear Mr. Ambassador, as a representative of many Malaysian students studying in the United States, I would like to invite you to a casual public debate about the possibility of recognizing U.S. university degrees in Malaysia. Your opinion is highly regarded by our community, and I am sure, as kind as you are, you won't say no to an opportunity to alleviate confusion and preoccupation from our fellow Malaysian students." The Ambassador agreed, and the group moved to the auditorium of the World Bank.

The Ambassador was completely unprepared for a policy debate but looking at the hundreds of pairs of eyes in the audience focusing on him, silently yet urgently asking for answers, he could not refuse. Despite the fact that Ahchu had initially caught the Ambassador off guard, they conducted a polite and fruitful conversation, with ample opportunities for questions from the audience.

Soon after this event, certain American degrees started to be recognized in Malaysia. Hundreds of Malaysian students could now finally return home to work in the roles they were qualified for and earn what they deserved. Today, American degrees are held in high esteem in Malaysia. Not surprisingly, having solved one of the largest Malaysian students' crises in the U.S., Ahchu was unanimously elected as the President of Malaysian Student Association for that year.

The annual convention the following year went equally smoothly, with Ahchu re-elected as president. He was so adored by his fellow Malaysian students that he didn't even need to do the usual networking. Everybody knew who Ahchu was, "Isn't he the student who fought for our rights?" However, just as he was getting used to this situation and expecting no more surprises, a new challenge confronted him.

In 1963, the annual conference of the Malaysian Student Association was held in Boston. Ahchu was excited to meet up with some of his old friends and joined them for an evening of fun the night before Election Day. He knew he had no need to network for the presidential election.

The next morning, when he walked into the auditorium where the voting would be taking place, he sensed that something was different. "Who are all these strangers?" Ahchu contemplated as he glanced at scores of Malaysian students new to the Association, "I must have a bad memory because I do not recognize most of them." Before he could completely cast his doubts away, the election result came in— he had not been re-elected. It wasn't until much later that he realized there had been a well-planned strategy against him: numerous new members had been dispatched to the conference promptly at 9 a.m. to cast their votes. And their sole purpose had been to elect someone other than Ahchu and relieve him of his position. Those involved had been working to usurp his leadership for the entire year.

To say the least, Ahchu was thoroughly surprised. He didn't hold a grudge against those responsible. He reflected, "It was me who had become too complacent with the status quo. Even with all the new people shuffled in at the last minute, I could have made the effort to talk to as many of them as possible before the voting, so that they at least would have an idea of who I am and perhaps change their minds accordingly." Ahchu learned a valuable lesson from this failure. A good leader has to have experienced defeat and failure, and a good leader should never be blindsided! On such occasions, Ahchu always takes the opportunity to reflect on his own actions, even if the outcome has not been entirely his fault. Surprises are like changes in the weather; you just can't avoid them. If it's sunny and pleasant, you go out and take a stroll. If it's not, you learn to watch the weather report closely and take an umbrella with you.

Chapter 11

HAVE I MET YOU BEFORE?

Coco Kejia Ruan

"Love is patient, love is kind. It does not envy, it does not boast, it is not proud."
– Corinthians 13:4

Chinese parents seem to have the most unrealistic expectations when it comes to dating, and Ahchu's parents were no exception. Ah Mah and Papa repeatedly warned Ahchu explicitly or insinuated implicitly, "Do not date at school, concentrate on your studies." Then as soon as Ahchu graduated from medical school, they wondered when the wedding would take place.

The conundrum of finding one's significant other is hard enough for anyone, but it was even harder for Ahchu, then an intern at St. Luke's Hospital, New York City with only eight hours off in a 48-hour shift.

Ahchu's love life was far less exhilarating than his academic and professional adventure. From a young age, he valued smartness combined with beauty. His first crush back in Malaya had been Rosemary, a straight-A student and a champion swimmer, good looking but not mesmerizing. A shy Ahchu never explicitly communicated his fondness and the closest the two had gotten was when Ahchu sometimes visited Rosemary's house on

Saturday mornings, sitting at least five feet from each other in the living room and chatting for hours. Ahchu dated a girl at Hunter College, but that did not work out either. Ahchu had a habit of lightly tapping his car horn to notify approaching pedestrians or another car trying to switch lanes. She didn't like it and repeatedly chastised him, even after Ahchu explained that he was not being rude but alerting others to avoid an accident. From then on, Ahchu composed a new list of criteria for his significant other— ethical, beautiful, smart, hardworking, always ready to pitch in, not overbearing, and religious; but it was difficult to spot this person in the crowd.

It seemed as if God was aware of Ahchu's frustration and set out to answer him. One late evening after 40 hours on duty, as he was taking a stroll across Columbia's campus, he saw a flyer on the bulletin board about an upcoming international student mixer at Vassar College. Ahchu was thrilled. He desperately wanted to go even if it meant he would not have any time to rest during his eight hours off. Younger readers may be wondering what the big deal was about a casual mixer, however, in those days, the rules of social conduct were different, and mixers were one of the few opportunities for young men and women to spend time with each other and meet new friends. So it really was a *big* deal.

"Hey, do you want to go together?" someone asked Ahchu. When Ahchu looked up from the flyer, he saw a psychiatric resident from Hungary standing right next to him and staring at the same flyer. The two immediately formed a pact, and Ahchu offered to drive them both to Poughkeepsie, where Vassar College is located.

This was December 5, 1965. To his dismay, after the two-hour drive in the dead of winter, Ahchu did not find any girl particularly attractive at the mixer. Unlike the psychiatrist resident who managed to hold many girls' hands because he supposedly could read palms to tell their fortunes, Ahchu did not receive a particularly warm welcome. However, things took a sudden turn when, halfway through the evening, in walked Linda.

As if manipulated by some divine intervention, Ahchu hastily walked towards her and introduced himself, "Hello, my name is Ahchu. Have I met you before?" While this may have seemed an overly hackneyed pick-up line to Linda at the time, 53 years into their marriage, Ahchu still insists that he really thought they had met before. She looked so familiar. Believing in reincarnation, Linda's explanation is that they were together happily in a previous lifetime.

They quickly became acquainted, and Ahchu asked Linda out on a date the next day. Linda was so attractive that she had already been asked out on a breakfast date by an Indonesian-Chinese student from Columbia, and on a dinner date by a Caucasian. Short on time but not wanting to let this opportunity slip through his hands, Ahchu boldly proposed, "How about lunch?," to which Linda said yes.

Ahchu took Linda to the only Chinese restaurant in town, and they had a good time. When they came back, he suggested a game of ping pong, which he won; no big deal. Time flies when people are happy, and soon Ahchu had to leave and go back to St. Luke's Hospital, and Linda was off to meet her next date.

A Chinese meal followed by a game of ping pong— perhaps not the most fancy or romantic combination, but these simple pleasures fostered their mutual affection. Sometime later, Ahchu discovered that Linda's other date had taken her to a French restaurant, trying hard to impress her. However, Linda was not as impressed by her other suitors as she was by Ahchu, "You were humble, and you didn't try to impress me while the others did. That's why I thought you were more reliable, and it turned out I was right." Another secret that Ahchu uncovered much later, was that Linda was much better at ping pong than he was, indeed she was an undefeated champion in high school. During their 53 years of marriage, Ahchu has never beaten Linda at ping pong again. To this day, she swears that he won fair and square the first time around. She would not have let any man win unless he earned it.

Back at St. Luke's Hospital, Ahchu, an intern with a meager income, used the hospital phone to call Linda from time to time, as cell phones had not yet been invented. Long-distance calls were expensive, and the hospital administration soon tracked down the source of this huge increase in telephone charges. One day, the chief of the telephone department called Ahchu out, "Young man, I could make you pay this large sum of money, but I will not. Can you tell me who you were calling so frequently?"

Ahchu, although bashful, decided that 'honesty was the best policy', and confessed to the hospital administrator. The woman was a kind, motherly figure in her fifties, and was sympathetic to the wishes of this young man in love to stay in close contact with his long-distance girlfriend, so she considerately did not make him pay. Instead, they made a deal that as long as Ahchu called Linda no more than once a week for under 10 minutes, he could continue using the hospital phone.

The busy couple got the chance to meet face-to-face again when Linda's host family in Buffalo invited Ahchu to visit them over Christmas. Upon knocking on the door, Ahchu was welcomed by the host family father reading out a social commentary article. Ahchu assumed the article was describing the current government, and although he wasn't expecting this 'test' of his political acumen, he eloquently commented on the state of war in Vietnam, the most hotly debated issue in the freezing winter of 1965. "Did you know that this article was written in Julius Caesar's time?" Linda's host father informed Ahchu playfully, and the usual family reunion resumed, leaving Ahchu astounded by the recurrent themes of history. Humans have not changed much; the same problems that existed in Julius Caesar's time existed in 1965 and still exist in 2020. Even though this episode was overshadowed by Ahchu's euphoric mood at being with Linda, it lingered in the back of his mind. He is the kind of person who is concerned about public welfare even in the midst of his most vital personal affairs.

On New Year's Day, 1966, Linda came to New York City to celebrate with Ahchu. He took her and his friend Fumiko to an annual New Year dinner hosted by a Malaysian Chinese doctor in Chinatown. "Nice to see you Dr. Wang, let me introduce you to my fiancée," thus spoken, Ahchu tightened his arm around Linda and nodded at his doctor friend.

"Congratulations!" Dr. Wang was in utter shock because Ahchu had brought a different girl as his companion to the dinner every year, but none of them had been his girlfriend, and all of sudden he was getting married to this previously unheard-of girl. "Let us see the ring!" Dr. Wang said. Ahchu smiled coyly into Linda's eyes and answered, "My mom is having it made back in Malaysia."

Circumspect as Ahchu is, it was not characteristic of him to be engaged without a ring, nor was it characteristic of him to propose to a girl he had just met three weeks ago! In truth, it had all been a split-second decision. Ten minutes earlier, Ahchu pulled up smoothly in front of the home of his host and kindly dropped off Fumiko, saying, "It's too long a walk from the parking lot to the house in this weather, you should go in first." However, when Linda tried to get out as well, Ahchu stopped her. Puzzled, Linda teased him, "If you wanted to be a gentleman and let the ladies get out first, why didn't you let me go with Fumiko? It doesn't make sense for me to come all the way to the parking lot with you." Ahchu hesitated to reply. As he drove, thoughts were flying around inside his head. "IQ (intelligence quotient): she is as dedicated to her studies as I am, and she is doing well at Vassar — 9 out of 10. BQ (beauty quotient): she's gorgeous (and still is 53 years later) — 9.5 out of 10. EQ (emotional quotient): I remember when I drove from New York City to Vassar one weekend and almost drifted into the opposite lane of the highway because of my fatigue, which could have resulted in a serious accident. Linda begged me seriously, "You can't drive to see me anymore. This is not safe for you." While other girls may stubbornly insist on seeing their boyfriends frequently, she always puts my well-being ahead of herself. Also remembering that ping pong match on our first date, I have not met a single person more considerate than she is— 9 out of 10. Family background: she comes from a decent family who believes in integrity— 9 out of 10. That adds up to 36.5 out of 40 in total." No one is perfect, but Linda's score triumphed over the scores of the other girls Ahchu was dating. "I think that is as high a score as I am likely to get. I am convinced. It's her! I want to marry her."

You may laugh at Ahchu's methodical approach, even at supposedly the most romantic moment in his life; evaluating his future spouse as if he were hiring an employee or admitting a student to college. But this is the way Ahchu has always been. The more important a decision is, the more methodical he needs to be. No wonder he is a staunch Methodist, President of the Senior Methodist Fellowship when he was barely 16, youngest member of the Fellowship. The 'Methodist' denomination is so called because its founder, John Wesley, organized the church governance in a very methodical way. Clearly Ahchu is extremely well-suited to the Methodist way of life.

"Linda, may I introduce you to my doctor friend as my fiancée? I want the host to know you are special to me." Ahchu finally gathered up the courage to utter the question. *Is this a true proposal?* The reader might wonder; regardless, they have been happily married for 53 years. "Sure," Linda replied casually, and they walked into the house hand-in-hand, as if nothing significant had just happened.

The young couple planned to get married in August 1966. All seemed to proceed smoothly except for one incident. In late April, Ahchu opened his mailbox to find a long letter from Linda that read, "... I don't think we should see each other anymore. After careful consideration, I think I am only 20; too young to get married. I have made plans to attend medical school, and I think I should wait at least until after that. My father expects it of me."

Although he was startled, Ahchu knew that frustration without action is fruitless, so without further ado, he dialed Linda's number and appealed to her with all his reasoning. He worked his persuasive magic, and by the end of the one-and-a-half-hour phone call, their wedding plans were back on track. Linda's father once said, "Ahchu can talk a bird down from the tree." This was the one and only time that Ahchu violated the deal he made with the kind-hearted hospital administrator about telephone usage, but fortunately, he wasn't punished for it.

Following Chinese tradition, the wedding was to take place in the groom's home, in this case Malaysia. Ahchu and Linda planned to travel first to Hong Kong to meet Linda's parents, then to Malaysia to get married, returning to Hong Kong, and eventually back to the U.S. the day after Labor Day in order for Ahchu to continue his residency.

On a balmy August morning, Ahchu boarded the plane that would take him to Hong Kong to meet Linda's parents. Linda has a huge family: her father has 12 siblings, not to mention an abundance of cousins. They all approved of Ahchu in their own manner. As an example, as soon as he spotted Ahchu walking into the room, Linda's oldest uncle approached him with a grim smile and asked him to open his mouth, "Please let me see your teeth." This elderly gentleman held the traditional belief that good teeth signified good health, examining his future nephew-in-law in the same way he might a horse!

Ahchu and Linda traveled to Malaysia to get married and spent their honeymoon in a small room at the local swimming club, similar to a YMCA. The bathroom, sink and toilet were down the hall, one for males, one for females. The floor of the bathroom was wet and dirty. It was all Ahchu could afford. After the honeymoon, thrilled and ecstatic, they boarded their flight and flew back to the U.S., on time for Ahchu to resume his residency.

Ahchu and Linda have now been married for 53 years. Thinking about all the miracles and coincidences they went through to become a couple, it's hard not to believe that they are meant to be together, mandated by some divine force. They get along so well, as if they knew each other in previous lives and have been reincarnated into this world to be together again, as Linda firmly believes. That is not to say they never have disagreements. As soon as they returned from Malaysia, Ahchu had to go back to work, leaving Linda to clean up their dirty, shabby fifth floor walk-up, subsidized apartment near St. Luke's Hospital. When Ahchu came back home from the hospital, he asked Linda, "What have you done all day?" Linda, having endured a long day of cleaning, took this as an insult to her hard, domestic work. She shot back angrily, "I have been scrubbing the bathroom and the floors all day while you gloriously saved people's lives!" Ahchu soon realized his mistake and retreated quickly to the other end of the apartment.

Such incidences of small bickering might seem insignificant in the face of all the challenges Ahchu and Linda have faced together, but love is never easy, and a successful marriage takes patience and compromise. Their best piece of relationship advice is to never go to bed angry. And throughout the years, through conflicts large and small, Ahchu always remembers his ecstatic feelings when he first saw Linda and asked, "Have I met you before?"

Chapter 12

'K.J.' WAS COINED

Coco Kejia Ruan

"Whatever you do, work at it with all your heart, as working for the Lord, not for human masters."
– Colossians 3:23

The word 'intern', now established as the term for 'person in training', originates from the French word *interner*, which means "to send to the interior, to confine." This sense of confinement adequately described the lives of many medical interns in Ahchu's era, working prolonged hours every day in the confined environment of the hospital. Ahchu was no exception. However, despite this physical confinement, his pursuit of professional excellence had no limit. To break free from this confinement, Ahchu cites two ingredients in his magical formula: proaction and resilience.

After graduating from medical school, Ahchu started his surgical internship at St. Luke's Hospital in New York City in July 1965. He began his internship as Dr. Keat-Jin Lee, his real name. He ended his internship as Dr. K.J. Lee. His given name at birth in Malaya was Lee Keat Jin, Lee being the family name which preceded the two-syllable given name, Keat Jin.

There was no hyphen between Keat and Jin, but the two syllables were not to be separated. As you may remember from Chapter 1, Ahchu is his nickname. At Harvard and Columbia, he was called "Keat" which annoyed him no end. He therefore added a hyphen between Keat and Jin. This proved to be a mistake, as people commonly made Keat his last name, or sometimes mistook Jin as his last name. When he started his internship, the operator paged him through the hospital public address system: "Needed or wanted Dr. Kitchen Lee." That was the straw that broke the camel's back. He immediately changed his professional name to K.J. Lee.

Along with the 'birth' of his new name, 'K.J.', he developed his *modus operandi*. His intern experience was all about proaction, and he would later proudly profess that, "the way I function is to accomplish every task in a medically correct and efficient manner, so that everything is already in place by the time the attending doctor comes around." In a U.S. hospital setting, the attending doctor is ultimately responsible for the patient's care. He or she is the doctor whom the patient engaged to render care and hold accountable.

In St. Luke's Hospital, the surgical attending doctors usually made their rounds to check on their patients at 6.30 in the morning. In the field of surgery, it is an open secret that good doctors make their rounds before going into the operating room, unlike certain doctors who make their rounds after their operations. While the duration of an operation (on average two or three hours) does not seem long to the doctors, it makes a huge difference to the well-being of the pre- or post-operative patients waiting in their rooms while the doctor carries out other operations. In the worst-case scenario, a patient's medical condition could deteriorate drastically in a short period of time, while the doctor remains completely unaware in the operating room. This could potentially put that patient's life in jeopardy. At the other end of the spectrum, patients who have recovered need to wait for the attending doctor to sign their paperwork before they can go home. The hours waiting for the doctor to come are usually spent in dreaded impatience and idleness. Patients are trapped in a place they do not want to be in, gazing at the world outside and waiting to be 'freed'.

To avoid these scenarios, Ahchu decided that, "if I make my rounds at 5.30 in the morning, a whole hour before the attending doctors who make their rounds at 6.30 a.m., routine matters will be taken care of and serious medical conditions could be noted in preparation for the attending doctors." Of course, this was easier said than done, considering the number of hours he worked every day, sometimes way past midnight. Furthermore, as an intern on-call, his sleep was often interrupted by nurses with questions about the patients.

A typical shift for an intern was less than 10 hours off duty in a 48-hour rotation. If you asked Ahchu what color the sky was in Upper West Side, Manhattan in the 1960s, he would not give you the conventional answer, "blue," or even the poetic answer, "burnt orange mixed with lavender and a trace of mulberry." He would tell you, "it was starry on a black background," or rather, the more Ahchu-esque answer, "I don't know." The reason is simple— he went to work before the sun had risen, and he never got out of work before the sun set.

In addition to his meticulous approach to ward rounds, Ahchu made sure that the attending doctors on whichever floor he was assigned to that day would have all the necessary equipment and supplies prepared, and that patients' medical records were always up-to-date.

For Ahchu, the key to being a good surgeon is not only a calm and precise approach in the operating room, but also paying attention to the most minute task. Any effort is worthwhile when it makes a difference to the patient's experience.

It is no surprise that Ahchu successfully completed his training as an intern with distinction and moved on to become a resident. However, his magical formula for success now needed a new twist. Ahchu had set his mind on becoming an otolaryngology surgeon before he started his internship and one year of compulsory general surgery residency, but he was equally interested in facial cosmetic surgery. For some reason, most fortunately for Ahchu, the resident assigned to the plastic surgery department for the year never arrived, and the hospital was urgently looking for another resident to fill the gap. Ahchu was thrilled to take on the task, but the rules had it that if he didn't fulfill one year of general surgery residency, he could not go on to be a resident in otolaryngology the following year.

Passionate to learn, Ahchu would have taken on both roles if time permitted. But given the situation, he could only pick one. If he had found the decision easy, then he would no longer be the thoughtful, persistent 15-year-old who didn't take no for an answer back in Penang, Malaya.

Challenging unreasonable conventions was in his blood. In high school, prefect meetings were always held during school hours. Unwilling to miss classes, Ahchu suggested holding the meetings after school hours to the prefect master, who arrogantly responded, "If you don't like it, don't be a prefect!" To be chosen as a prefect was an honor. Prefects were the top students with leadership skills. Out of respect for the prefect master and not wanting to cause a public commotion, Ahchu swallowed the hard rejection with a polite smile and went home. That night, he called up the principal at home and explained the situation diplomatically. Starting the next day, a new school rule was in place: all extracurricular activities, including prefects' meetings, would henceforth be held after school hours. Ahchu won the silent battle with proaction.

However, a proactive response didn't always work out. Life threw him a curve ball when he applied to medical schools. His interviewer from Harvard Medical School told him, "If we don't accept you, Harvard is betting on the wrong horse." On a Friday evening in early winter, Ahchu ran into his jubilant classmate, Marty Feldstein. Marty had just been accepted into Harvard Medical School.

Ahchu wondered when his acceptance letter would arrive. Since a proactive approach had served him well in the past, he made the foolhardy decision to dial the home number of the assistant dean who interviewed him. Ahchu was a little too 'proactive' to realize this was a huge mistake. This was the United States, not a small town in Malaya where he had a close relationship with his teachers. What was more, he did not realize that it was against all etiquette to call a superior or even an acquaintance at home on a Friday night. For this, or perhaps other reasons, Ahchu was rejected by Harvard Medical School. He was accepted by Columbia University College of Physicians and Surgeons and other schools. As hard as it was to admit, his impulsiveness could have sealed his rejection from Harvard Medical School.

Like others, he had stumbled and fallen, but he always climbed back up and learned from his mistakes. This time, he was determined to use his proactive attitude, minus the impulsiveness, to defy convention in order to achieve his goal. After rounds of negotiations, Ahchu eventually agreed with the hospital that he would spend six months in general surgery training and another six months as a plastic surgery resident, fulfilling both his desire to learn and the program requirement.

Ahchu maintained his adventurous and resilient spirit throughout his residency at St. Luke's, making new friends and devising new procedures. He met frequently with the chief of plastic surgery who used to work in Vietnam and loved to talk about Vietnamese cuisine. Coincidentally, Ahchu's wife, Linda, was born and raised in Vietnam by a Hong Kong family. This shared connection naturally fostered a friendship between Ahchu and the chief of plastic surgery. Ahchu also became friends with the Fellow in plastic surgery (a position higher than resident). At this time, the conventional procedure to tighten one's facial skin was a 'facelift'. This involves making incisions on the skin, stretching it, and getting rid of the extra tissue before closing the incisions. The Fellow wanted to try a chemical peel procedure to tighten the skin. Instead of making incisions on the facial skin, a chemical peel entails spreading acid over the face. After a couple of weeks of what looks like a terrible sunburn, the skin will tighten itself to give a more youthful appearance. The Fellow had read about chemical peels but never performed one.

One day after work, the Fellow tapped Ahchu on the back and surreptitiously said, "Ahchu, let's go to the library to look up the procedure for a chemical peel, then you can help me do one!" Ahchu was always curious to explore new procedures, but he hesitated, "what if the procedure is unsuccessful? How much risk is involved? Does the patient know what she is getting into?" After much deliberation, the quest to learn overcame his doubt and uncertainty, so Ahchu consented to research the chemicals involved, the proportions, and duration of the procedure. He was already confident in his dexterity from his practice as a medical student and his early days of knitting and needlepointing at an all-girls pre-school. Even before becoming an intern, as a fourth-year medical school student, Ahchu had his surgical rotations at Bellevue Hospital in New York City where he performed and assisted in minor surgeries. Needless to say, practice makes perfect, and Ahchu had trained his hands 'fast and well' at Bellevue Hospital; now he was ready to put his experience and dexterity into practice and innovation. Not wanting to attract attention, unbeknownst to the nurses and doctors, the Fellow scheduled the 'chemical facelift' plastic surgery procedure for their first patient after dark in a private treatment room. Ahchu carefully read the protocol and mixed the chemicals like an alchemist, while the Fellow performed the procedure. Two weeks later, the patient returned to the hospital looking more beautiful and more youthful than before. Ahchu gave a sigh of relief on witnessing the success. He never allowed himself to imagine what would have happened if the result had turned out otherwise.

His year as a resident at St. Luke's wasn't always worry free. On one occasion, a serious accusation caught him off guard. When Ahchu and his new wife came back to New York after spending two weeks on honeymoon in Malaya, he opened his mailbox and was astounded to find a letter of accusation. Ahchu checked the envelope several times just to make sure that it was addressed to him. Unfortunately, the name "K.J. Lee" was printed in the middle of the envelope as well as on the header of the letter. He was even more perturbed when he finished reading it:

> "Dr. K.J. Lee,
> I was thoroughly disappointed at your decision to sublet your cheap, hospital-subsidized apartment for higher rent. This is both legally and ethically wrong... Furthermore, I cannot believe that while you sublet the apartment, you stayed overnight in the on-call room with a nurse..."

The signature belonged to a junior hospital administrator. Ahchu was so flabbergasted by this unfounded accusation that he did not know where to start to right the wrong.

Before his trip to Malaya, he had been assigned a resident-subsidized apartment on 115th Street and Amsterdam Avenue near St. Luke's Hospital.

There was a reason why the rent for the dirty fifth-floor walk-up apartment was a mere $90 per month. Ahchu recounts that his weekend entertainment was watching the drug dealers and drunkards across the street drop empty liquor bottles to see which would hit the pavement first. Furthermore, Ahchu's wife remembers the instance when someone tried to climb in through the fire escape while she was cooking in the kitchen on a sunny August evening.

Two newly arrived nurses at St. Luke's had nowhere to stay for two weeks while their rented apartment was being renovated. These two weeks coincided with the two weeks Ahchu was in Malaya getting married and honeymooning. Always eager to help those in need, Ahchu offered his apartment to the nurses for free. The "nurse in the on-call room" mentioned in the junior administrator's letter was his wife, Linda. Since the apartment was unsafe, Linda would accompany him to the on-call room while he was on-call at the hospital.

After drawing a deep breath in and slowly breathing the air out, Ahchu calmed his rage and started composing a reply. Plan A, he could find the administrator and explain the truth. It sounded like a reasonable idea, however, within the hospital system, residents were always looked down upon by administrators, So Ahchu was in no place to argue with him, let alone ask for an apology.

Having learned from the school of hard knocks, Ahchu chose Plan B. He took time to collect the relevant evidence and sent it in a 'registered return receipt' envelope to the chairman of the Board of Trustees. This meant the chairman had to sign his name upon receiving the letter. Furthermore, Ahchu copied all members of the Board of Trustees.

Four days later, Ahchu received another letter in his mailbox. This time it came from the chairman of the Board of Trustees, politely inviting Ahchu to have lunch with him. In the end, the Board of Trustees not only issued Ahchu a written apology, but also reprimanded the junior administrator who had wrongly accused him.

Ahchu's **magical formula** had worked again, and in this case the key ingredient was resilience. Despite the difference in hierarchy, Ahchu knew that as long as he was on the side of the truth, he could defend himself in such unjust situations. It simply took forbearance, perseverance, resilience, and smart moves.

Many would imagine that the years of training after medical school (between graduating from medical school and becoming an attending physician) are purely routine. In Ahchu's case, it couldn't have been more different. He not only broke free from surgical traditions, but also defied the intern's confinement from the outside world. To him, living a just life is as important as practicing medicine and having a strong work ethic. A person should never solely focus on improving one side and thereby stymie development of the other. Through all the obstacles that he encountered and all the lessons he learned, Keat Jin morphed into Dr. K.J. Lee at St. Luke's Hospital, ready to take on further challenges in life, for himself and for his patients. 'Curveballs' along the way are indeed the mentors of life.

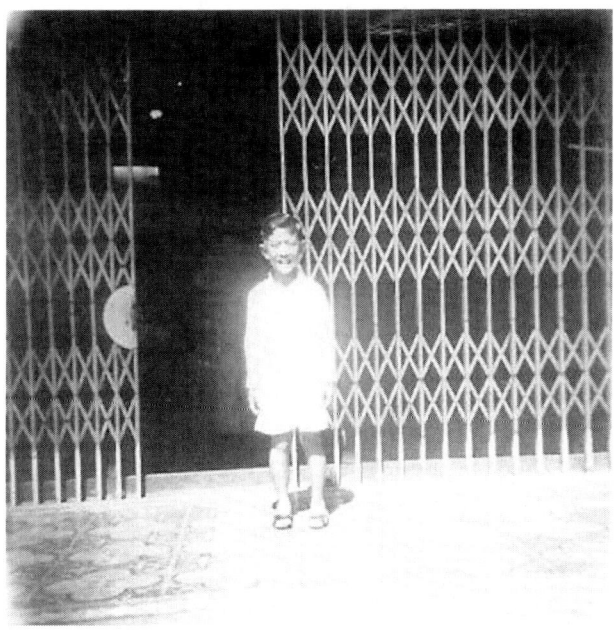

Image 1. Seven-year-old K.J. at 38th China Street, Penang, Malaya, his birthplace and first home. (Chapter 1).

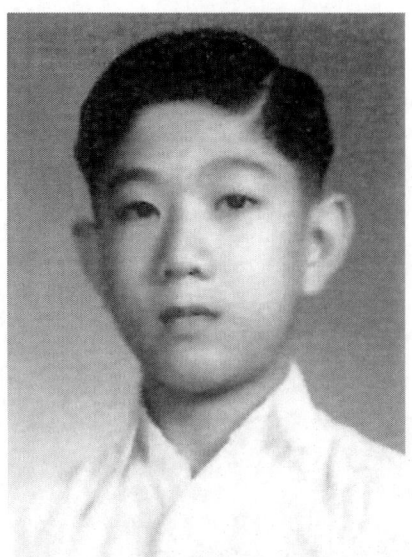

Image 2. K.J. aged 12, pictured for his ID card, 1952.

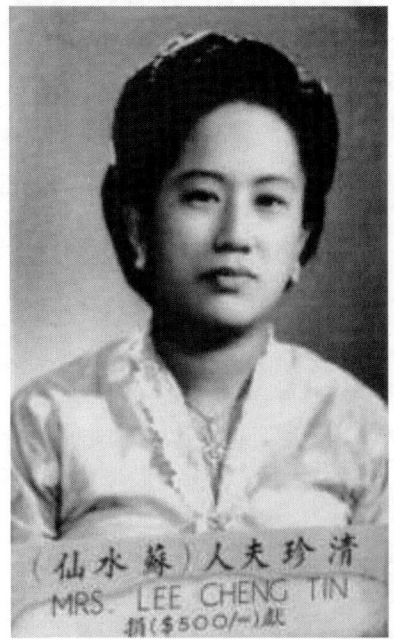

Image 3. K.J.'s mother, Saw Chooi Sean, 1973.

Leeway: Reaching Beyond Expectations 95

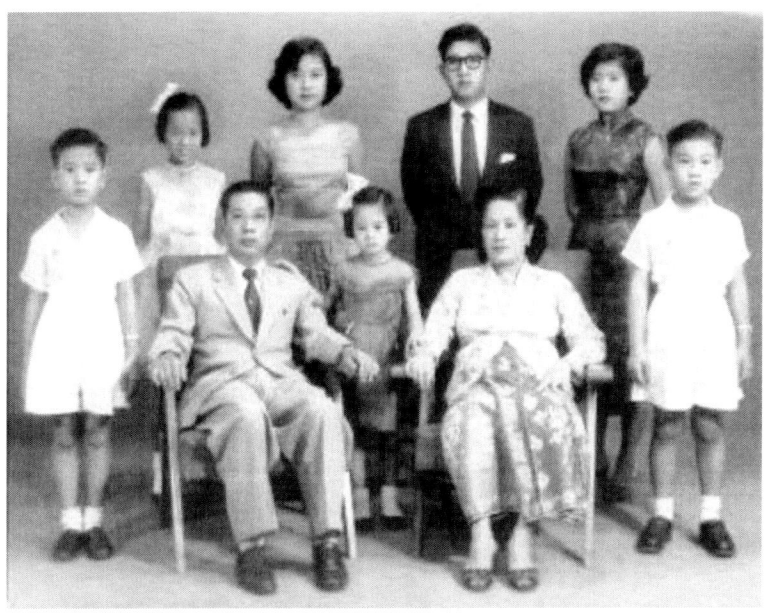

Image 4. Lee family photo (K.J. is in the backrow in a dark suit), 1957.

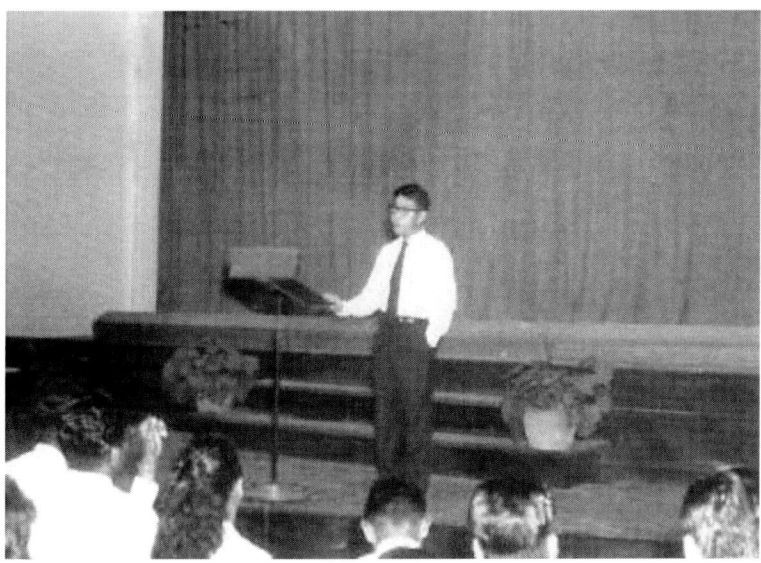

Image 5. K.J. at a debate at the age of 16, 1956.

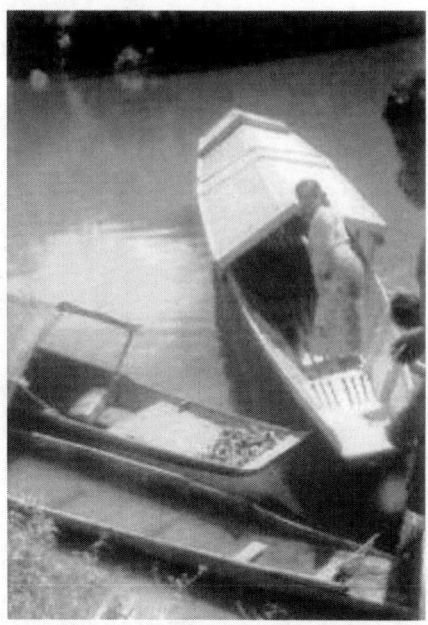

Image 6. K.J.'s mother sending him off to the U.S., 1958. (Chapter 4).

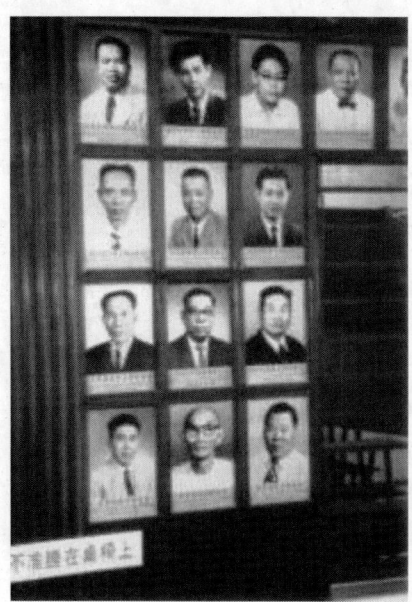

Image 7. The Lee Clan, 1958. K.J.'s father is in the centre of the second row from the bottom.

Leeway: Reaching Beyond Expectations 97

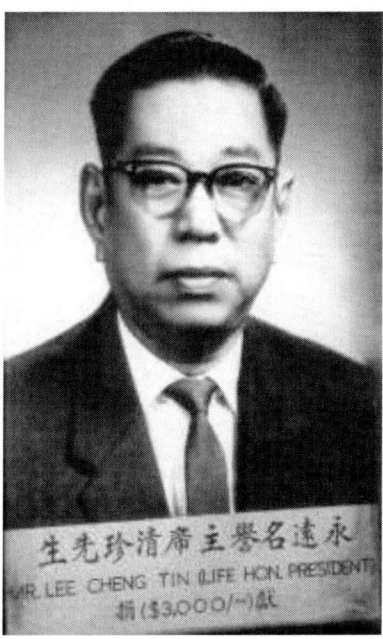

Image 8. K.J.'s father, 1958.

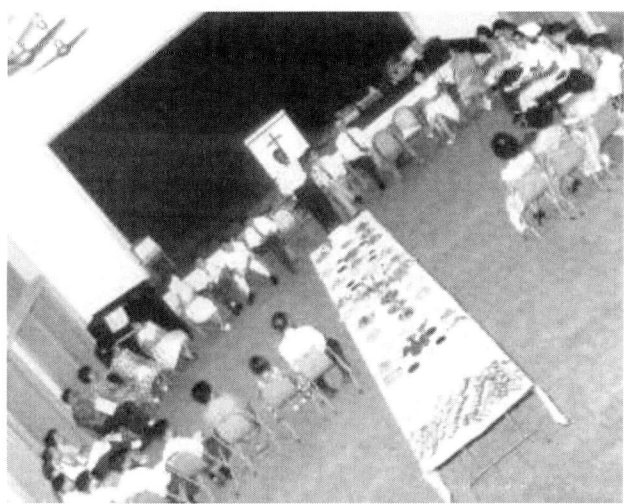

Image 9. Penang Methodist Youth Fellowship Farewell Party for K.J., July 1958. (Chapter 6).

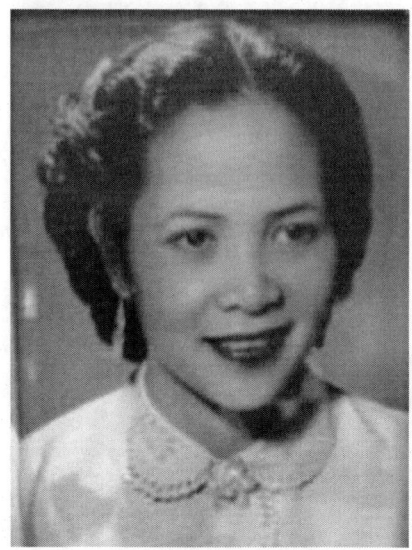

Image 10. Linda's mother, Mrs. Leontine Ho, 1948.

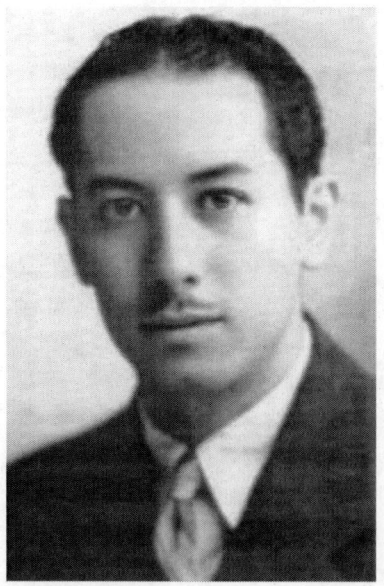

Image 11. Linda's father, Mr. John Ho, 1948.

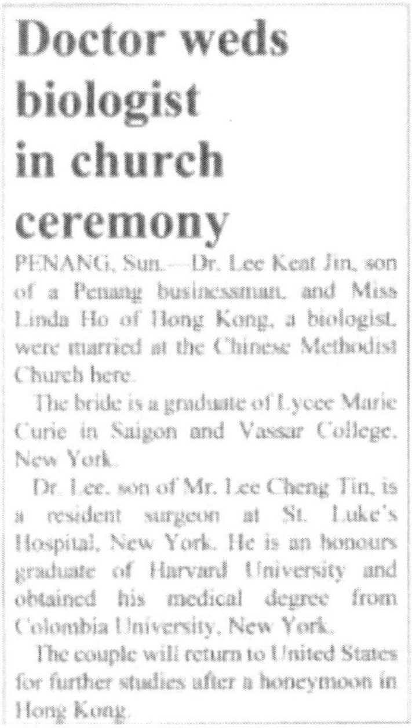

Doctor weds biologist in church ceremony

PENANG, Sun.— Dr. Lee Kent Jin, son of a Penang businessman, and Miss Linda Ho of Hong Kong, a biologist, were married at the Chinese Methodist Church here.

The bride is a graduate of Lycee Marie Curie in Saigon and Vassar College, New York.

Dr. Lee, son of Mr. Lee Cheng Tin, is a resident surgeon at St. Luke's Hospital, New York. He is an honours graduate of Harvard University and obtained his medical degree from Colombia University, New York.

The couple will return to United States for further studies after a honeymoon in Hong Kong.

Image 12. K.J. and Linda's marriage announcement in the Straits Times, Straits Echo, August 21, 1966. (Chapter 11).

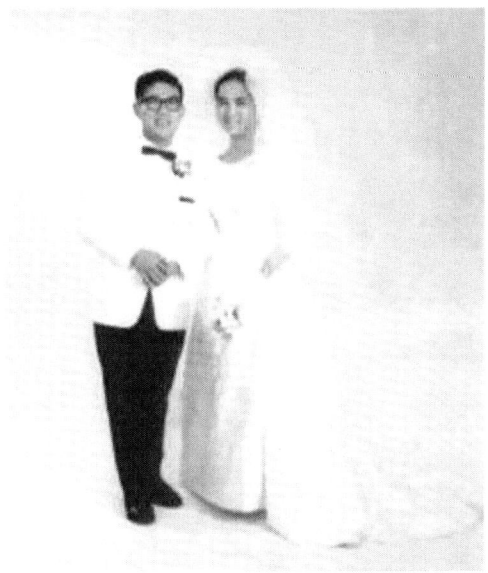

Image 13. K. J. and Linda on their wedding day.

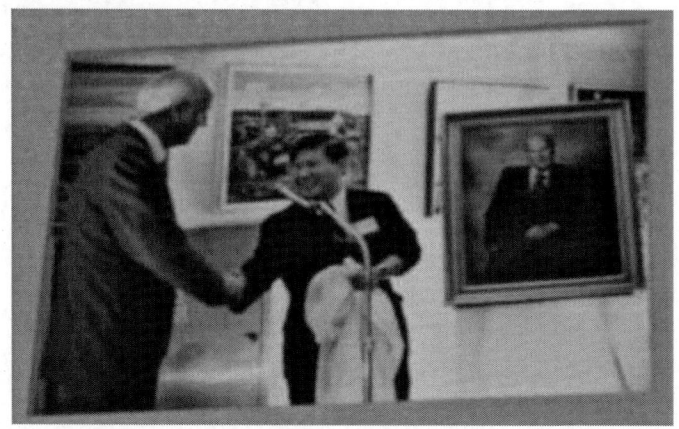

Image 14. K.J. unveiling the portrait of Professor Schuknecht at Harvard, 1978. (Chapter 13).

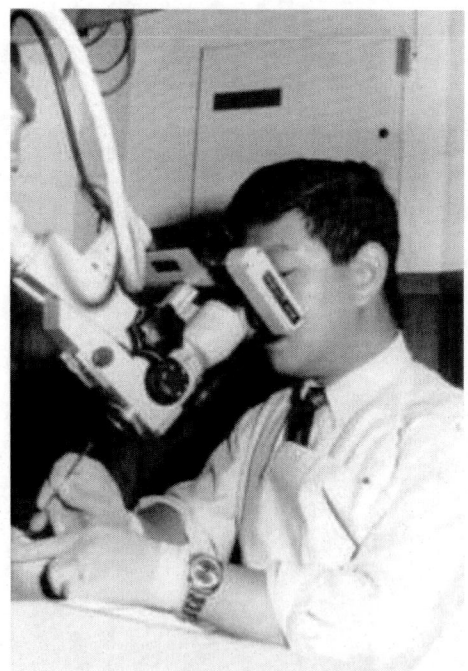

Image 15. K.J. at the House Ear Institute Temporal Bone Dissection Laboratory, 1971. (Chapter 14).

Leeway: Reaching Beyond Expectations 101

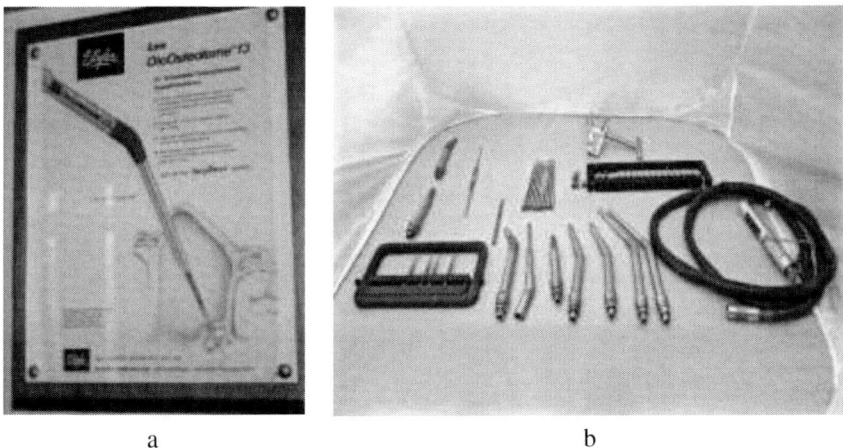

a   b

Image 16 a, b. Some of K.J.'s surgical inventions, for approaching the pituitary and skull base. (Chapter 16).

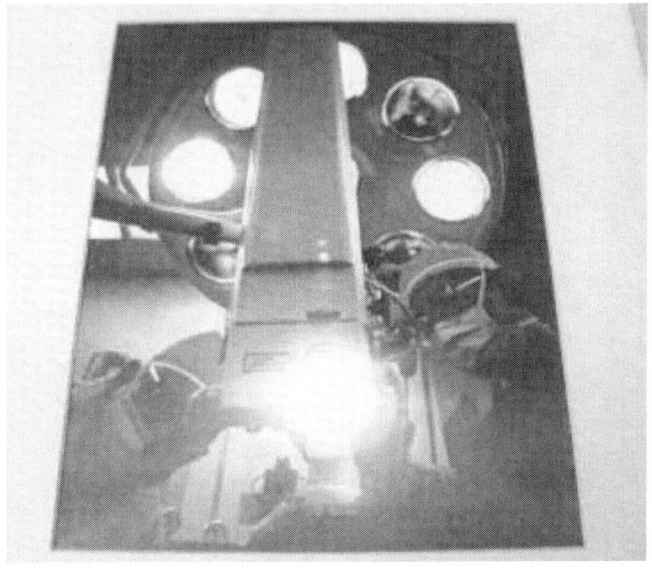

Image 17. K.J. developing laser surgery for ENT, 1975. (Chapter 17).

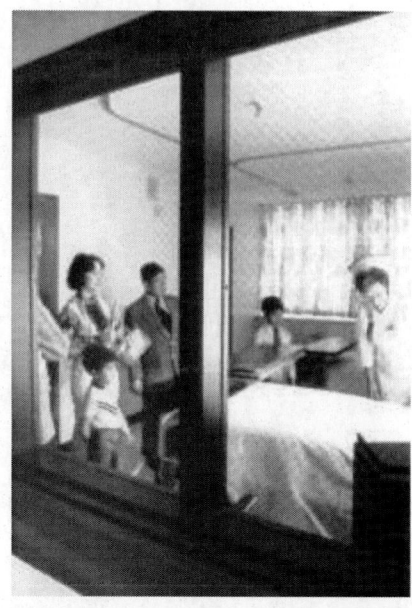

Image 18. K.J., Linda, Ken and Lloyd, inspecting the new Verdi Building at the Hospital of St. Raphael, 1976, the year K.J. was operated on for fibrosarcoma of the back.

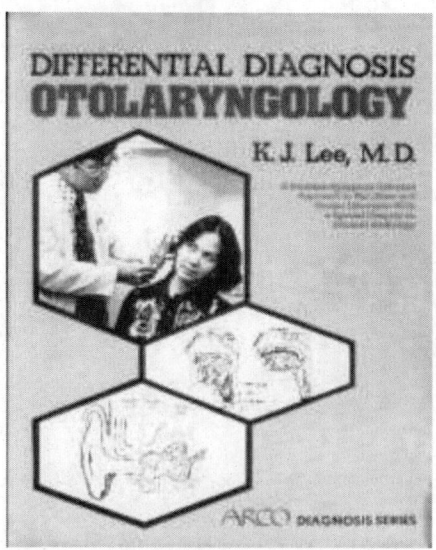

Image 19. K.J.'s 1978 otolaryngology book for lay people.

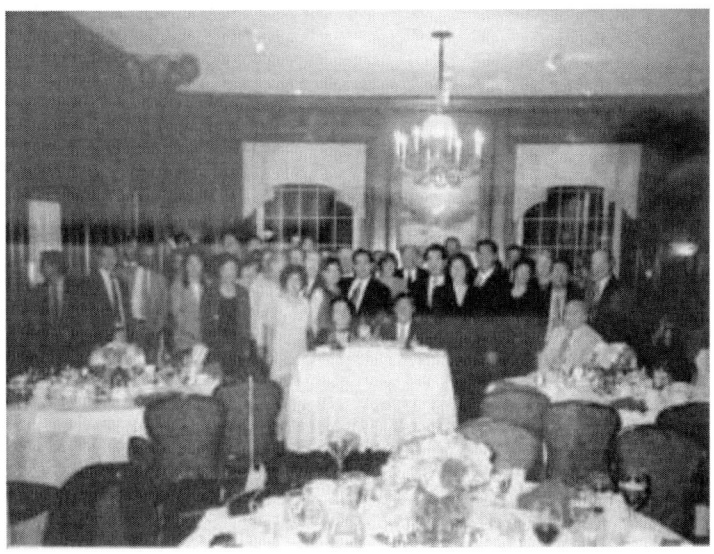

Image 20. K.J.'s 60th birthday party, 2000.

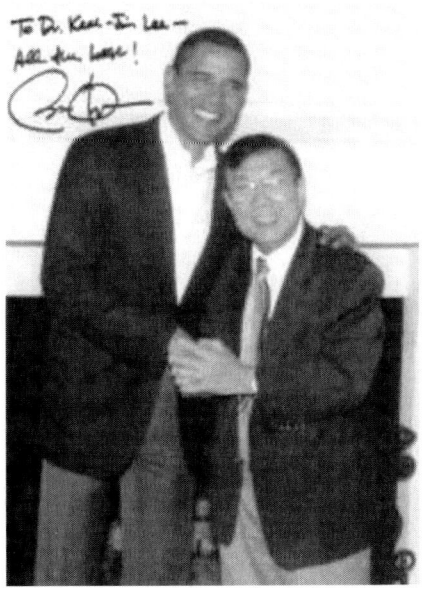

Image 21. K.J. with President Obama, 2007. (Chapter 22).

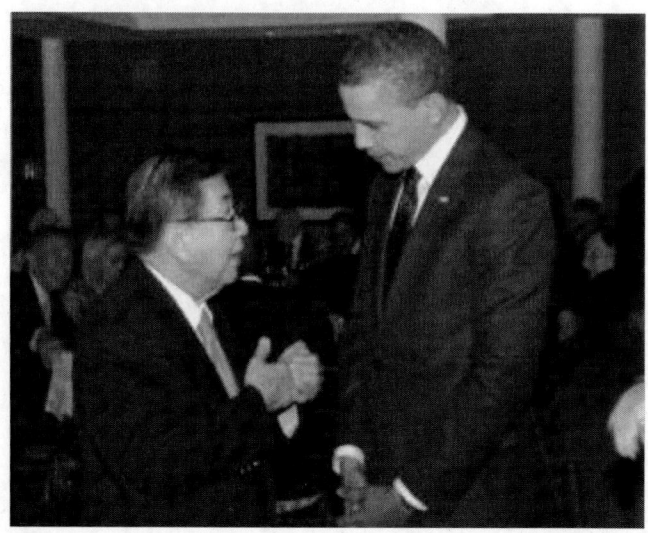

Image 22. K.J. with President Obama, 2008. The pair worked closely together to introduce Electronic Health Records (EHR), a concept which is yet to realize its full potential, and which K.J. is still working on. (Chapter 22).

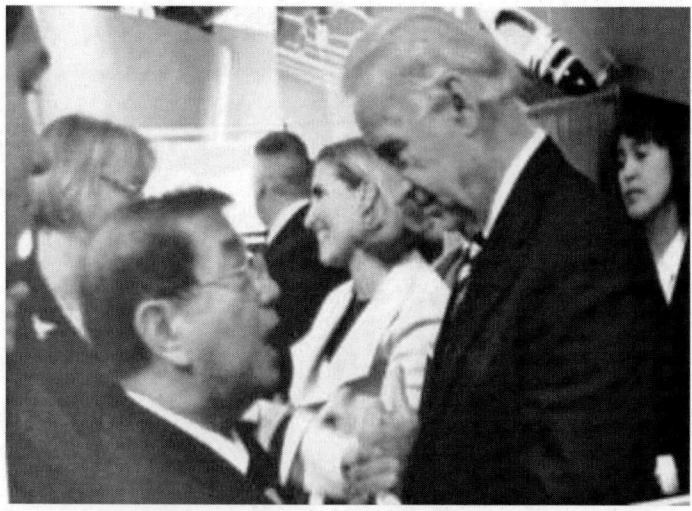

Image 23. K.J. with Vice President Biden.

Leeway: Reaching Beyond Expectations 105

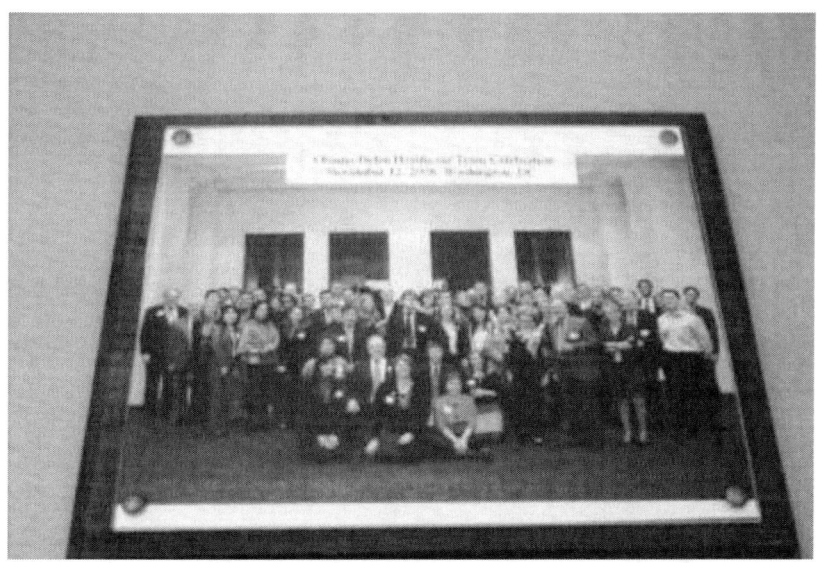

Image 24. Obama-Biden Healthcare Team Celebration, 2008. (Chapter 22).

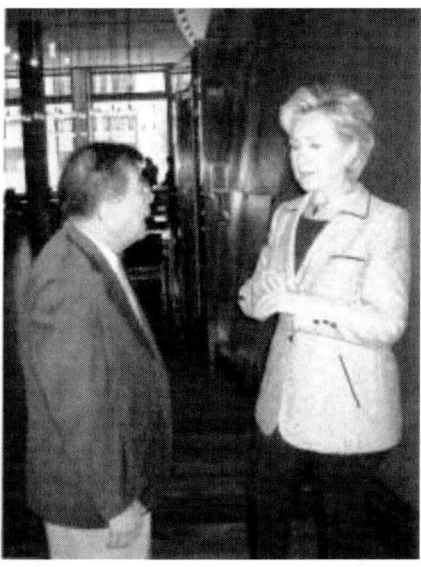

Image 25. K.J. with Hillary Clinton, 2008, with whom he collaborated on the original health savings account idea in 1993, as well as efforts to reduce wastage in healthcare funding during her 2008 presidential campaign. (Chapter 22).

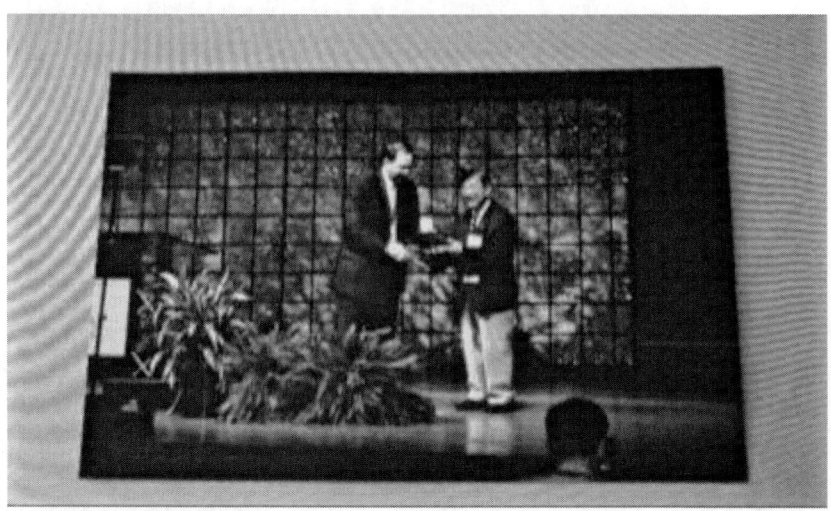

Image 26. K.J. receiving the American Academy of Otolaryngology - Head and Neck Surgery presidential citation from Dr. Denneny in 2008.

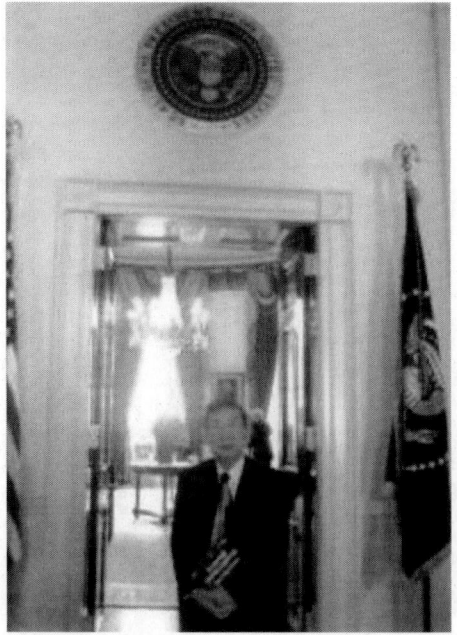

Image 27. K.J. at the White House Christmas Party, 2011.

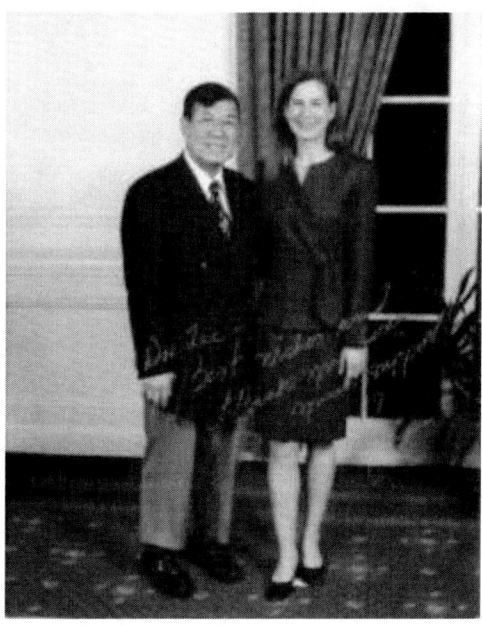

Image 28. K.J. with Lt. Governor Bysiewicz.

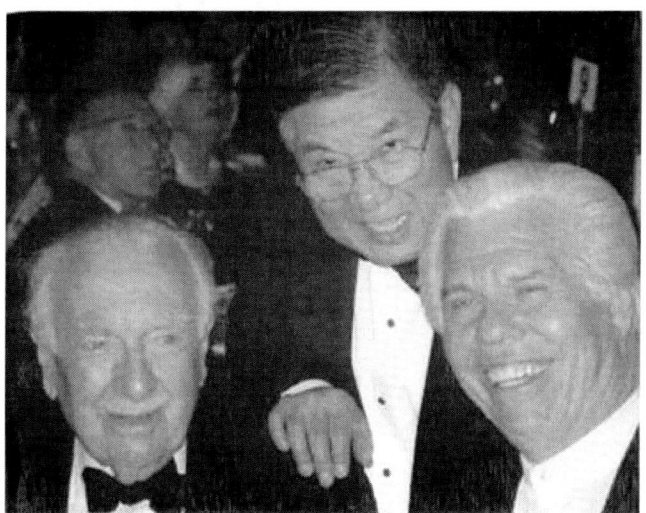

Image 29. K.J. with Walter Cronkite and Bill Austin.

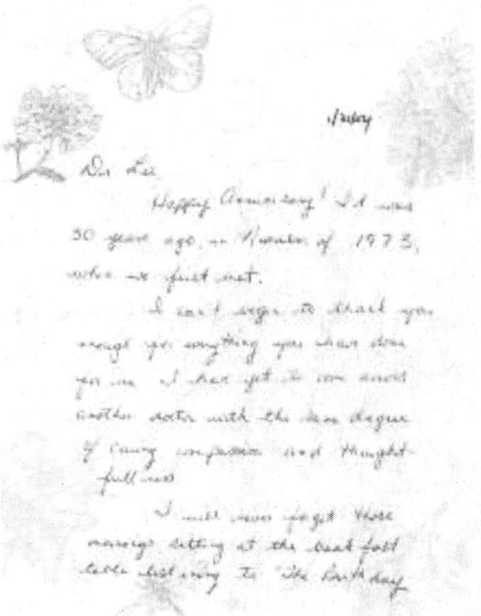

Image 30 a, b, c. A note from a patient.

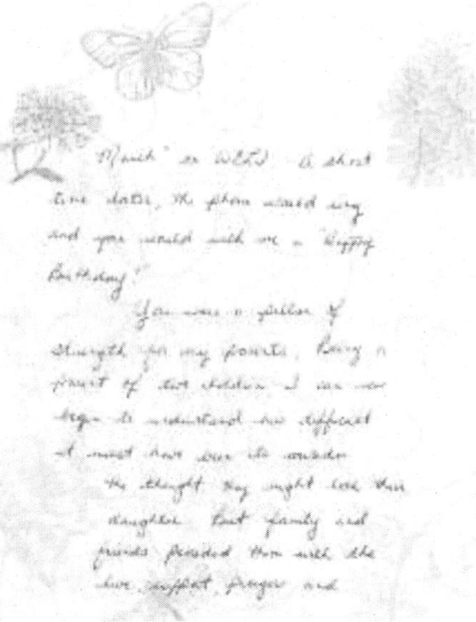

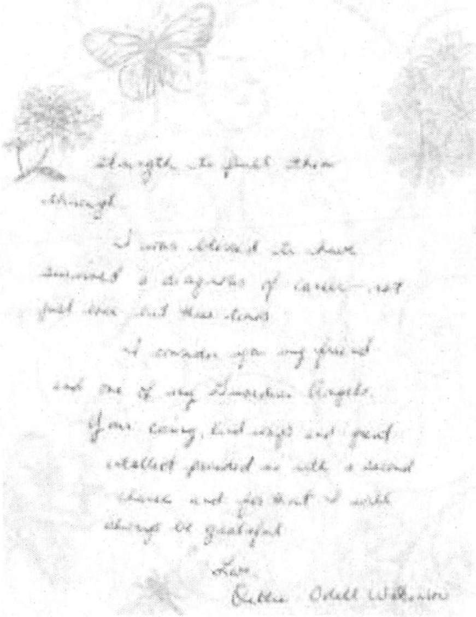

Leeway: Reaching Beyond Expectations 109

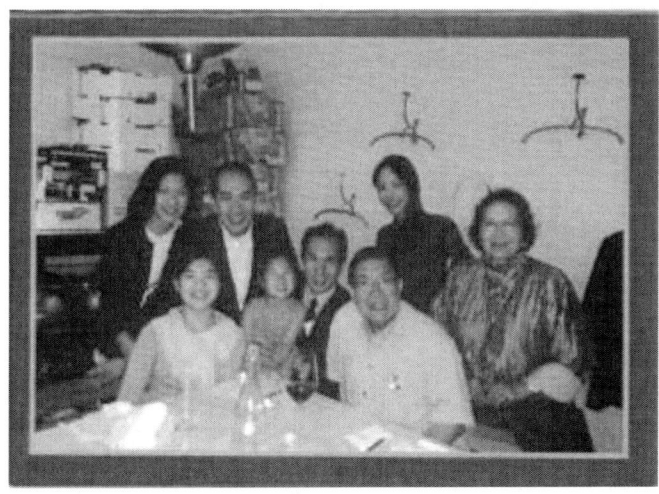

Image 31. K.J. and Linda, Ken, Susan, Morgan, Olivia, Lloyd and Chieko in London.

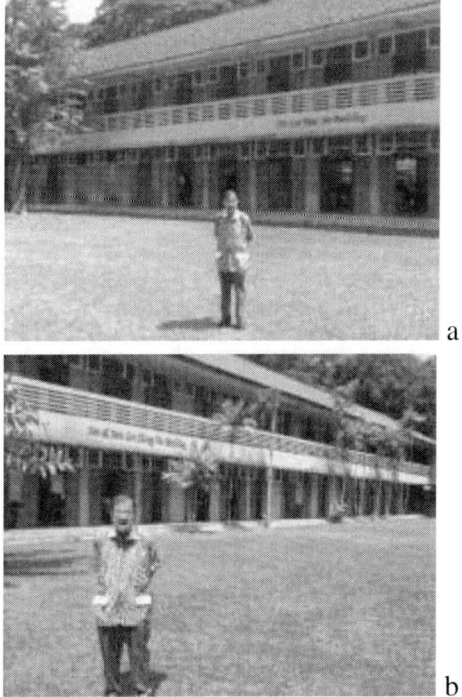

Image 32 a, b. Buildings at the Methodist Boys School in Penang, Malaysia named after the school's famous alumnus K.J. Lee and his parents.

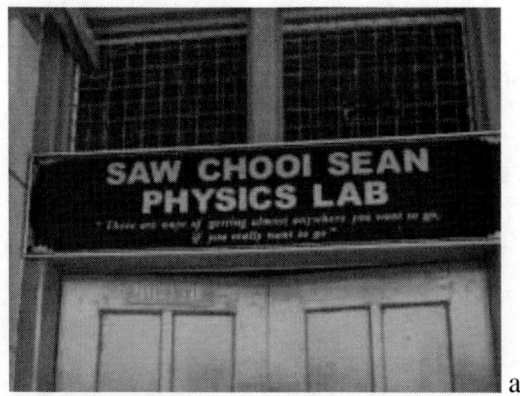

Named after K.J.'s mother (maiden name).

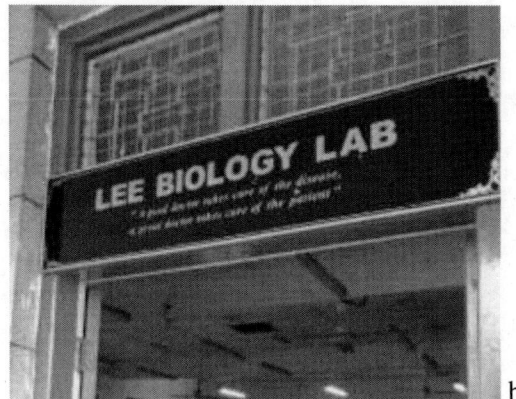

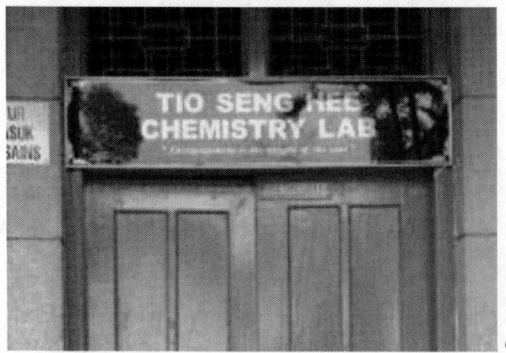

Image 33 a, b, c. The chemistry lab at K.J. Lee's high school, named after K.J.'s teacher/mentor.

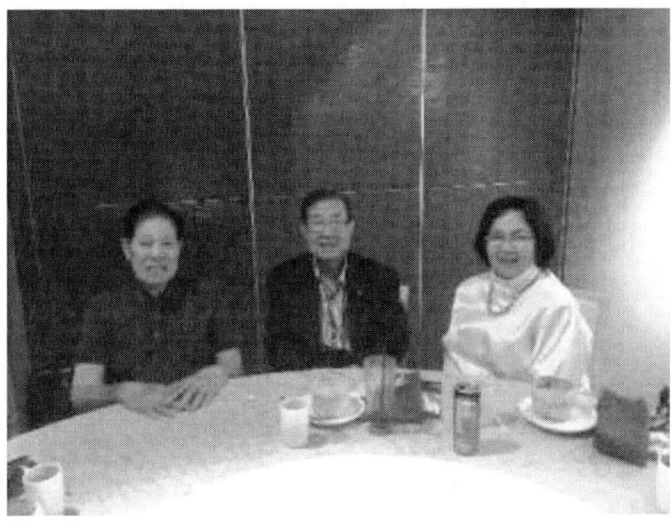

Image 34. August 3rd, 2019; dinner in Liang Court, Singapore, hosted by Mr. Goh Cheng Liang, illustrious patient and now good friend of K.J. Lee. (Chapter 16).

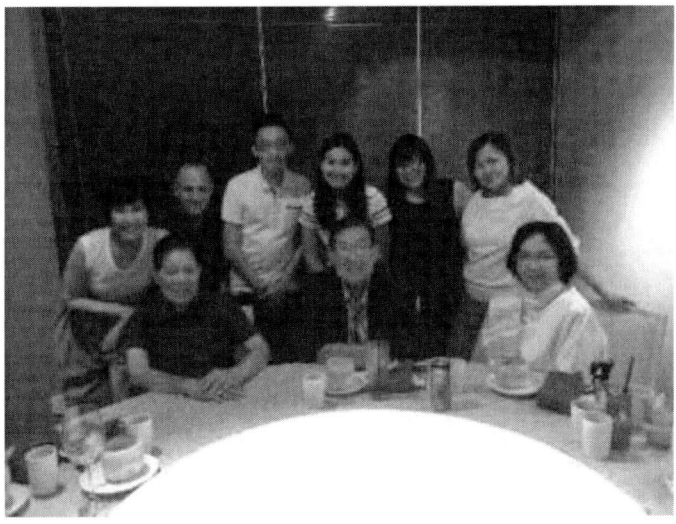

Image 35. August 3rd, 2019; dinner with Mr. Goh Cheng Liang, illustrious patient and now good friend of K.J. Lee, and his family in Liang Court. (Chapter 16).

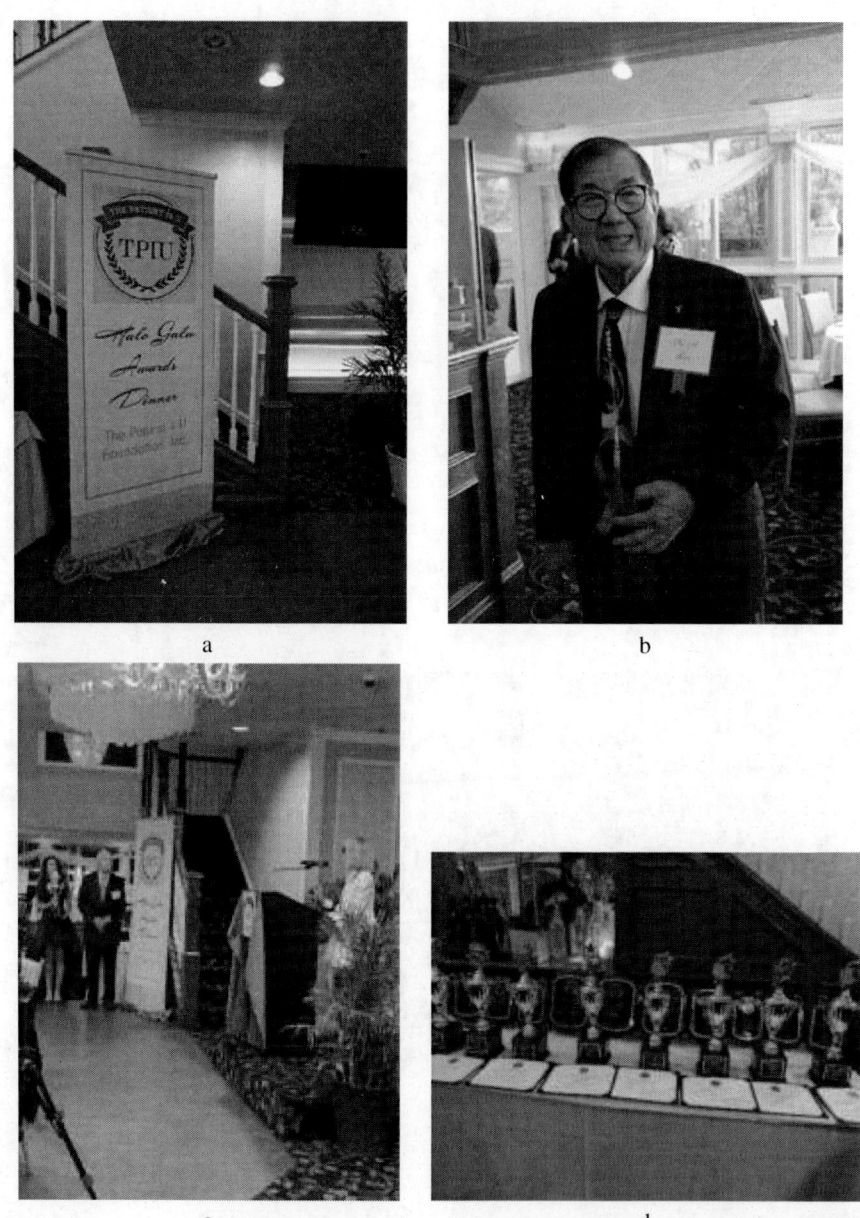

Image 36 a, b, c, d. The first Awards Gala Dinner of The Patient is U foundation, held on October 15th, 2019. (Chapter 23).

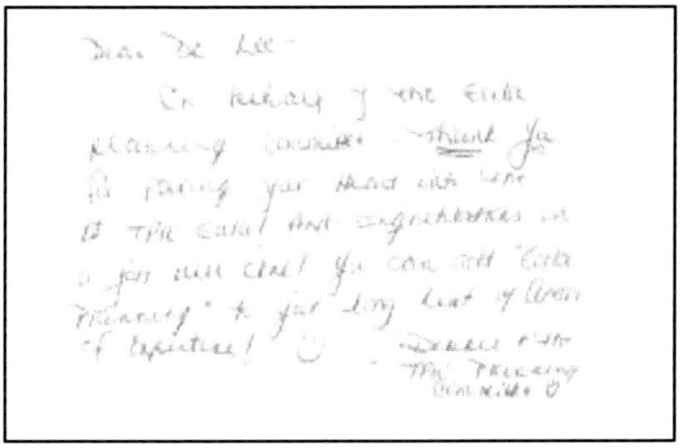

[Handwritten note]

Dear Dr. Lee –
On behalf of the entire planning committee – thank you for pouring your heart into what is Truly Grand and unprecedented in a few such that you can well take "meaning" to your long list of terms of expertise! 😊

— Deanne & the TPIU Planning Committee 😊

a

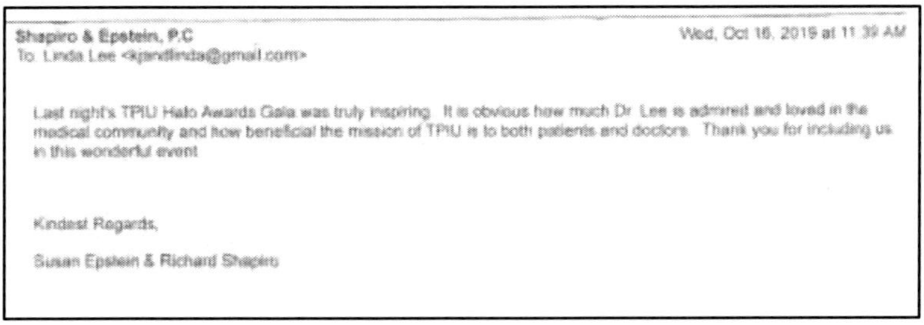

Shapiro & Epstein, P.C
To: Linda Lee <kjandlinda@gmail.com>
Wed, Oct 16, 2019 at 11:39 AM

Last night's TPIU Halo Awards Gala was truly inspiring. It is obvious how much Dr. Lee is admired and loved in the medical community and how beneficial the mission of TPIU is to both patients and doctors. Thank you for including us in this wonderful event.

Kindest Regards,

Susan Epstein & Richard Shapiro

b

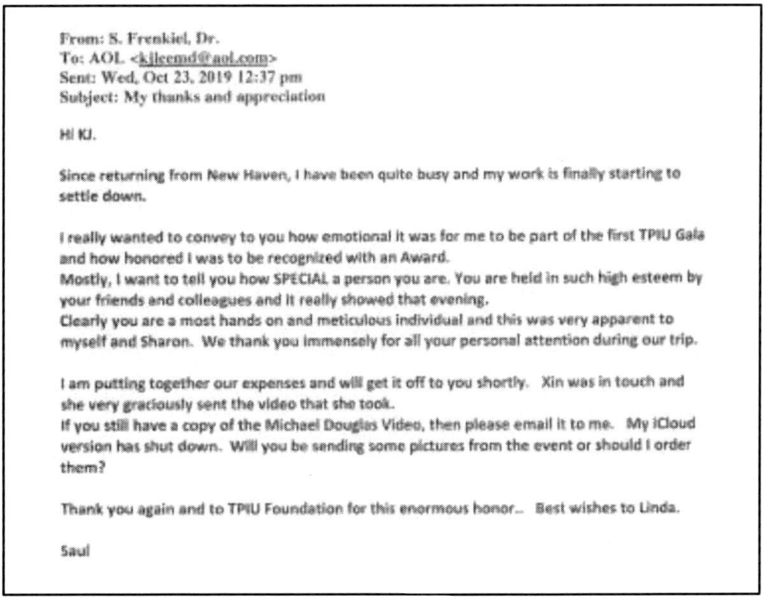

From: S. Frenkiel, Dr.
To: AOL <kjleemd@aol.com>
Sent: Wed, Oct 23, 2019 12:37 pm
Subject: My thanks and appreciation

Hi KJ,

Since returning from New Haven, I have been quite busy and my work is finally starting to settle down.

I really wanted to convey to you how emotional it was for me to be part of the first TPIU Gala and how honored I was to be recognized with an Award.
Mostly, I want to tell you how SPECIAL a person you are. You are held in such high esteem by your friends and colleagues and it really showed that evening.
Clearly you are a most hands on and meticulous individual and this was very apparent to myself and Sharon. We thank you immensely for all your personal attention during our trip.

I am putting together our expenses and will get it off to you shortly. Xin was in touch and she very graciously sent the video that she took.
If you still have a copy of the Michael Douglas Video, then please email it to me. My iCloud version has shut down. Will you be sending some pictures from the event or should I order them?

Thank you again and to TPIU Foundation for this enormous honor... Best wishes to Linda.

Saul

c

Image 37 (Continued).

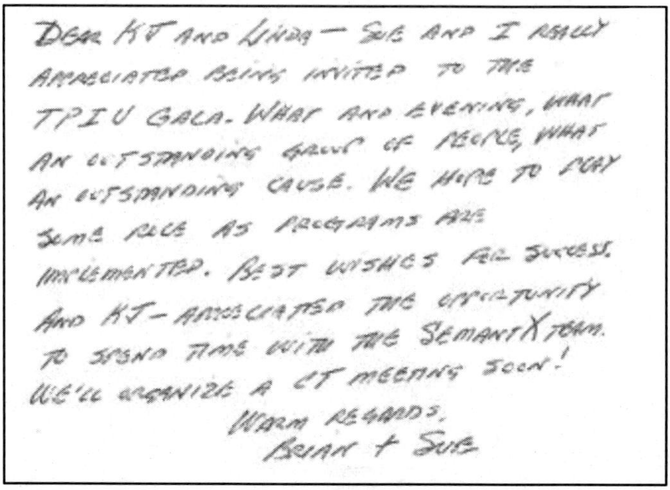

> Dear KJ and Linda — Sue and I really appreciated being invited to the TPIU Gala. What an evening, what an outstanding group of people, what an outstanding cause. We hope to play some role as programs are implemented. Best wishes for success. And KJ — appreciated the opportunity to spend time with the SemantX team. We'll organize a CT meeting soon!
> Warm regards,
> Brian + Sue

d

Image 37 a, b, c, d. Letters of appreciation from honorees and attendees at the first Awards Gala Dinner of The Patient is U foundation. (Chapter 23).

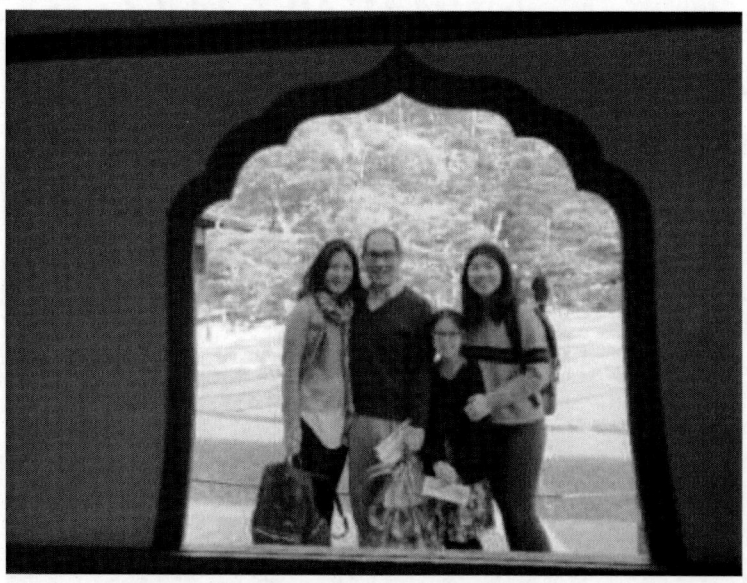

Image 38. K.J. Lee's oldest son, Ken, and his family. L-R: Susan, Ken, Olivia and Morgan.

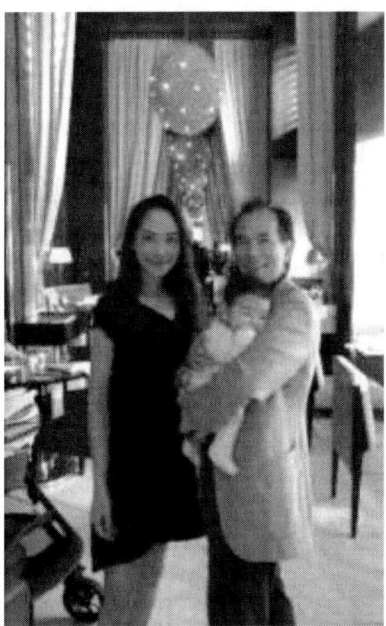

Image 39. K.J. Lee's middle son, Lloyd, with his wife, Chieko, and son, Elias.

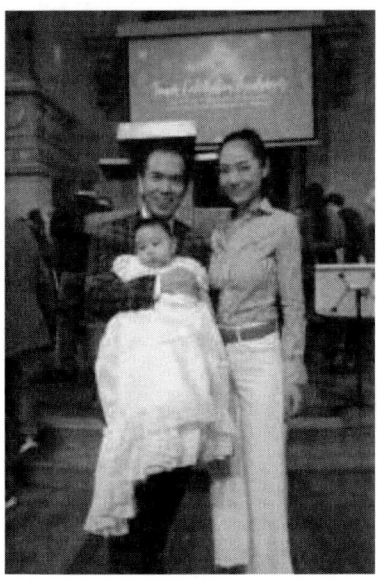

Image 40. Christening of Elias in London on September 29, 2019. The christening gown was made by his grandma, Linda.

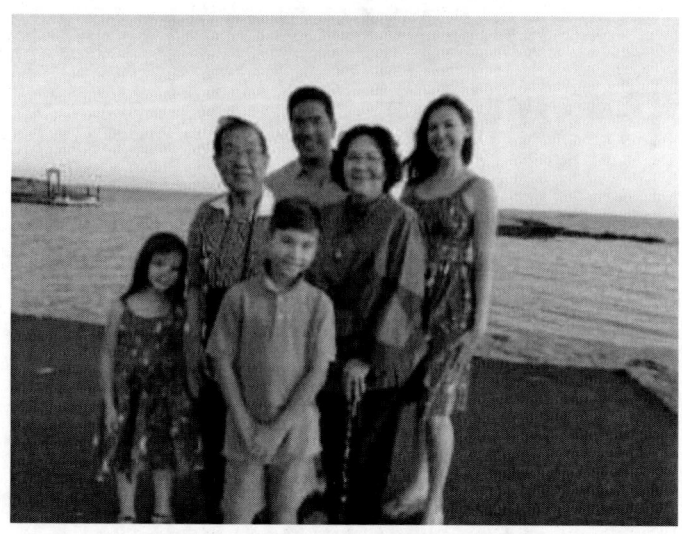

Image 41. K.J. and Linda Lee with their youngest son, Mark, and his family in Sachem's Head, Connecticut, in July 2019. Front, L-R: Juliet and Mason Lee; Middle, L-R: K.J. and Linda Lee; Back, L-R: Mark and Jennica Lee.

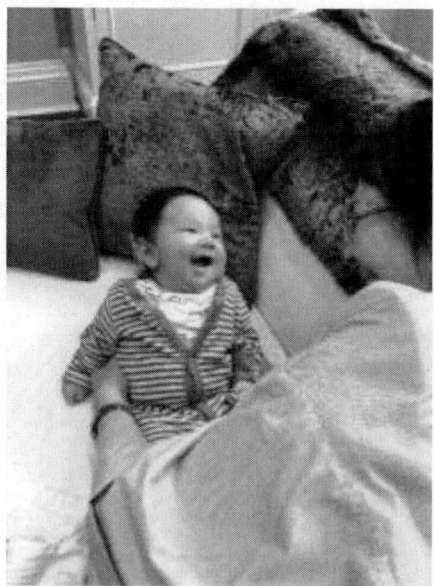

Image 42. K.J. and Linda's youngest grandchild, Elias Lincoln Lee, pictured with his grandma in August 2019.

Leeway: Reaching Beyond Expectations 117

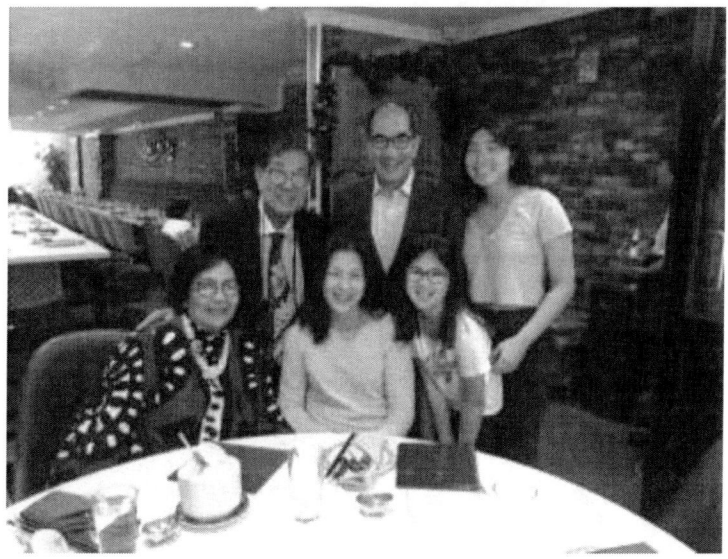

Image 43. K.J. and Linda at their 53rd anniversary dinner with their son Ken and his family, Susan, Morgan and Olivia.

Chapter 13

RESIDENCY

Sally Hyun Jung Jee

"The price of success is hard work, dedication to the job at hand, and the determination that whether we win or lose, we have applied the best of ourselves to the task at hand."
–Vince Lombardi

"I'm telling you, K.J. You'll only get told off," Michael said. K.J. shrugged. "You never know until you try." "Let him do it, Michael," Paul said, "maybe we'll get to see a dejected K.J. for once." K.J. had just finished medical school, his surgical internship, and one year of general surgery. His current post was at the Massachusetts Eye and Ear Infirmary, Harvard Medical School's teaching hospital for otolaryngology - head and neck surgery, where he would spend the next three years as an ENT (Ear, Nose, and Throat) resident. Michael and Paul, both southerners, were two of K.J.'s five colleagues in his residency group.

"You're really going to do this, aren't you?" Michael asked. Michael had met K.J. only a few months before, but he had spent enough time with K.J. to know that once he had set his mind on something, he wasn't going to take no for an answer. K.J. glanced up at the sixth floor of the Infirmary building, where the office of Dr. Schuknecht, the chairman of otolaryngology - head and neck surgery at Harvard Medical School, was located. "Yes," K.J. said. "I need to do this."

As K.J. climbed the five flights of stairs to Dr. Schuknecht's office, his mind was racing. He did not want to come across to the chairman as insolent in his very first year as resident. But neither could he receive a subpar diploma after 13 years of painstaking work after high school.

The shock K.J. had felt when he first laid eyes on the diploma for the Massachusetts Eye and Ear Infirmary was still fresh in his mind. The diploma, which hung in the office of one of his older friends, was absurdly large and paper-thin. The texture reminded K.J. of a badly printed newspaper rather than a certificate for a physician's expertise in ENT. What's more, 'Harvard Medical School' was not on the diploma. Instead, 'Massachusetts Eye and Ear Infirmary' was printed across the flimsy paper. "No one down south knows where Massachusetts Eye and Ear Infirmary is," Michael said. "They won't believe me when I say I've done my residency at Harvard." K.J. knew he had to do something. However, redesigning the diploma wasn't something he could do on his own, he first had to gain Dr. Schuknecht's support.

School pride wasn't the only thing on K.J.'s mind, when he decided to try and change the diploma. He cared deeply about ENT, and he wanted the design of his diploma to reflect his pride in the discipline.

A circumspect man, K.J. had picked his field in medicine after meticulous research and careful thought. From his medical school days, he knew he wanted to go into one of the surgical specialties— he had an agile mind and equally deft hands to match. Surgery also suited K.J.'s personality. He was a doer, a man of action, and liked getting quick results for his treatments. Disciplines such as internal medicine and psychiatry, where it took much longer for the physician to see a clear result, would not have suited him.

Once K.J. narrowed his scope of attention to surgery, he surveyed each of the surgical disciplines. He immediately crossed out obstetrics and gynecology from his list. When labor started at night, the obstetrician would deliver the next day. Even if a woman went into labor in the early afternoon, the process of delivering a newborn may take the entire day and last well into the night. Urology was also off the list when he realized that the most common examination a urologist had to perform was a rectal exam.

Some of K.J.'s friends had chosen orthopedic surgery, but to K.J. the field seemed rather dull. Arthroscopies and hip or knee replacement surgeries were yet to be invented, so most of an orthopedic surgeon's work entailed wrapping up broken legs in plaster casts. The physician would then suspend the leg using a pulley system hung from the frame of the bed. This process required strength which K.J. wasn't sure he had, at 5'3" and weighing 140 pounds. He then briefly considered becoming a neurosurgeon, but in those days, the success rates of neurosurgeries were low.

Finally, K.J. looked into ENT and found himself the perfect match. ENT surgery handled a variety of structures in the head and neck— the nose and the sinuses, the throat, and the ears. So naturally, the scope of surgeries was much greater than most other disciplines. An otolaryngologist could be performing facial plastic and reconstructive surgery, including cosmetic surgery, while also excising cancerous lesions and performing the reconstruction. He could also diagnose and treat allergies of the ear, nose, throat and sinuses. An otolaryngologist dealt with both the pediatric and adult populations, both male and female, and both fine and large structures in the human head and neck. Stapedectomy, a very delicate surgery in otolaryngology that restores hearing, would be performed on the stapes— a structure in the middle ear that is the size of the letter *s* on this page. At the other end of the spectrum, treating tumors in the head and skull base would mean surgical procedures that involve the head, oral cavity, jaw, and neck. K.J. was good with his hands and loved fine surgery, but he also enjoyed learning about the other aspects of this broad and ever-expanding field. The sheer variety that ENT offered stimulated and challenged him. When K.J. discovered that the broad subspecialties in otolaryngology were yet to be fully developed, he was excited. He anticipated that he and his colleagues would work to help the specialty blossom into a stronger and even more encompassing one. K.J. explored the history of ENT as well as the huge potential of the specialty. He believed he could contribute vastly. Together with his professors and colleagues, he could help transform it into a well-respected and highly sought-after specialty.

Another added advantage of becoming an otolaryngologist was that when K.J.'s hands become less adept due to age, he could choose to practice in the office instead of retiring. A neurosurgeon wouldn't have the same option, since neurologists and not neurosurgeons take care of most office work, including diagnosing ailments.

In the 1960s, a major problem that deterred many residents from choosing ENT was that otolaryngology had fallen into disfavor since the advent of sulfa drugs in the 1930s and penicillin in the 1940s. Prior to this, when antibiotics didn't exist, patients with sinus infections or ear infections would need an ENT doctor to operate on them. When sulfa drugs became widely commercialized in the 1930s and penicillin in the 1940s, a large number of infections could simply be treated with antibiotics. Though antibiotics were an important leap in the history of medicine, they meant that less and less ENT surgeries were being performed. K.J., however, knew he could make a difference in the field and help make ENT a popular discipline again. At the time of writing, otolaryngology-head and neck surgery is one of the most highly sought-after residencies, accepting only medical students with stellar academic records.

After completing two years of general surgery training, K.J. attended a graduation dinner where all those who were leaving the hospital stood up and announced where they were headed. "Orthopedics," some said. "Obstetrics and Gynecology," said others. As his turn to speak approached, K.J. felt his mouth turn dry. It was the first time he had attended such an event, and he had not prepared what to say. He knew that since ENT was far from a popular discipline at that time, many assumed that only foreign medical graduates and those who graduated from subpar medical schools specialized in it. Everyone in the room would be astounded if K.J., a graduate of the prestigious Columbia University College of Physicians and Surgeons, told them he would be going into ENT. As K.J. stood up to announce his specialty, he had a thought— or rather, a vision.

"I'm going to Harvard to do a head and neck surgery residency," he said. He quickly sat back down and avoided the curious, even confused, gaze of the others. He did not want to answer any questions they might have. There was no such head and neck surgery residency. Years later, when ENT became a much stronger specialty, the leadership of the American Academy of Otolaryngology tried to come up with a new name for the discipline. Eventually, they decided on Otolaryngology - Head and Neck Surgery. Now, every otolaryngology department uses this name. That night, at the graduation dinner, K.J. unknowingly coined a term that would be used by generation upon generation of otolaryngologists in the U.S. and around the world.

As K.J. recalled the reasons he had chosen otolaryngology over other specialties at his graduation dinner, he knocked on Dr. Schuknecht's door. "Come in," Dr. Schuknecht said. Dr. Schuknecht was, to say the least, a good-looking man. He was tall, towering over most of the Infirmary staff, and blue-eyed. He could be charming and suave when he wanted to be, though his piercing blue eyes always betrayed the no-nonsense scientist in him.

(At times, Dr. Schuknecht was even quite blunt. In 1969, while still a resident under Dr. Schuknecht's tutelage, K.J. developed Ménière's disease, a disease of the inner ear that causes vertigo and substantial hearing loss. Naturally, his wife, Linda, was concerned. When K.J. and Linda were invited to dine with Dr. Schuknecht at an associate professor's house, Linda asked Dr. Schuknecht about her husband's illness. "We don't know what causes Ménière's disease, and we also don't know of any cure," Dr. Schuknecht replied, "if it comes to it, we'll just have to destroy the ear." Linda burst into tears at the dinner table, and the associate professor gave Dr. Schuknecht a reproachful glance. Dr. Schuknecht immediately challenged his colleague. "Herb, do you know a scientifically proven cure?" he asked. Of course, Dr. Schuknecht never meant to hurt Linda, but his scientific mind didn't allow him to believe in anything that wasn't experimentally verified. There was no known cure for Ménière's disease, and he didn't want to beat around the bush. In this way, Dr. Schuknecht drummed his belief in the scientific method into his residents, including K.J.)

"What can I do for you, K.J.?" Dr. Schuknecht asked. "I'd like to discuss the diploma I'll be receiving at the end of my residency," K.J. said. K.J. explained that most residents were dissatisfied with the design of the diploma, especially since there was no mention of Harvard Medical School on it. All the while, Dr. Schuknecht's keen blue eyes pierced into K.J.'s deep brown ones. K.J. tried not to be intimidated. "Well spoken, K.J.," Dr. Schuknecht said, when K.J. finished talking. "I agree with you completely." Before he became chairman at Harvard Medical School, Dr. Schuknecht worked at the Henry Ford Hospital in Michigan. Now, as a Harvard professor, he wanted the diploma he signed to read *Harvard Medical School*.

"My wife, Linda, is an artist and an architectural student at MIT. I could ask her for a first draft of the design for your critique," K.J. offered. That night, K.J. related what had happened during his meeting with Dr. Schuknecht to Linda, who was very enthusiastic about taking on the diploma project. Linda designed the first draft and the subsequent drafts, which ultimately led to the diploma that is still in use today. Unlike the previous version, which was almost the size of half of a newspaper, the diploma she designed was elegantly sized. Most importantly, it read *Harvard Medical School* in one corner and *Massachusetts Eye and Ear Infirmary* in the other.

The diploma enterprise was far from the last project K.J. undertook as a first-year resident in ENT. One day, about nine months into his residency, he overheard Dr. Schuknecht and another professor chatting in the elevator. The subject of their conversation was how to improve on the system of 'chart review', a standard research method in which the physician would survey the outcomes of surgery by reading patients' medical charts. This method, though convenient, depended on others' appraisal of the patients' conditions.

"I don't believe in chart review," Dr. Schuknecht said to his colleague, "we should call every patient to come to the clinic and examine each one if we're going to do proper research on surgical outcome." "That's impossible," the colleague said, "there are over a thousand patients. We can't possibly reach that many people or have the time to examine them." "That's the only way it should be done," Dr. Schuknecht said.

Dr. Schuknecht's words resonated with K.J. Chart review was definitely the most convenient way to analyze patient data, but K.J. knew that the most convenient method wasn't always the best one. To ensure accuracy of the data, following up on every patient was something a scientist had to do. That very afternoon, K.J. visited Dr. Schuknecht's office once again. "I heard your conversation with Dr. Gasik the other day," he said, "I want to volunteer for the mastoidectomy-tympanoplasty outcome research." "Would you have the time, K.J.?" Dr. Schuknecht asked. Dr. Schuknecht's concern was well founded, since the residents barely had time to sleep or eat. "I'll make the time," K.J. answered.

Dr. Schuknecht's eyes widened. He had never seen a resident as passionate as K.J. was about both patient care and research. "This young man is going to make it big someday," Dr. Schuknecht thought. (This same passion would lead K.J. to perform 25 rhinoplasties while most other residents did five to 10, and over 30 stapedectomies while others did 10 to 15.)

Dr. Schuknecht hired a part-time social worker who would track down the patients and a part-time secretary to help organize K.J.'s work. He then volunteered his own time to supervise K.J. in his research project, which took many evenings a week over the course of a year and a half. For statistical analysis, K.J. worked with the newly established Harvard Computer Center. This collaboration was one of the earliest uses of computers for 'big data' analysis of outcome studies.

The resulting research paper, 'Results of Tympanoplasty and Mastoidectomy at the Massachusetts Eye and Ear Infirmary', was published in April 1971[12]. The milestone paper was widely praised within the medical community and established the standards for 'chronic ear' surgery, the same standards that are still in use today by younger generations of otolaryngologists.

It would have been customary to name Dr. Schuknecht, a well-established professor and chairman, as the first author of the paper. But Dr. Schuknecht refused to do so, insisting on putting K.J.'s name first. "I've had my moments of fame," he told K.J. "Now it's your turn, K.J. You did most of the work." K.J. received no monetary compensation for this immense extra undertaking but is forever grateful to his giant of a mentor in surgery and research.

---

[12] K.J. Lee, H. F. Schuknecht, "Results of Tympanoplasty and Mastoidectomy at the Massachusetts Eye and Ear Infirmary," *The Laryngoscope*, vol. 81, no. 4 (1971): 529-543. Available at: https://onlinelibrary.wiley.com/doi/10.1288/00005537-197104000-00004.

Dr. Schuknecht was a devout atheist. He held one of his best teaching conferences every Sunday from 10 a.m. to noon. The residents used to refer to them as 'Sunday school'. K.J. had to switch his hour of worship in church so as to attend. He held the man in such high esteem that he would never have considered missing it.

As a first-year resident at the Infirmary, K.J. was allowed to operate on patients under supervision. He performed relatively simple surgeries such as tonsillectomies, while all stapedectomies, which involved more complicated and delicate procedures, were referred to the chief resident, Dr. Reynolds. Dr. Reynolds, in addition to being a skilled surgeon, was a dashingly handsome man. One day, after being evaluated by him for a stapedectomy, a patient asked him how many stapedectomies he'd performed. "Ms. Watson, I hate to tell you the number I have done," Dr. Reynolds quick-wittedly answered, as he swiftly exited the room with his usual flair. K.J. couldn't help but smile— the stapedectomy that Dr. Reynolds had just scheduled would be his very first one. "Dr. Lee, thank you so much for referring me to Dr. Reynolds," the patient exclaimed, her eyes dreamily following Dr. Reynold's graceful figure as he walked out into the hallway.

Dr. Reynolds' smooth manners didn't end here. Once, while K.J. was talking to him on the phone from his apartment, Linda dropped some dishes on the floor. "K.J., could you ask Linda what I could do to help?" asked Dr. Reynolds, who lived eight miles away from the Lees, in his suave voice.

As chief resident, Dr. Reynolds would summon the first-year resident to see a patient in the middle of the night while he was on call. "Who's the patient?" K.J. would ask. "Jimmy," Dr. Reynolds would answer, sighing heavily. Everyone knew who Jimmy was. A man in his late forties, Jimmy had Osler-Weber-Rendu Syndrome, hereditary hemorrhagic telangiectasia that causes frequent nosebleeds. These nosebleeds were so uncontrollable that to stop them, doctors had to pack his nose, putting gauze in both nostrils as tightly as humanly possible. Sometimes they would have to inject medicine into Jimmy's nose to stop the bleeding.

Jimmy would come in day and night, sometimes even three times a day. Doctors in the Infirmary, of course, felt sorry for him. The process of packing the nose was extremely painful for Jimmy, and it wasn't entirely painless, even for the most experienced doctors, to see the patient suffer every time. In fact, Jimmy's nostrils were one big cavity since he didn't have a septum, the part-cartilage and part-bone structure that separates the right and left nostrils. Years and years of packing his nose had destroyed it.

Doctors are, however, only human. Whenever they were on call, they dreaded hearing that Jimmy was in the emergency room, since that meant that they were faced with another sleepless night. It would take hours to stop the nosebleed. However, by the end of their residency, the residents regarded Jimmy not only as a patient but also as an instructor. Jimmy taught every doctor in the Infirmary how to treat the most difficult nosebleeds. What's more, he taught them what it takes to be a true doctor: having compassion for patients and maintaining that compassion even when woken up at 2 in the morning.

K.J. further proved his diligence and commitment in his attitude towards the additional responsibilities assigned to first-year residents at the Infirmary. In the late 1960s, there was no 'audiovisual' department staffed by professionals to support morbidity and mortality conferences, clinical pathology conferences or visiting professor lectureships. Dr. Schuknecht therefore charged the six first-year residents with being responsible for the audiovisual (AV) 'cart'. Each took responsibility for two months. Most of the residents complained that working as an AV technician was not what they had signed up for and performed the job haphazardly. However, in his usual way, K.J. took it seriously and even solicited his wife's help to transform an instrument cart on wheels into an AV cart on wheels. The new and improved cart included specific sections for an 8mm movie projector, a 16mm movie projector, a projector for the 2x2 slides, a projector for the old-fashioned lantern slides, a box of different colored chalk and an eraser, a three-foot-long wooden pointer, and extra bulbs for the different projectors. This was all organized like a surgical instrument cart, ready for any eventuality. K.J. would always arrive at the lecture hall 15 minutes ahead of schedule to check the AV cart and its contents were in full-working order.

K.J. also helped organize and streamline the Infirmary's 'crash cart', which contained all the equipment necessary to deal with cardiac arrest situations. When K.J. assumed his position as chief resident, the cardiac arrest cart was in disarray and could never be found in the same location. He organized and stocked the cart and found a convenient and permanent place to store it. That very night a member of the hospital board had been admitted as a patient and suffered a cardiac arrest— the cart was put to good use, saving his life.

Chapter 14

THE ARMY

Sally Hyun Jung Jee

"There is no love without forgiveness, and there is no forgiveness without love."
– Bryant H. McGill

March, 1970: K.J. was four months away from finishing his residency, and the nation was still at war. The year before, on November 15th, the largest anti-war protest in American history had taken place in Washington, D.C. There was palpable tension in the air. Nevertheless, the Vietnam War continued, and many of the drafted men came back dead or maimed.

K.J., like many other young men in the country, was drafted and terrified of going to Vietnam. He was married with a baby son. "If I die in the war, what's going to happen to my family? And my parents back in Malaysia?" These thoughts, among others, kept him awake at night as he tossed and turned in bed. Some of his friends spoke of dodging the draft by crossing the border to Canada. But K.J. had already left home once at the age of 17. Since then, he had given his all to build another one in the United States. He couldn't simply walk away from his second, newly adopted home.

There was nothing K.J. could do but wait. And wait he did until Colonel McMaster, the Chief of Otolaryngology at Walter Reed Army Medical Center, came to visit Dr. Schuknecht. Walter Reed was the main Army hospital of the time, and Colonel McMaster was tasked with the crucial mission of assigning doctors to different Army hospitals around the globe.

K.J. was in the operating room with Dr. Schuknecht, preparing for the next surgery, when he learned that the visiting surgeon who would be watching the surgery was Colonel McMaster. "Dr. Schuknecht, could you please put in a good word with the Colonel, so he doesn't send me to Vietnam?" K.J. asked. By this point in his residency, K.J. and Dr. Schuknecht were close colleagues having collaborated for a year and a half on the groundbreaking outcome research paper, 'Results of Tympanoplasty and Mastoidectomy at the Massachusetts Eye and Ear Infirmary'. Dr. Schuknecht certainly knew what kind of doctor K.J. was. "Of course, K.J.," Dr. Schuknecht said, "you're a great and industrious young surgeon. You should be an academician."

After the operation, Colonel McMaster, who was planning to start a residency-training program at Madigan Army Medical Center in Tacoma, Washington, approached Dr. Schuknecht. The Colonel was looking to recruit a young otolaryngologist who could help develop this residency. "The guy would have to be a good teacher, a skilled surgeon, and an academician. Do you know anyone finishing residency this year who'd fit the bill?" Colonel McMaster asked Dr. Schuknecht. "I know just the guy you need," Dr. Schuknecht answered. On June 30th, when K.J. graduated from the Massachusetts Eye and Ear Infirmary, he was assigned to the Madigan Army Medical Center.

When K.J. reached Tacoma, Washington, on July 1st, he realized that he would have to wait another three months before he could check into his assigned Army quarters. Until then, he had two options: rent a cheap motel room or live in a makeshift apartment. Choosing the latter, he moved into the tiny apartment with his wife and two-year-old son. Unable to afford shower curtains, K.J. and Linda had to mop the floor every time they used the shower. So when K.J. and his family finally moved into Army quarters, their living accommodation seemed almost luxurious. They had three tiny bedrooms to themselves, and most importantly, their bathroom wouldn't flood every day.

In their new home in Army quarters, K.J. discovered the PX, the Army's version of a large grocery store. On the day K.J., Linda, and their baby son Ken moved in, K.J. felt 'rich' and went to the PX to buy huge succulent strawberries for Linda and Ken. The strawberries were exquisitely delicious. The next visit to the PX, however, proved to be a disappointment in human nature. K.J. was there to buy confectioners sugar, and unable to find it, he asked the storekeeper where it was. The storekeeper quickly and confidently announced that the Army had not carried it for years. As K.J. was walking out, he bumped into a neighbor's wife who escorted K.J. to an aisle where there were boxes of confectioners sugar, stacked up against one another. That day, K.J. learned from the storekeeper that in life, one has to watch out for careless and lazy people.

K.J. had vowed not to make any enemies in the Army, to keep a low profile. At the time, most Army hospitals operated in a relaxed, non-academic fashion, and Madigan was no exception. Some doctors made rounds before going into surgery, but others simply didn't. While military doctors were paid more than a normal resident, they had neither strict office hours nor a boss to impress. Since most of the medical personnel would be leaving the Army in two years, working at Madigan seemed like a temporary stint. Realizing that they may never have such a laid-back schedule again, many doctors were determined to relax.

Encouraging these doctors to stay in the vicinity while on call at night proved difficult. In principle, the physician on call couldn't leave the general area of the medical facility they worked in. The doctors, however, would often be in Seattle, an hour-and-a-half's drive from Tacoma.

To K.J., the duty of a doctor was something sacred. A doctor's care could determine whether someone lived or died. "We've got to make rounds twice a day and take calls seriously," K.J. told the residents and colleagues, keeping his tone as conciliatory as possible. He knew that making enemies wouldn't help him achieve anything. While K.J. was the acting director of the residency-training program, his authority was marginal at best— the doctors knew they would most likely never see K.J. again after he was discharged from the Army. Despite his best intentions, the disgruntled looks from many of his co-workers told him he had already made a few enemies. "What's this guy talking about? He sure has a big mouth," the angry faces seemed to be saying. K.J. took a deep breath. "Use your hearts, please," K.J. pleaded, "every patient here is someone's beloved son, maybe even someone's father. Try to think about that." [Little did K.J. know, this was the seed that would blossom into The Patient Is U Foundation (TPIU) in 2017, 47 years later]. K.J. saw the eyes of his coworkers soften and knew, instinctively, that this was his one chance to get his message across. "Take calls at night, please. I'm not asking you to be in the hospital, but at least be in the same town," he added.

The change didn't happen overnight, but after a few weeks, K.J. noticed that things were improving. As K.J. led by example, practicing medicine as conscientiously as he always had, his fellow surgeons started making rounds to check in with their patients. Those on call became more responsive. There was, however, another issue.

One night, while K.J. was in the emergency room, he saw a psychiatrist treating a surgical trauma patient who had been in a car accident. K.J. knew the man enough to recognize that he was a good psychiatrist. He also knew that psychiatrists should never be on surgical trauma call, suturing up patients. "We've got to excuse that guy from surgical trauma calls," K.J. told his surgical colleagues. "Psychiatrists shouldn't be treating surgical trauma patients." His colleagues laughed at him. Are you crazy, K.J.? There are only seven of us on surgical trauma call. If we take the psychiatrist off, each of us would end up taking more calls," one surgeon said. "What are you going to do, K.J.? Talk to the commander? You'll get court-martialed," others told him. "You'll be sent to Vietnam as punishment," added another colleague.

K.J. felt a sudden chill. Like many men, he had only narrowly missed being sent to Vietnam. If they had been a little less lucky, they would have been holding M16 rifles in the middle of a thick tropical jungle or in the rice paddies, fearing for their lives.

But K.J. refused to let the matter rest. Using a psychiatrist, who has no surgical training, to treat surgical trauma victims could jeopardize the patients. K.J. was determined to persuade the commander, using the best of his reasoning skills. When he finally managed to arrange a meeting, he explained that having a psychiatrist on surgical trauma call could seriously endanger the outcome of the patient's treatment. The commander remained silent. "Please, just imagine that one of the patients is your little girl," K.J. said, "would you want a psychiatrist to suture up the lacerations on her beautiful face?" The commander didn't make any promises, but K.J. saw a glimmer of hope. Within a few months, psychiatrists had been taken off surgical trauma calls.

In 1972, K.J. felt a lump in his back. Of course, he couldn't possibly treat or operate on himself, so he visited a specialist at Madigan. "It's nothing to worry about," the specialist told K.J., "it's just a little cyst." After a quick surgery to remove the lump, K.J. was back on his feet the very same afternoon, caring for his patients.

K.J. left the Army shortly thereafter, on June 30th, 1972. A few months later, however, he realized that another lump had formed at the same spot. By 1976, the lump had grown to the size of a golf ball. A Johns Hopkins trained surgeon in New Haven excised the lump and told K.J. it was cancer. K.J. traced the cancerous lesion back to the original specimen that the Madigan specialist had removed from his back in 1972. That specialist had not only misdiagnosed cancer as a cyst but also failed to remove the 'cyst' in its entirety. "You have to file a lawsuit against that specialist," K.J.'s friends told him. "That man has to pay for his sloppy practice." Though K.J. didn't know whether he would live or die, he refused to bring the matter to court. He didn't want to penalize another human being for making an unintentional mistake.

K.J. had faced many crises in life, most of which he had turned to opportunities. This time, his own life was at stake. Still, he wanted to use the moment to forgive rather than hate. "My life is out of my hands now," K.J. thought. "It's in God's hands." "[A]nd forgive us our trespasses as we forgive those who trespass against us…"

K.J. survived his cancer, and in 1997, he received a call from the Chief of Otolaryngology - Head and Neck Surgery at Madigan Army General Hospital. K.J. returned to Madigan once more, this time as a visiting professor and invited speaker, rather than as a drafted soldier, for the 25th anniversary of the residency that he had helped start.

Chapter 15

K. J. Lee's Essential Otolaryngology

Sally Hyun Jung Jee

"The Chinese use two brush strokes to write the word 'crisis.' One brush stroke stands for danger; the other for opportunity. In a crisis, be aware of the danger— but recognize the opportunity."
– John F. Kennedy

In 1970, when K.J. started writing *K.J. Lee's Essential Otolaryngology – Head and Neck Surgery*, he was just a graduating resident preparing for his own board exam. By the 1980s, he was the author of the most widely read and celebrated ENT book in the world.

After finishing their residency, all otolaryngologists were required to apply to the American Board of Otolaryngology and take the oral and written exam to become a Board-certified otolaryngologist. This was often a traumatic experience. It was rumored that in one exam, a candidate had punched the examiner in the nose, convinced that he was making the exam excruciatingly hard only for him. Otolaryngology is a broad discipline with many subfields, and in the 1970s, there was no common curriculum— every residency taught its residents differently. Residents learned from the 'apprenticeship' method rather than from organized lectures, as if they were technicians rather than scientists. If the chairman of the residency program was more inclined towards rhinology (treatment of the nose and associated diseases), the residents' training would be geared towards this area of ENT; if the chairman specialized in otology (treatment of the ear), the residents would study more about the ear. Dr. Schuknecht at Harvard, an otologist, offered extra lessons in otology and otopathology every Sunday, from 10 a.m. to 12 p.m., which the residents would jokingly refer to as Sunday school. Many hospitals, however, did not have an organized lecture system. The so-called 'Home Study Course' was inadequate. There were no basic science lectures for residents, therefore by the time the board exam came around, many residents felt insecure and unsure of what they should be studying. In fact, it was not uncommon for graduating residents to get a part-time job and take a year off to study. One of K.J.'s friends spent a year away from his family living in a trailer in order to prepare for the exam.

Thanks to Dr. Schuknecht and his other teachers, K.J. was well prepared for the Board exam in November of the year he graduated from residency and knew he would pass. He had been taught well by his professors, especially in otology. K.J., however, felt that he had not done enough studying. He wanted to read every textbook in otolaryngology and every journal published in the last five years. He also knew that the exam was in many ways unfair, as other residents were much less fortunate than him in terms of preparation and teaching. He felt strongly that Board exams shouldn't be such traumatic experiences, especially for young otolaryngologists who have already trained for three to five years. The field of otolaryngology needed a core curriculum and a Board exam that focused on what everyone had to know. K.J. considered talking to the American Board of Otolaryngology or the chairman of residency programs, but he knew they wouldn't listen to a young doctor fresh out of residency. So he came up with his own way to resolve the dilemma: he decided to write a text encompassing the entire field of otolaryngology – head and neck surgery for young otolaryngologists. To do so, he needed more than a few months.

In Chinese, the word *crisis* is a combination of words that mean *danger* and *opportunity*. While other graduating residents saw only danger as they faced the board exam, K.J. saw the perfect opportunity. But when K.J.'s

Army supervisors at Madigan General Hospital learned of his decision to skip the exam that year and take the one offered a year later, they were alarmed. "K.J., you're the one resident I know that would definitely pass the board exam this year. Why would you do something like this?" they asked him. K.J. told them that he was planning to write a textbook that would help otolaryngologists prepare for the board exam. His supervisors and colleagues laughed. "You're 20 years too young to be writing a book," they said. "If you don't take the board exam this year, I'll send you to Vietnam," a colonel added. But K.J. wouldn't take no for an answer. "I want to solve the crisis that every graduating resident in otolaryngology faces," he told his supervisors.

In the end, K.J. managed to persuade his supervisors to let him take the exam the following year, in his usual polite but tenacious way. When he finally had their approval, K.J. started working on his book, organizing all the key information on 5×8 index cards. This work would be the basis of his book, *K.J. Lee's Essential Otolaryngology - Head and Neck Surgery*. Across the globe, the book remains the most widely read text in the field to this day, translated into several languages.

K.J. started his preparation for the book in July, 1970. By the date of the next board exam in October, 1971, he had read every ENT textbook there was in the English language, encompassing both American and British texts. He also read all the ENT journals that had been published in the last five years. He made notes from all of these texts on 5×8 index cards, which he catalogued and organized by topic. He then stored them in shoeboxes, which fit the cards perfectly. His wife, Linda, helped him a great deal and was unfailingly supportive of his endeavor.

If K.J. ever had any treasures of his own, they were his index cards. At this time, K.J. was stationed in the Army and living in Army quarters with his wife and two young sons, one aged three and the other an infant. While the family's main living space was on the first floor, the second floor housed two bedrooms as well as a small study room for K.J., where he kept the shoeboxes filled with index cards. "If there ever is a fire while I'm not here, the first thing you should do is to grab the shoeboxes and throw them out of the window," K.J. told his wife, "Then you grab our sons and run out." K.J.

is a devoted father and husband, but even when those he loves most could be in danger, he is able to apply his usual logic— shoeboxes can be thrown out of the window, but children can't.

After K.J. passed his board exam in 1971, other residents asked him if they could borrow his index cards. Of course, K.J. said yes; he had made the cards to share with others. Copy machines were hard to come by in those days, and only big libraries had them. What's more, the charge for using them was around 10 cents per page, so it would cost a small fortune to copy all of K.J.'s index cards. The residents therefore ended up borrowing the original cards. The problem was that if they borrowed 10 cards, they would usually give back eight. None of them were stolen, but index cards were, by nature, easy to lose. Feeling the pressure of the impending exam, residents would carry them everywhere they went— to restaurants, to their beds, even to the bathroom. At the end of the day, it was hard to keep track of all 10.

After losing his index cards one too many times, K.J. decided that it was time to publish them so that they would be accessible to a wider audience. In 1973, he went to his professor, hoping he would help him to find a suitable publisher. "Why are you trying to publish a book, K.J.? Why don't you just read my book?" his professor asked him. It was unthinkable to the professor that someone as young as K.J. could be publishing a book. When K.J. went to his colleagues, they reacted in the same way. "No publisher is going to accept a medical book written by a 31-year-old," they told him.

K.J. decided to go directly to the publishers and found out that his peers weren't wrong. When he approached the big-name publishers in the medical field, they wanted to see his résumé. When they realized that K.J. had passed the board exam only a year or two ago, they didn't even bother to take a look at his index cards.

K.J. would not take no for an answer. Broadening the scope of his search, he finally found a small publisher in Long Island that was willing to publish his work. The company was not a medical textbook publisher but one that printed mimeographed ring binders for nurse's aides. Its operation was, to put it mildly, humble and low budget, considering the owner of the company published from his garage. "There's one condition to publishing your book," the owner said, "I get to keep every penny from the sales." "It's a deal," K.J. answered. Later, some of K.J.'s colleagues asked him why he had agreed to such a terrible deal when he had spent so much time and effort on the book. The reason was simple: K.J. wasn't in it for the money.

Soon afterwards, K.J.'s index cards were mimeographed and made into three ring binders. The first edition was small enough to fit into the pocket of a doctor's white coat. The book was an instant success. Overnight, every ENT resident rushed to the stores to buy *K.J. Lee's Essential Otolaryngology – Head and Neck Surgery*.

The same company in Long Island printed the second edition, and by the time K.J. was planning for the third edition, the owner had retired, having earned a significant amount of money from K.J.'s book. This wasn't a problem, since by now, the big medical publishing companies that had initially turned the book down were clamoring to get hold of it. Instead of having to send his resume and beg the established medical publishers to take a look at his index cards, K.J. could now pick and choose any publisher he wanted.

The problem came from an unexpected direction. When a big company took over publication of K.J.'s book, the publisher's in-house editors wanted to tamper with the style of the text. *Essential Otolaryngology*, in its entirety, was written in short sentences that resembled study notes. These sentences reflected the origins of the book and provided the shortest distance from one essential fact to another. The publisher, however, wanted to convert K.J.'s notes into full paragraphs. K.J. had written the book for residents to read on the run; he didn't want them to spend unnecessary time deciphering long texts while their board exam was just around the corner. Since the change that the publisher suggested would destroy the spirit of the book, K.J. fought back. Once again, he didn't take no for an answer, and the book remained the way it was.

To this day, every ENT trainee reads *K.J. Lee's Essential Otolaryngology – Head and Neck Surgery*. Instead of using its full title, most doctors endearingly refer to the book simply as *K.J. Lee's*. "When we face a situation in the emergency or operating room that we don't know how to handle, we talk to one another and say, 'Let's see what *K.J. Lee's* says.'

Then, we look into your book," numerous doctors have told K.J. over the years.

On one occasion, a newly wed young doctor who had just passed the board exam came to New Haven. At a dinner party, he introduced himself and his wife, Mary, to K.J. As soon as Mary heard K.J.'s name, her eyes widened. "Wow, you're the guy!" she exclaimed, pointing her index finger at him. K.J. was baffled. "Have we met before?" he asked Mary. "Sure we have. You're the guy who was in bed with us! During our honeymoon, all that my husband wanted to do was read *K.J. Lee's* in bed," she said, half-joking and half-serious.

K.J. is well-known by young otolaryngologists around the world, as the board exams in many countries list his book as compulsory reading. The book has been translated into Chinese, Portuguese, Spanish, Ukrainian, Turkish, and many other languages that K.J. himself has never learned to speak. Some of these translations abided by copyright laws while others pirated the book. K.J. didn't mind this and has never considered taking legal measures. "Imitation is the sincerest form of flattery," Oscar Wilde once said, and K.J. agreed. He was happy that his book was so widely read, helping otolaryngologists across the globe for four decades. In awarding K.J. the Presidential Citation, Dr. Richard Holt, President of the Academy of Otolaryngology - Head & Neck Surgery, said, "K.J. through this book has taught more otolaryngologists around the world than anyone else."

Most medical textbooks last three editions if they are successful. In 2016, the 11th edition of K.J.'s book was published with the help of dedicated co-editors, Yvonne Chan and John C. Goddard, who updated the text with cutting-edge discoveries made in recent years. The same co-editors are now preparing the 12th edition. The two, both in their forties, have promised K.J. that as long as they live, they will continue to publish new editions of his book every three to four years. When they retire, others will take on the job. The book will carry on, long after K.J.'s lifetime, perhaps long after the lifetime of anyone living in this world today. In 2018, *K.J. Lee's* celebrated its 45th anniversary. In honor of this landmark achievement K.J. himself has added a prologue describing the evolution of otorhinolaryngology into one of the most respected and sought-after specialties by graduating medical students.

Chapter 16

THE MAN FROM TIMBUKTU

Sally Hyun Jung Jee

"The enlightened ruler is heedful, and the good general full of caution."
– Sun Tzu

The man reached into the jar and took the embalmed head out, cradling it in his arms as if it were his infant child. "Pretty, eh? It's the freshest we've got." He chuckled. The man took a step towards K.J. and his lab technician, Laurel, who instinctively took a step back. He smiled again. "Where do you want me to put this?" he asked. "Over there would be fine. Thank you," K.J. said, pointing at the dissection table across the room. He then realized that the man wasn't wearing gloves. "Just put it down for now. I'll get you some gloves," K.J. said. "Nah, I don't need 'em. I work with these every day." Laurel winced visibly as the man started walking to the table, carrying a full human head with his bare hands. Her wide eyes darted back and forth between the man and K.J., whose expression was, as usual, pensive. His coworkers often marveled at how he never seemed to lose his cool. Of course, he had his moments of panic and sorrow in his private life, but when he was at work, operating on a patient or doing research in his lab, he always kept a cool head.

The secret to his composure was a system that K.J. dubbed 'risk management'. A cautious man by nature, a quality most likely inherited from his parents, he meticulously charted all eventualities and prepared for as many of them as he could. Before each surgery, he rehearsed in his mind the protocol to follow in case of unexpected patient complications, including cardiac arrest. Fortunately, in more than 50 years of K.J.'s surgical experience, no patient has ever had a cardiac arrest. There were occasional complications, but none that he couldn't successfully handle. Some told him it was a waste of time to prepare for events that may never happen, or happen only rarely. But K.J. never wanted to be blindsided, especially when lives depended on him. No variable, even a highly unlikely one, was ever ignored.

The first step to this risk management system was to observe the situation at hand. So as the man moved across the room, K.J.'s keen eyes followed him. He looked to be in his mid-twenties. He was tall, slender and towered over both K.J. and Laurel. Clothes that most men his height would have filled out hung loose on his frame. Pale, bony arms protruded from his sleeveless t-shirt, so faded that K.J. couldn't tell its original color. His jeans were not only frayed but coated with grime— especially around the two back pockets, as if he had been sitting on a street corner for days or, perhaps, had a habit of wiping his ungloved hands on his pants. The man's most distinctive feature, however, was his bushy beard and an equally expansive head of hair to match. Forgotten bits of food were suspended in his beard like unfortunate flies caught in a spider's web. "Please tell me you'll keep an eye on him," Laurel whispered to K.J., glancing at the man nervously. K.J. gave an almost imperceptible nod. Then, he put on his gloves and got to work.

K.J. was studying an alternate pathway through which otolaryngologists like himself could remove a pituitary tumor, which is located at the base of the skull. At the time, the dominant method for pituitary surgery was a craniotomy, which required a surgeon to open up the patient's skull and move the brain, allowing the surgeon to reach the pituitary. While it might take as little as 30 minutes for a surgeon to excise the tumor, the process of shifting the brain could take an hour or longer. Even for a small tumor, craniotomy meant major surgery. Major surgery, in turn, meant a higher risk of post-surgery complications and, at worst, death.

As K.J. prepared a CAT scan for the embalmed head, he recalled a conversation he'd had with a colleague several months ago— the conversation that ultimately led to his experiment in fine-tuning a safer surgical route for pituitary tumors. "This is absurd," K.J. remembered telling his colleague. "We're doing these pituitary surgeries in the most invasive, roundabout way possible." "Well, could we devise another way?" The colleague had asked, pouring his third cup of coffee into the mug. "We could go through the nose. That way, we'd reach the pituitary more directly." "That approach was an epic failure, K.J. It's been, what? Fifty years since the last time someone's actually used it." "Times have changed. The reason doctors back then failed was that they didn't have antibiotics and the right technology: microscopes and cautery. We have them all now." "Even if that's true, we still don't have the equipment for surgery like that." "Someone's got to make it," K.J. said. "Sure." The colleague stared at the bottom of his mug, empty once again. "I'm gonna get more coffee." Lost in thought, K.J. didn't notice him leave. "Someone's got to make it," he said to himself.

To make such equipment while mapping out a new pathway to the pituitary, he needed a whole head specimen. This he acquired from Timbuktu, Ohio, where many of his colleagues also bought their cadavers and temporal bones for dissection. K.J. was preparing to make the trip to Timbuktu when the man who sold the specimen told him not to worry. He would deliver it, in person, to K.J.'s lab.

Trying to ignore the man from Timbuktu, who continued to fix his gaze on the specimen, K.J. spent the day plotting an X-ray correlation of the head. His goal was to develop a kind of GPS system that would take him to the pituitary tumor. This work, along with a dry skull dissection that he later performed on his kitchen table, would provide the anatomical basis for his acclaimed dissertation[13]. K.J. would then go on to design a self-retaining

---

[13] K.J. Lee, "The Sublabial Transseptal Transsphenoidal Approach to the Hypophysis," *The Laryngoscope*, vol. 88, no. 7 (S10) (1978).

speculum, a modified air drill, and other dissecting instruments best suited for his new surgical approach. The dissertation, including both the anatomical procedures and the equipment he developed, would revolutionize pituitary surgery. Until endoscopes came into fashion, K.J.'s surgical route would remain the dominant method of pituitary surgery.

This success, and the ensuing publicity, would attract people from all walks of life to K.J.'s practice. During the early years of practicing his new surgical method, K.J. had a patient whose hospital wing was swarmed with grave-looking men in suits. Sometime after the patient's surgery, a government representative asked to meet with K.J. At first, K.J. refused, and his secretary conveyed the message that he was not available. But on his second visit, the representative would not take no for an answer. So K.J. came face to face with him requesting details about the patient's condition, all the while curious if K.J. had conspired with the patient. The patient, it turned out, was a high-profile businessman who had committed a 'white-collar misdemeanor'. While imprisoned, the man found out about his pituitary tumor and specifically requested that he be sent to K.J., for he had heard of K.J.'s new method and its outstanding success rates. The conventional transcranial route to remove a pituitary tumor at that time required days in the intensive care unit and weeks in the hospital. Using K.J.'s new transnasal route, the patient stayed one night in the intensive care unit and was discharged from the hospital after only a few days. The representative was, therefore, concerned that the surgery was 'fake'—a ploy to delay the patient's prison sentence. Luckily, the representative who came to K.J.'s office quickly realized that other than carrying out the surgery itself, K.J. had nothing to do with the "white collar misdemeanor" patient.

K.J.'s future success would also see him treat many celebrity patients, one of which would be a billionaire listed at one time by Google as the richest man in Singapore. One day in the 1980s, K.J.'s nurse alerted him that there was a patient in the waiting room surrounded by an entourage which included a cardiologist and an anesthesiologist. This patient and his doctors had heard about K.J. and his diagnostic and surgical skills on the opposite side of the globe. K.J. treated him, and besides periodical checkups, the two remain close friends to this day. On August 3rd, 2019, this patient invited

K.J. and Linda to join him and his family for dinner in Singapore. Despite his status and wealth, he is a humble, kind, sincere and down-to-earth individual.

However, back in the dissecting lab, K.J.'s future success was the farthest thing from his mind. Now that the day's work was over, K.J.'s thoughts inevitably turned to the man from Timbuktu. Before closing the lab and heading home, K.J. ordered pizza. He and Laurel removed their gloves and scrubbed their hands fiercely, trying to rid themselves of the pungent smell of preservatives. The man, however, seemed utterly disinterested in such basic sanitary measures. When the pizza arrived, he grabbed a slice and started wolfing it down. K.J. couldn't help but stare at his unwashed hands— the same hands he had used to carry an embalmed human head without gloves earlier that day.

"Hey, you're gonna put me up in your house, right?" The man asked K.J., after he had eaten his fill. He had flown all the way from Ohio to deliver the head. (Readers may wonder how he got through airport security with a human head; but this was the 1970s, over 20 years before full airport security checks were in place.) K.J. couldn't possibly say no. An alternative option was to book the man a hotel room. But as a young surgeon just starting out in his career as an otolaryngologist, K.J. had very little, if any, money to spare.

K.J. felt his basic sense of human decency and his very human sense of fear colliding within him. His wife, Linda, and his two boys would be home. What would they think when he brought a complete stranger home unannounced?

Trying to keep his cool head, K.J. recalled the second step to risk management: survey all possible options. The living room sofa or the porch— attached to a separate bathroom— were the two accommodation options he could provide. The third step was to select the option that minimizes risk. K.J. chose the porch.

The Lees had recently set up an alarm system to protect the house from potential break-ins. The porch, however, was not yet included in the system. If someone were to cross the porch and step into the living room at night, the alarm would sound. The renovated porch with beautiful large glass windows overlooking the swimming pool, temperature controlled and with access to its own bathroom was the ideal guest room.

That night, K.J. couldn't fall asleep. Half-expecting to hear the alarm any minute, he listened to the even breathing of his wife lying next to him. As a doctor, he had managed risks his entire life, but none of them had involved the safety of his family. "I'll protect my family no matter what," he thought. "If the alarm goes off, I'll be ready."

But the alarm didn't go off. At 4 a.m., when K.J. finally drifted into sleep, it was as heavy as his many responsibilities in life. The man from Timbuktu was a gentlemanly, kind and helpful guest. K.J. learned that one should not pre-judge a person.

Chapter 17

THE ITEMS HE LEFT BEHIND

Sally Hyun Jung Jee

"The greatest legacy one can pass onto one's children and grandchildren is not money or other material things accumulated in one's life, but rather a legacy of character and faith."
– Billy Graham

The waves rise and fall, reaching their crests and troughs in rapid succession. Though they lack the elegance of the perfect sine or cosine graph in a math textbook, their movements are fluid and, to those who can see it, full of life. Few people would find human brainwaves aesthetically appealing, but K.J. has often felt that there is a peculiar beauty in these waves, especially in those of newborns, whose brains are so amazing and brimming with possibilities.

It was the early 1980s, K.J. was investigating the Auditory Brainstem Response (ABR) machine supplied by the Southern New England Telephone Company. It recorded brain wave activity in response to sound. Using these brainwaves, the machine collected information about the inner ear— called the cochlea— and related brain pathways, detecting hearing loss in both children and adults. In the research K.J. was conducting, the ABR machine was used to screen for hearing disabilities in newborns. First, K.J.

pasted small electrodes the size of M&M's on the infant's forehead, and the rest was the job of the 1980s ABR machine. By today's standards the machine was fairly crude, but at the time it represented a shining example of frontier technology.

As the machine picks up the brain waves, the infant falls asleep in his mother's arms. The mother's brow furrows, and worry lines cross her forehead. She looks back and forth between the peaceful sleeping face of her young son and the poker face of K.J., who is interpreting the ABR results. "What if my baby can't hear? What do I do then?" A million thoughts race through her head. When K.J. finally announces that her son has normal hearing, she lets out a sigh of relief. "Thank you so much, Dr. Lee," she says, shaking K.J.'s hand heartily as she leaves the examination room.

Most parents, like this one, hear good news. Unfortunately, some discover that their infants have been born with severe hearing loss. The newborn hearing screening, however, is not the final word on a child's hearing ability, since hearing can be rehabilitated if the child is treated within the first three years of life. After that, rehabilitation is less successful.

This is precisely why early detection of hearing disabilities is so important, and K.J.'s research— one of the many projects he took on after publishing his world-renowned text, *Essential Otolaryngology - Head and Neck Surgery*, and his monumental thesis on an alternative pathway to pituitary tumors— does just that. K.J. recalls the day when the Southern New England Telephone Company approached him with a research proposal. The company wanted to test the efficacy of the ABR machine in newborn hearing screening and needed the help of a medical professional. K.J., a competent doctor and research scientist, fit the bill perfectly. He was also known to conduct research without requesting payment, a quality that the company probably looked most favorably upon.

K.J. was, of course, on board the minute he heard the proposal. It didn't matter to him that he would be working without pay. He understood the importance of the ABR test and wanted to play his part in promoting infant hearing screening on a national level. He didn't want another child to miss the valuable but narrow window in which their hearing loss could be rehabilitated. After receiving permission from the administrators, obstetricians, and pediatricians of the Hospital of Saint Raphael in New Haven, Connecticut, K.J. started a clinical trial to test the hearing of every baby born at the facility. "I don't understand how people ask about the payment first. When I was doing research, the payment never even crossed my mind," K.J. would later recall.

Today, thanks to the work of K.J. and many other medical professionals, 43 out of 50 states in the U.S.A. have hearing screening requirements for newborns, which mandate the screening of every newborn for hearing loss before he or she leaves the hospital.

Another research project that K.J. took on was developing a new line of voice prostheses for patients without a larynx, more commonly called the voice box. If a patient has advanced cancer in the voice box, the doctor may have to remove the entire voice box in an operation called a total laryngectomy, which would treat the cancer but leave the patient without the ability to speak. During a total laryngectomy, the windpipe (trachea)— which conveys air to and from the lungs— and the esophagus are separated. The patient, therefore, has to breathe through a hole in the neck, which externalizes the windpipe. The voice prosthesis, placed in an opening made between the windpipe and the esophagus, enables speech by closing this opening and rechanneling air into the esophagus.

In 1980, a well-known voice prosthesis invented by a doctor and a speech pathologist was introduced to the market as the first commercially available voice prosthesis. While the device was undoubtedly a brilliant invention, it had two minor problems: the price and an involved 'installation' process. K.J. addressed precisely these two problems in his model of the voice prosthesis. He named it the Blaise-Raphael prosthesis after Saint Blaise, a physician and guardian saint of the throat, and the Hospital of Saint Raphael, where he conducted his trials for the prosthesis. Unlike the well-established model, the Blaise-Raphael prosthesis was very simple to install and very cost effective. And while the other prosthesis had to be replaced every few months, K.J.'s model worked well for years. Sadly, in a capitalist world, the value of an invention is often determined by its commercial potential rather than by its objective quality. After a couple of years, the company that manufactured the Blaise-Raphael prosthesis notified K.J. that it had decided to discontinue the model.

"Why would you make such a decision? My prosthesis costs much less and it lasts much longer than the other models," K.J. contested. "That, Dr. Lee, *is* the problem," the executive told him. Since K.J.'s prosthesis cost less and functioned too well for too long, patients didn't have to repurchase it frequently, and the company couldn't make much profit. So history was ultimately shaped by the forces of capitalism.

Capitalism, however, couldn't stop K.J. from leaving his mark in the medical world. Throughout the 1980s and 1990s, K.J. pioneered and developed laser surgery in Connecticut, giving lectures and workshops for his colleagues, many of whom were not well versed in laser technology. At that time there were three main types of lasers used in otolaryngology - head and neck surgery: the argon laser, the YAG laser, and the carbon dioxide laser. The argon laser removed hemangioma, a type of birthmark, in the face and neck area, while the YAG laser treated large vascular lesions. The carbon dioxide laser, now the most frequently used laser in the field of otolaryngology, removes benign and cancerous lesions from the voice box.

Among the many laser surgery patients K.J. has operated on, there are some who are especially dear to his heart. The first was a teenage girl who had been in a car accident and was brought to the emergency room. Her voice box was severely damaged, and the doctors told her that she would never speak again. Even for seasoned healthcare providers, delivering bad news to a patient is emotionally taxing. Watching the teenage widen her eyes with disbelief, transition to angry tears for having to suffer a misfortune she never deserved, and finally resign herself to the fact that she had lost her voice forever, must have been painful for every medical staff member involved. The worst moment, many doctors say, is when they see the light go out of a patient's eyes, leaving a dull, petrified glaze.

When the teenager came to K.J. with such a sad glaze in her eyes, K.J. tried to keep a cool head, and instead of giving up on the patient he commiserated with her. "I will try my best to restore your voice," K.J. told the patient as he looked directly into her eyes. He saw a faint glimmer of hope return to them. Using the carbon dioxide laser, K.J. successfully reconstructed the patient's voice box. In a few months, the teenage patient, who was once told that she would never speak again, was able to speak just as fluently as she always had. Now 60 years old, she still keeps in touch with K.J. and gives him updates on her condition. "No one notices that I'd lost my voice and had to restore my voice box to speak again. When I tell others, they're absolutely shocked," she says.

In his later career, K.J. taught not only the practice but also the business of medicine. In the early 1980s he became interested in the concept of a management service organization (MSO), an entity that guides doctors on the administrative side of running a medical practice. K.J.'s philosophy was that an MSO should stand behind and beside doctors to help them practice medicine conscientiously *and* gain business acumen. Thereby boosting physician morale and decreasing stress. According to K.J., the manager of an MSO must stand behind the clients rather than walk ahead of them: and while the manager's job should be to provide useful ideas that support physicians, he or she should never order them around. With this philosophy in mind, K.J. started lecturing both nationally and internationally to his colleagues, developing courses on the practicality of medicine, increasing efficiency and customer service. "Knowledge to treat, heart to care, at a sensible cost." He has lectured frequently in many countries including Australia, Chile, China, Hong Kong, Malaysia, Mexico, New Zealand, the Philippines, Portugal, Singapore, South Korea, Thailand, Turkey and the United Kingdom. He has also led delegations of otolaryngologists to Australia, China, Hong Kong, Malaysia, New Zealand, Singapore, Thailand, and the United Kingdom.

One of the things K.J. always addresses in his lectures is the importance of thoroughly reading any contract that one signs with an insurance company. If a doctor signs the contract blindly and neglects to read the fine print, he or she may find themselves locked into an agreement they cannot get out of. The dilemma is that most doctors, trying to juggle long hours in the office with their obligations at home, don't have time to go over an agreement with a fine-tooth comb.

"I really can't make the time to read everything, and if I hire a lawyer to go over the contract, I'll have to pay a lot of money," many doctors tell K.J.

He offers a simple solution to this problem. "In every household, there is a room similar to the small room in every airplane. And we all have to use the room every day. We relax, and we read a magazine or newspaper in there," K.J. tells his fellow doctors, "When you get the 20-page agreement from the insurance company, bring it into this room." At this point in the lecture, everyone bursts into laughter at the thought of the "room similar to the small room in every airplane." K.J., however, goes on with his speech with a serious expression on his face, because reading a contract carefully is no laughing matter. K.J. emphasizes that the reading process can, and should, take a week or two, even three.

"Don't think of it as urgent. Just bring three highlighters with you, and make sure to read a little bit every time you use this room. Use red highlights for the clauses you absolutely can't accept, green for those you have no problem with, and yellow for the items you're willing to negotiate with the insurance company," he says. He then does a simple calculation: "Assuming that you visit this small room at home on average twice a day, there are at least 42 occasions in the span of three weeks to relax, highlight the contract, and figure out what to negotiate."

Another topic K.J. frequently lectures on is investment. Of course, K.J. is no investment banker and has no law degree or MBA. Everything he teaches is based on common sense and learned from the school of hard knocks, and K.J. always notes at the beginning of his lecture, "I may be right, or I may be wrong."

When one buys a stock, it can go up or down. If it goes up, the stockholder is happy, but the stock is just a piece of paper until it is sold. If the stockholder decides not to sell it, it may go back down. If the stock were sold, and its price keeps increasing, the stockholder would regret the sale. To deal with the complexities of the stock market without extensive financial knowledge, K.J. introduces what he describes as "a little naïve way," or a "home-made rule" for the average person: "When the stock goes up, sell a percentage of it. If you sell half and make a profit, but the stock price keeps increasing, you still have the other half. If the stock price falls, you've made money on the half you sold."

On the subject of real estate investment, K.J. lays down three rules of thumb. The first rule is, as every real estate agent would say: "location, location, location!" The second is that land is far less trouble than buildings, since no one can steal or really damage a piece of land, and there is less property tax. The third is to find a location one knows well.

If someone decides to purchase a building, K.J. advises against residential real estate, which is generally more of a headache than commercial real estate. Unlike commercial real estate, (which is non-residential property rented to businesses), the success of residential real estate depends solely on an uncontrollable variable: how responsible the individual tenants happen to be. "Some people say that if you rent a residential building to professionals, such as doctors and lawyers, you won't have any trouble. This may be true by and large, but there are always people who defy common sense," K.J. explains, "I know someone who had a doctor couple as tenants in an upper middle class home. The two doctors tied a rope in the living room ceiling to hang a tire and let their children swing in it inside the house." Strict eviction laws can also be a problem if the residents are utterly irresponsible, since it is extremely hard to evict tenants from a residential property, even if they destroy the building and don't pay rent.

The advice that K.J. likes to close his lecture with is to keep a checklist. "Besides making a checklist, you have to look at the checklist at least three times a day," says K.J., "I have at least 20 items per day, and whatever is not done, I carry onto tomorrow's checklist." K.J. is blessed with a near-perfect memory. Even in his seventies, he seldom needs notes for the hundreds of lectures he gives.

Of the many things K.J. has imparted to the younger generation, the importance of keeping a checklist may be the most valuable advice he will leave behind. Without his fierce attention to the details in life, K.J. would not be the man he is today. Along with his checklists, K.J. has some other personal habits that have helped him through the highs and lows of life.

Wherever K.J. goes, whether it is an academic conference or a friendly dinner with colleagues, he always brings his briefcase with him. "If I go to meet a colleague and that person is late to the meeting, I won't waste 15 minutes doing nothing but waiting," K.J. says.

This habit started during his high school days in Penang, Malaya, a place known for its unpredictable bursts of rain during the monsoon season. If K.J. happened to be outdoors during one of these showers, he would be forced to suspend his bicycle journey and take refuge under something that would cover his head. While most other boys waited for the rain to pass without much thought, K.J. refused to waste time. He carried around his school bag and notebook at all times, so that if he were to take shelter somewhere during a shower, he could go over his class notes and rehearse his physics and chemistry formulas. To this day, K.J. is proud that he has never let natural phenomena get in the way of his studies or his work.

Since high school, K.J. has been a workaholic who takes his work home, as well as anywhere else he visits. He understands however, that driving himself without any reprieve is counter-productive and so he makes sure to 'de-stress' after a busy week. For the past six years, after working late, at 1 a.m. he curls up in bed and pulls a blanket over himself. He then plays a thriller film on his iPad. After two restful hours immersing himself in the world of 'cloak and dagger', K.J. feels energized and ready to bear through another grueling day ahead of him.

Another strategy that K.J. uses to relax dates back to his high school days in hot, humid, tropical Malaya. After a day at high school, he would always change into comfortable pajamas when he got home. In college and medical school, he would do the same as soon as he got back to his dormitory. His roommates thought he was unwell! Now, he changes into his pajamas when he gets home or, if he is traveling, back in his hotel room. "I can think better when I feel comfortable," K.J. says.

Some of K.J.'s other habits may seem rather peculiar to those who don't know him. But if you ask him, he will happily give you a clear explanation for each and every one of them.

First of all, K.J. doesn't like lending people money. This in itself is not unusual— the world is full of swindlers and betrayers, even among those you know and trust. But while K.J. refuses to lend money, he chooses to give money to those who deserve it, without expecting to be repaid. "Lending or forwarding people money is the way to ruin friendships," K.J.'s mother told him, time and again. (Another piece of her advice, "Good arithmetic makes good friends.") K.J., however, is not a man who can simply ignore the hardships of those around him. Though he has been deceived and let down many times in his life, he remains trusting of others, willing to give them second chances and hopeful of discovering the good in them. The only way K.J. can reconcile his own caring nature with his mother's sensible advice is to give freely and unconditionally, but wisely, not to lend. That way, he will never lose a friend over money.

Another of K.J.'s seemingly incomprehensible habits is that whenever he charges his phone in a hotel room or in someone else's office or a restaurant, he takes off his shoe and puts the phone inside it. Again, K.J. has clear reasoning behind this. "If you have your phone inside your shoe, you'll never be able to walk away and accidentally leave the phone or the charger," he explains. A clever way of avoiding a common and costly mistake.

In the height of the coronavirus (COVID-19) pandemic, K.J. wrote an op-ed: *"With the onslaught of coronavirus upon humanity, perhaps we can create a silver lining. In this day and age of fear, can we as humans reenergize ourselves to be more compassionate to each other. When another shopping cart bumped into us at the supermarket, we utter: "not a problem, you go ahead" with a genuine smile. Likewise, on the highway, lining up at the post office, work place and at home, etc. Be more tolerant of our fellow human beings. There are good aspects in everyone. Republicans have good and poor ideas. Similarly, Democrats have good points and not so good ones. When one Party does something good, the other Party should acknowledge the good points when criticizing the other's flawed policies. May this coronavirus crisis teach us to be a kinder and gentler nation, thus a kinder and more gentle world."*

K.J. analyzes all the habits that have shaped who he is today, using the same keen, scientific mind with which he examines his patients. He then imagines himself as an infant in Penang, Malaya, safely nestled in his mother's arms and drawing his first breath in this world. There were no ABR machines back then, but if there had been one, it would have recorded K.J.'s brain waves, no different from those of any hearing infant K.J. has screened. Like all other infants, K.J.'s small infant brain was full of possibilities—possibilities that blossomed into visions, then into actions. "Vision becomes thoughts, thoughts become words, words become actions, actions become networking, networking becomes results, and results become success," K.J. says.

Chapter 18

"Dr. Lee, Please Pray before You Operate"

Coco Kejia Ruan

"Heal me, LORD, and I will be healed; save me and I will be saved, for you are the one I praise."
– Jeremiah 17:14

"K.J., I am so disappointed in you. I thought you were a real scientist," said K.J.'s patient, a fellow Yale Professor, upon visiting K.J.'s office, "I will not be coming back to you anymore." Professor Beardsley was so agitated that his pointed index finger was trembling. Following the imaginary trajectory line from his fingertip, one could see a decently sized print hanging on the wall of K.J.'s office. The slightly faded print was kept in a well-polished glass frame. It featured three surgeons surrounding an operating table, focusing on the patient. The patient's exposed abdomen, instead of his face, is shown. Tiny spots of blood are on the drapes, the surgeon's gloves, and surgical equipment. It is not a typical picture that one would find in a medical office.

Silence permeated the room for the next 15 seconds. Given the impeccable nature of K.J.'s academic achievements, research, publications, and technical dexterity, he has seldom been criticized, if ever, throughout his career as a surgeon. On the few occasions he has been questioned, he always made sure to clarify and resolve the misunderstanding. But this time, he didn't speak. He stood up and raised his right hand to shake Professor Beardsley's hand. When asked how he could maintain his calm in this situation, K.J. replied, "I knew he would come around somehow."

K.J. glanced at Professor Beardsley as he stomped out of the office, while holding the door for him as a gesture of courtesy and appreciation of another's opinion. As soon as Professor Beardsley had left, K.J.'s glance returned to the picture. He was not looking at the three surgeons, nor the patient, but instead at the figure whose hand gently taps the back of one of the surgeons and whose eyes affectionately look at the patient's open wound. This figure does not wear a light blue sterile gown because he is not a surgeon. It is, in fact, an image of Jesus Christ.

The first time K.J. (then known as Ahchu) saw a version of this print was in a small make-shift hospital in Penang, Malaya with less than 20 beds. The occasion was so distressing that he only caught a glimpse of the image before moving on. He didn't even have time to count how many surgeons there were in the painting.

It was 9 p.m. on a November evening in 1954, and Ahchu's memory is disjointed and incomplete. Urgent footsteps on the wooden floor, distorted shadows of people reflected on the glaringly white wall, and frustrated, insistent voices: "Hurry up! He doesn't look well." "Be gentle. Don't shake the stretcher too much. The patient is too weak to suffer more discomfort." "Watch out for the corner! We need to make a turn there." "Watch out for the IV pole!"

There was no elevator in this small home converted into a hospital. The doctor and staff were carrying the patient on a flimsy stretcher down the stairs for an X-ray. As an apprehensive 14-year-old, Ahchu cluelessly tagged along with the doctor and his team of staff surrounding the stretcher, trying to poke his head in to get a clear view without obstructing their harried movements. The person on the stretcher was none other than Ahchu's father, the then 44-year-old Papa Lee.

Papa had been severely ill for years. He weighed only 80 pounds on his 5'4" frame, and he was as jaundiced and yellow as a piece of wrapping paper. Before moving him to the Seventh-day Adventist Hospital, they had tried both Chinese herbal medicine and Western antibiotics to no avail, and none of the doctors could diagnose exactly what was wrong with Mr. Lee.

Papa went through a series of three surgeries and almost did not survive. Every day after school at 1 p.m., Ahchu would go to the hospital as quickly as possible because the doctor and one registered nurse (RN) at the Seventh-day Adventist Hospital spoke only English, and Papa needed someone to interpret for him. Interpreting for Papa was not an easy task. In spite of the fact that he was an orphan and had only eight days of primary school education, he was extremely intelligent, careful, thorough, and analytical. Because of the complexities of his illness with no end in sight, Papa grilled Dr. Bruski politely and thoroughly with extreme precision. While searching for the right words to interpret for his dad, 14-year-old Ahchu was subconsciously taught to be polite, thorough, precise, and analytical, and to never take no for an answer. By Papa's bedside, Ahchu also fetched whatever he needed. He remembers doing his math homework at the bedside till dark and scribbling down the probability of Papa's recovery according to the doctor. "20%. What does that mean?" As he mindlessly wrote the slash and two tiny circles on each side, Ahchu murmured to himself, "what about the remaining 80%?" The odds distracted Ahchu from his homework. He also remembers falling asleep on the hospital chair and waking up suddenly to the gleaming moonlight in a cold sweat. As he stared at the vacant ceiling, vacant white wall, and vacant white hospital sheets, he was afraid that when he woke up next, Papa's bed would be vacant too. He remembers waiting helplessly outside the operating room and praying, "How I wish I could be a surgeon and operate on Papa, so I could be certain of his condition."

Miraculously, under Dr. Bruski's care and God's grace, Papa recovered. After weeks of accompanying Papa and interpreting for him, Ahchu became familiar with the small hospital and its only doctor, Dr. Bruski. In the same room as Papa one patient had a craniotomy, another had pneumonia, and yet another had fractured bones. It seemed unbelievable that one doctor could take care of such a variety of illnesses.

Impressed by his medical skills and boundless compassion, Ahchu (K.J.) remained in contact with Dr. Bruski long after Papa was discharged from the hospital. Later, when K.J. became a doctor, he contacted the now retired Dr. Bruski and inquired about his place of training. K.J. expected Dr. Bruski to say Massachusetts General Hospital, the best hospital in the US for training general surgeons. Dr. Bruski smiled amiably and answered, "No, I never had one day of surgical training. I am a general practitioner. I only had surgical atlases and the Bible. We prayed before each operation." Stunned by the answer, the young doctor, K.J., did not yet fully grasp the significance of Dr. Bruski's answer. K.J. also remembers the only nurse (RN), a Seventh-day Adventist missionary, gathering her nurses' aides every shift to evaluate the patients. She always started and ended with a prayer.

Entering the field of medicine didn't make K.J. feel more empowered when dealing with diseases, but rather more humbled. In the summer of 1965, while K.J. was an intern at St. Luke's Hospital, he heard bad news from home that his mother, Ah Mah, had suffered a stroke. Disease simply would not spare his family. Upon hearing the news, all K.J. could think of was Ah Mah's tears when she sent the 17-year-old Ahchu abroad to Harvard. To a woman who had never attended one day of school and had no real concept of distance, sending her first born son 12,000 miles away was akin to sending him to Mars, with the possibility that they'd never meet again.

Now on the other side of the globe, it was K.J. who worried, "will I ever be able to see Ah Mah again?" While agonizing over his mother's health, K.J. couldn't simply book an airline ticket and fly home the next day. He was an intern. In the sixties, interns worked more than 36 hours in a 48-hour shift and had hardly any vacation time. Earning $500 per month as an intern, supporting a family of his own, and helping two younger siblings through school, flying back was not financially or physically feasible. All he could do was worry himself sick day and night and feel helpless. In distress, K.J. and his wife Linda prayed. Reality once again hit K.J. hard in the face. He thought to himself, "Having medical training is not enough to ensure my family's well-being, I need to work harder and do more."

K.J.'s family came from humble beginnings, but both of his parents were hard working and wanted the best for their children. K.J.'s parents educated all seven of their children well. After years of diligent and careful saving, Ah Mah bought a shop house in the Chinatown District of Singapore in the 1950s. Papa meanwhile expanded his business as a bicycle repair man to a sales distributor for tires. When his business was not doing well and he got into debt, he forced Ah Mah to sell her shop house in Singapore to help him settle the debt. Willing to do anything for the family, Ah Mah quietly agreed, but that night she had a stroke.

It is said that when a healthy person suddenly has a stroke, it is because he or she is traumatized psychologically. Ah Mah didn't have it easy, and she had always lived with trauma. When K.J.'s maternal grandparents separated, Ah Mah went to live with her mother, while her brother went to live with their father. This family breach had always disturbed Ah Mah, to the extent that one night she dreamed of her father crawling on the wall in her bedroom. Appalled, she was not sure if the skeleton with a thin layer of saggy skin was just a dream or her father's ghost. K.J. would never forget the mixture of sorrow, fear, and insecurity in Ah Mah's eyes when she retold the dream to him, and he imagined Ah Mah looking the same way when she had to sell the shop house. Luckily, it turned out that the crawling figure was only a dream. Eight years later, K.J. found his uncle in Singapore after a long search, and when he inquired about his maternal grandpa, his uncle told him, "My dad passed away a year ago." Using basic arithmetic, K.J. was relieved to conclude that the crawling figure that had bothered Ah Mah for years was simply a dream and not a ghost, because at the time Ah Mah had the dream, her father had not yet died. Nevertheless, Ah Mah had always treasured family ties with her parents and children, and K.J. felt painfully guilty for not being able to even give her a hug when she most needed it.

Ah Mah gradually recovered her speech and ability to walk and started to function almost normally, but the enormous sense of loss and despair lingered for decades after this misfortune. With his meager savings, K.J. decided to invite his mother over to live with him for a year with his wife and two young boys, hoping that the family reunion would improve Ah Mah's outlook. He would later recall this precious year spent with his mother as God's blessing. His wife was kind enough to help take care of Ah Mah.

K.J.'s eldest two sons were able to get to know their grandmother. (K.J. and Linda's third son was born five years later.)

Life went on, and K.J. continued conquering challenges medically, emotionally, and financially, while hoping no further misfortunes would befall him and his family. Contrary to his hope, K.J.'s life has always been plagued by major and minor discomfort and illnesses. At the age of 16, he developed facial paralysis. Although it was not too serious, he had to be hospitalized in case of medical emergency. In 1963, as a third-year medical student, K.J. underwent a right ear mastoidectomy. When he was a senior resident at age 29, he developed Ménière's Disease. At the age of 31, K.J. developed cancer in his back. It was diagnosed and treated, but the treatment was inadequate, and it recurred five years later. It was an obvious case of malpractice, but K.J. decided to forgive. Fortunately, and through God's healing, the cancer was successfully treated the second time. K.J. was frequently confronted by minor medical conditions. When he was a toddler, he would wake up in the middle of the night and vomit. Even now, he suffers from indigestion around once every six months, requiring him to travel with medicine wherever he goes.

A common misconception is that doctors **don't contract illnesses** as easily as lay people, but this is far from true. In addition to witnessing first-hand life, death, and everything in between on the operating table, surgeons suffer from many afflictions themselves. Challenged by daily ordeal, either vicariously or directly, they have to hold on to their steadfast belief in science and, perhaps more importantly, hope and God's grace. In the grimmest valleys of life, the allure of giving in to doubt and vulnerability is ever looming. Nevertheless, K.J. always tries his hardest to grab hold of the divine essence, something stronger than himself. For this reason, he always prays before performing a surgery. He firmly believes that doctors and all healthcare providers are instruments of a supreme healing being, God, to "cure sometimes, treat often, comfort always" (Hippocrates). One day, when he happened to see in a catalog the print with Jesus standing behind three surgeons in an operating room, he bought it without hesitation. It has been hanging in the most conspicuous spot in his office ever since.

He didn't know then that this print was the exact same one he had seen at the Seventh-day Adventist Hospital where Papa Lee was cured decades ago in tropical Penang, Malaya. In fact, he didn't discover this until years later when his consulting network referred a seriously ill cardiac patient to the headquarters hospital of the Seventh-day Adventist Health System in Orlando, Florida. At that main hospital hung the original portrait of Jesus standing behind the surgeons. When K.J. saw this original painting, he finally made the connection between the print hung in the stairwell in 1954 in a tiny makeshift hospital in Penang and the one in his office. In a flash, it finally made sense why Dr. Bruski made possible the seemingly impossible.

Fast forward another decade into K.J.'s medical career. Sitting in his office one day, K.J. saw the last name Beardsley on his patient roster, although he didn't immediately make the connection. This was 10 years after Professor Beardsley from Yale had criticized K.J.'s decision to hang a print of Jesus in his office as unscientific, and K.J. had long forgotten about the unpleasant exchange.

The next day, Mrs. Beardsley walked in with her husband to be evaluated by K.J. She unfortunately had throat cancer. Professor Beardsley didn't say anything about his prior awkward encounter with K.J. years before, and K.J. treated Mrs. Beardsley like he would any other patient—with full dedication and compassion.

On the morning of Mrs. Beardsley's surgery, as she was wheeled into the sterile operating room, her stretcher was stopped momentarily by Professor Beardsley. K.J. waited patiently for Professor Beardsley to say his words of comfort and encouragement to his wife, but to his surprise, Professor Beardsley turned and looked K.J. straight in the eye, appealing: "Dr. Lee, please pray before you operate." God is K.J.'s closest teacher, friend, guardian, and savior.

Chapter 19

K. J.'s Cardinal Rules

Coco Kejia Ruan

"Blessed is the man who walks not in the counsel of the wicked, nor stands in the way of sinners, nor sits in the seat of scoffers; but his delight is in the law of the Lord, and on his law he meditates day and night."
– Psalm 1:1-3

"Thank you, Dr. Lee. See you next week!" K.J. nodded and smiled genially at his patient, "I hope your condition gets better soon." As his last patient walked out of the clinic, K.J. took a deep breath. He finally had time to admire the beautiful autumn view outside his window in Watertown.

It was a peaceful Saturday morning in October 1977. K.J. had settled in this clinic for five years, and everything seemed to be right on track. So far, the biggest issue (if it could even be called an issue) was that there were too many patients who wanted to see him. He was very popular. Word had got around that K.J. was not only an excellent diagnostician, but a skilled and compassionate surgeon who doubled checked every detail.

In the room adjacent to K.J.'s office, his secretary took a phone call. She picked it up before it rang three times. Her hurried action was incongruous with the tranquil Saturday atmosphere, but that was K.J.'s cardinal rule Number One— the telephone shall ring no more than three times.

The secretary rushed to the phone, put the receiver between her right ear and her shoulder, and fetched the appointment book from the table, "Good morning. Which date are you looking for an appointment?" "Let me see, Wednesday 4 p.m. ... Please hold on." There was a substantial break in the conversation. This was not because the patient had a long or unique last name that took a while to spell. Rather, it was because there simply was no space on the page to fit in another patient.

The secretary put down the receiver and put on her glasses. As she brought her eyes closer to the page, she was progressively more overwhelmed by the jam-packed marks written in different colors of ink: black, blue, and red. The black ink especially reminded her of groups of ants crawling slowly but steadily on a white background. She flipped to the next page to see if there were any open spots left. And the next page and the page after that. They all looked the same. In the end, she gave up and flipped back to the original page.

"Thank you for waiting. Yes, you can come at 4 on Wednesday." While she was talking to the patient, she selected her pen in yet another color of ink to write the appointment down.

"Did you say it was an emergency? If it is, you can feel free to come now." The definition of *emergency* differs widely between people working in medicine and laypeople. To the former, it means a life-or-death situation: unstoppable severe bleeding, swallowing a poisonous substance, heart attack, or difficulty breathing. To the latter, it might mean discomfort and anxiety caused by fear and uncertainty. To doctors like K.J., restoring the patient's psychological well-being is as important as keeping them physically safe. So, here comes K.J.'s cardinal rule Number Two— "A good doctor takes care of the disease; a great doctor takes care of the patient." In other words, as long as the patient finds it necessary, he or she has the right to see the doctor soon. [K.J. co-founded a not-for-profit foundation, an NGO, some years later named TPIU (The Patient Is U) to spread and emphasize this value of compassionate care. Empowering caregivers to treat patients as if they themselves are the patient.]

The secretary collapsed into her chair and sighed deeply after answering the phone. There was a time when she was too scared to answer any call because each one equated to another patient in the fully-booked doctors' schedule. Each patient adds work not only for doctors, but for secretaries as well. Sometimes she would ignore the calls to 'help' the doctors.

When K.J. found out, he was moved by his secretary's attempt to ease his workload, but to him, nothing was more important than the patients. After some deliberation, K.J. came up with his cardinal rule Number Three— for each new patient registered, he gave one dollar to his secretary.

In this way, K.J. conquered the greatest 'challenge' the clinic had to face. Even so, he felt blessed to work there because his fellow doctors were so considerate. K.J. had four colleagues: Dr. Jones who had started the group practice, Dr. Kobeyama, a goodhearted fellow whom K.J. rarely talked to outside of work, Dr. Campbell who was equally taciturn and dedicated, and Dr. Edward, whom K.J. helped to recruit. Dr. Edward was not quite the stereotypical, softly-spoken doctor. While working at Madigan Army Hospital K.J. became friends with Dr. Edward, then a 'post-doc' surgeon at the University of Washington. When the clinic decided to expand and hire a fifth doctor, K.J. immediately recommended Dr. Edward to work there under the same financial arrangement: doctors took 55% of the revenue, while Dr. Jones, the owner of the group practice, took 45% which covered the 40% overheads, leaving 5% as the owner's profit.

K.J. felt satisfied about the financial arrangements with Dr. Jones. He never had to worry about having a clean lab coat, nor worry about billing and collection. Whenever he arrived at the clinic in the morning, everything was always prepared to accommodate his preferences. He could solely focus on his work and his patients. "Dr. Jones totally deserves the 5% profit," K.J. thought. (Dr. Jones was the originator of the 'Super MSO' idea, which we will return to later in this book.[14])

Someone was knocking on the door. "Who could this be? I thought my last appointment for this Saturday was over," K.J. said to himself as he walked over and opened the door. It was Dr. Jones who was standing at the door, smiling at him, "Hi K.J., do you want to grab lunch with me today? Come, I will drive you to the restaurant." "Of course," K.J. willingly agreed.

---

[14] K.J. Lee, "Super Management Service Organization – MSO." Available at: http://kjlee.world/biography/uploads/reforms-5ba92b1873fcd.

Dr. Jones was not only professionally capable, but also kind and approachable in private settings. And after all, who could reject a kind boss's invitation to lunch?

Dr. Jones took K.J. out to a Chinese restaurant and ordered Kung Pao chicken and fried rice. When the food came, Dr. Jones didn't start eating right away, but rather looked at K.J. thoughtfully as he ate. "Is everything okay for you at the clinic?" Dr. Jones asked K.J. and squinted to check his watch. K.J. nodded and thought to himself, "Why is Dr. Jones being extra nice to me today? Am I his favorite doctor-employee out of the four?"

Dr. Jones picked up the chopsticks, stuck them in his bowl of rice, and moved tiny bits of rice to his mouth from time to time. He ate so slowly that his bowl remained full, and he remained silent for the next few minutes. In the polite and slightly awkward silence, K.J. thought of his co-worker Dr. Edward's recent accusation against Dr. Jones. According to Dr. Edward, Dr. Jones had secretly been taking 25% of the total income for himself instead of the mere 5% he was supposed to. The overheads were not 40% but 20%. "How could this be?" initially K.J. was in total disbelief, but Dr. Edward had concrete evidence from looking over the book-keeper's records. "But again, what can we do other than remain silent, even if this is true? Maintaining harmony is always better than quarreling or making enemies, especially over money, isn't it?" K.J. was deep in his thoughts when Dr. Jones suddenly put down his chopsticks. "Are you happy working with the other three doctors?" Dr. Jones asked. He followed up by saying, "If you do not like one of them, I can get rid of him." K.J. was flabbergasted, and he quickly finished his mouthful of food, and answered, "of course I am happy! They are all dedicated doctors."

Dr. Jones nodded absentmindedly, while looking at his watch again. It had only been 10 minutes since the food was served. K.J. couldn't help but wonder, "Is he in a rush to do something else after lunch? Or is it that Dr. Jones doesn't like Chinese food, and only came here to make me happy? Oh, Dr. Jones is such a nice man. He can't be the bad guy scheming behind all his loyal doctor-employees." Thinking of how kind Dr. Jones had been to him, K.J. felt glad that he had stopped Dr. Edward from spreading the rumor about Dr. Jones's scam. "Why couldn't Dr. Edward be as peace-loving as the rest of us? He must have been born defiant."

With unresolved conflicts in mind, K.J. finished eating in a hurry. Instead of driving him back to the clinic, Dr. Jones drove K.J. to his own house to have tea. As soon as K.J. sat down on the sofa, Dr. Jones stepped out again to "run an errand" and asked K.J. to wait till he came back. "What could Dr. Jones be doing at this hour of the day? Buying snacks to go with the tea? I honestly wouldn't mind just drinking tea." As K.J. remained in confusion, the door opened, and when Dr. Jones walked in, he was not alone. Dr. Kobeyama and Dr. Campbell walked in after him one by one. For a few seconds, K.J. waited for Dr. Edward to follow them, but there was no sign of him. After a few minutes, he did not think too much about his absence.

K.J. was in complete astonishment, and when his glance met Dr. Kobeyama's and Dr. Campbell's his bewilderment was echoed in their eyes. Before they could make sense of the situation, Dr. Jones reappeared in the living room, with no tea or food. He was holding a large portrait of himself in a frame gilded with gold. His polite smile vanished as he raised his head and looked the three doctors in the eye, one by one. With a serious and aloof expression, he announced, "I know you guys have all been talking about my taking more profit than I should have. Now I'm telling you that the rumors are all true. But it doesn't matter. This is *my* clinic. The patients are all *my* patients. You merely work here."

Dr. Jones stopped to catch his breath, awaiting the three doctors' reaction. Before anyone could form a coherent response, he pointed at his portrait and continued, "Now that you know the truth, I don't want to be the vicious person anymore. I intend to sell this clinic to you and collect 9% of the annual revenue for the next 10 years as the sale price. You have five minutes to decide to either take this deal or leave. If you choose to leave, as of Monday morning, my portrait will be hanging in the waiting room, and I'll lock the doors and change the keys to the clinic."

K.J. had not spent a longer five minutes in his life. Every second of the deliberation between a rock and a hard place was torture. Either he agreed to pay the high price to 'buy' the practice he had built, or he would have to start a clinic from scratch. Five minutes was not enough time for him to evaluate every single possible solution to the urgent dilemma. Yes, K.J. disliked deceitfulness, but what about his wife and two sons? How could he possibly find another job overnight to support his family?

"Dr. Kobeyama," Dr. Jones maintained his stern composure, "what do you think?" Quiet and conforming as he had always been, Dr. Kobeyama said yes. It seemed as if fear of authority ran in the Asian blood. "Dr. Lee, what about you?" "Yes, sir," K.J. reluctantly concurred. No other option was left to him. Two out of three; the majority had already said yes, leaving Dr. Campbell with no choice. He followed with a third "Yes." Although they weren't yet aware of it, Dr. Jones had cunningly started his negotiations with the three most docile and amenable doctors.

K.J. cannot remember how he walked out of Dr. Jones's house that day and was driven back to the clinic. Everything happened so fast that he could not even make sense of the situation. The kind boss that he had always looked up to suddenly turned out to be a schemer using the brutal technique of 'divide and conquer'. How could anyone have reacted calmly?

K.J. had plans to dine two hours away with some pediatrician friends in Worcester that evening. His wife later recalled that K.J. did not say a word on the two-hour drive there or back. Amidst the challenge and uncertainty of the future, K.J. chose to keep everything to himself and protect his family members from worrying.

Another meeting took place the following Monday between Dr. Jones and Dr. Edward. Dr. Jones was succinct and business-like, "Dr. Edward, here is the deal. Leave now if you disagree, and the other three doctors will see your patients." K.J. finally realized the extent of Dr. Jones' scheming. Dr. Edward was the most vocal, quick thinking and likely to rebut of the four doctors. Had he been at Dr. Jones's house last Saturday, he would have rebutted and resisted till the end, and Dr. Jones would not have achieved his high price. "Realistically speaking, Dr. Jones simply cannot find four substitute doctors overnight. It was all his ploy and maneuver!" It was too late for K.J., Dr. Campbell, and Dr. Kobeyama to realize their mistake.

It took months for K.J. to digest the consequences of his gullibility and to come to terms with the harsh reality. Nevertheless, out of love for his profession and his patients, K.J. was able to once again make lemonade out of lemons. He kept his head down and kept working. He gradually took over managing the clinic for free and used his negotiation skills to lower Dr. Jones's price down to 7% a year for all four doctors. At the end of the 10-year deal, Dr. Jones retired, and K.J. was elected by his colleagues unanimously to be the managing partner of the clinic. He served in that role until April 2012, a 23-year term. He was also appointed Chief of Otolaryngology - Head and Neck Surgery at the hospital for over two decades, when the term of office was three years. Through his skillsets and compassionate, empathetic care, KJ developed one of the busiest and most prestigious ENT practices in the U.S.

If K.J. has a weakness, it is his trust in other people. On this occasion he paid a painful price for this. But if you ask K.J. whether he would still choose to be kind and trusting of people if everything could start over, he would say yes, adamantly. But perhaps with a little more vigilance to "trust and verify."

Needless to say, K.J.'s last Cardinal Rule is— always be kind to others, regardless of the return. There have been moments in his life when compassion was repaid by wrongdoing, but K.J. chose to believe firmly in justice and light. When K.J. became President of the American Academy of Otolaryngology - Head & Neck Surgery, he awarded Dr. Jones the most prestigious Academy award, the Presidential Citation, recognizing him for advancing the sub-specialty of Facial Plastic Surgery and other contributions within the specialty of otolaryngology - head and neck surgery. To K.J., the cup is always half full and not half empty. He was pleased to have been associated with Dr. Jones. He learned much from his knowledge of the 'business of medicine'; some points K.J. would keep, others he would not.

Chapter 20

IT DOES NOT HAVE TO END THIS WAY

Clementine Xinyi Li

"[A]nd forgive us our trespasses as we forgive those who trespass against us…"
– The Lord's Prayer

The judge's hammer struck down on the pedestal with a swift thud, like a rock hitting the ground. To K.J., however, it sounded like a deafening roar that electrified his ear drums and numbed his senses, echoing off the hollow walls of the courtroom. He had to sit down, blink, and slowly bury his face in his hands. In his head, the attorneys' victorious cheers, his friends' congratulations, and the cold silence and shuffling of papers from the opposing party, all coalesced into a discordant, orchestral chaos. It played and played, until one clear teardrop slipped through his tightly clenched fingers, soon evaporating into nothingness.

When K.J. first formed the Ultimate Medical Group (UMG), he was filled with hopes of forming a group to anticipate the new 'pay for performance' or 'capitation payment' method in healthcare; he certainly did not anticipate an arduous, bitterly long legal battle that would prove to be one of the very worst experiences of his life. He would later reflect, "With UMG, the market wasn't ready for it, as pay for performance and capitation never arrived in the market, at least not yet."

In the mid-1990s, K.J. had a vision. A well-established surgeon and practitioner in his field by now, he increasingly regarded the payment system for doctors at that time as inefficient, and wasteful. Always a doer, K.J. quickly brought 124 like-minded Connecticut doctors together to form UMG, clasping hands as they prepared for a new payment format that he believed would be the next transitional step towards a better healthcare system.

How was this system different? At the time, when a patient visited the doctor, the doctor submitted a fee for each visit, so doctors were only paid when their patients visited them. With pay for performance and capitation, whether patients visited their doctor or not, the doctors would receive a regular payment from the insurance company, a 'per patient per month' method charging for each patient registered with the doctor instead of payment for each visit. This idea was ahead of its time in Connecticut. Though UMG in New Haven was ready to partake in it, the new payment system never came to fruition. Only very recently, almost 30 years after K.J. anticipated it, the government is finally preparing to reintroduce this method.

Now, to misquote Tolstoy, "Happy companies are all alike; every unhappy company is unhappy in its own way." When a venture is a success, happy shareholders with fattened wallets seldom complain and seek no trouble. However, where a new venture fails, it leads to a quagmire of complications and eventually, inevitably, legal conflict.

It all began when a certain Mr. X, the chairman of the board of UMG, was voted out. Mr. X's day job was running a huge Wall Street company with a revenue stream of approximately $2 billion, while also serving as chairman of the new startup UMG's board. He was unable to attend most board meetings. Understandably, he prioritized his former company, but the situation slowly worsened until the UMG board could not get anything done, always awaiting his approval, which seldom came. Therefore, at yet another board meeting which Mr. X did not show up to on time, he was voted out of office for practical reasons.

Mr. X's reaction to this decision was unexpected to say the least. He tracked the group of unfortunate doctors down over the phone, "I have a company with $2 billion in revenue, so just wait, I'm going to sue each and every one of you until you cannot put your kids through school!"

Among those accused was K.J. whose life became miserable thanks to Mr. X's aggressive approach. K.J. began to dread Fridays, when Mr. X and his team of lawyers would punctually send their weekly fax, each containing a fresh wave of accusations directed at the old UMG board members. One could not help but think that if Mr. X had only devoted half of this energy to managing UMG, perhaps he would not have been voted out in the first place. Nonetheless, K.J.'s life was seriously impacted by the incessant calls, mail, and abuse from Mr. X and his ferocious team of lawyers. Concerned about his family's safety and UMG's future, he began to lose sleep and could not eat properly.

Personal harassment was not the end of it, as Mr. X also sought to take UMG down. Not only did he stop funding it, he launched an investigation into UMG's finances. He hired a top accounting firm to look into potential inappropriate handling of funds. This team of accountants worked day and night for three days straight, and in the end, all they were able to find was one mistake in documenting $15.20 that UMG paid to a cleaning man for one hour of his undocumented service. Nothing else. They had no case.

Knowing that Mr. X was using everything at his disposal to collect enough evidence to file a court case against UMG, the remaining board members eventually decided that they would try to pre-empt Mr. X by gaining the upper hand in suing him first. It was not easy for K.J. to agree on taking this step, as he so disliked confrontation. Coincidentally, as K.J. hung up the phone after speaking to UMG's lawyer who informed him of the board's decision, his phone screen flashed again with an incoming call. The call was from none other than Mr. X.

"Listen, K.J.," Mr. X said, "let's have breakfast together, one-on-one. We need to talk things over." K.J. couldn't agree more, and gladly accepted the invite. All his doctor friends warned him against this breakfast meeting, saying that, "You are too naive, and he does not think like you. Do you think he's arranging this breakfast to let bygones be bygones? He's only going to have breakfast to intimidate you and chew you out!" But K.J. thought otherwise. "Maybe Mr. X has harangued us enough. Maybe he's ready to stop behaving aggressively and vengefully and start negotiating logically to come to a solution and reach a win-win for both parties."

The following day K.J.'s lawyers dutifully informed Mr. X's legal team that the law suit had been filed. Upon hearing this news, Mr. X instructed his secretary to cancel the breakfast meeting. As K.J. heard from the nervous secretary, he knew that the last chance for conciliation without bloodshed was dead and gone.

Thus began months of investigation, courtroom drama, angry phone calls, and ever-accumulating, unnecessary bad blood. K.J. has always said to his friends, his students, and everyone close to him, "Try not to make enemies in life. A man walking with friends beside him will walk far." Going to court is the very last resort for anyone, and he was in a state of disbelief that things had gone this far: why did UMG have to go through all this mess?

As the days dragged on, the issue was no longer about justice, nor even about right or wrong. The sharp pangs of anger dulled down to a throb, and all K.J. wished was for it to be over. The case was an ever-present, incessant pendulum of uncertainty hanging over the heads of all parties involved, swinging closer day by day but never quite reaching its target with its full explosive force, just inching threateningly closer. "It was probably one of the worst periods of my life. It was so stressful, and there was so much ill feeling going about. It was very, very unhealthy to live this way," K.J. later reflected.

At long last, the day of judgment arrived. K.J. dressed in his regular slacks and a jacket, but had to steady his hand to fasten his tie the way he had done every morning for over 40 years. The UMG board members accompanied K.J. to court, their eyes focused downwards in intense concentration, nothing crossing their minds besides a dull sense of finality and anticipation.

As the judge began to speak after the testimonies had been given, he closed his eyes and clasped his hands together in a gesture that resembled prayer. He pronounced, "From the records that we have examined, Mr. X failed to carry out his duty as chairman of the UMG board, and it was within the board's right to relieve him of the chairmanship. Mr. X also failed to fulfill his duty to continue funding UMG and breached the initial agreement between the two parties." The court ruled at 5 p.m. that Mr. X owed UMG all the unpaid funding, plus 5.5% interest, effective 5.01 p.m. That was when K.J. wept with relief and joy, while his colleagues were jubilant and cheered.

Revenge is an ugly word, and one that fails to describe this situation appropriately, as it was neither the intention nor the outcome. K.J. and UMG were pushed beyond their limits, and regardless of the result, they felt sorry that this happened in the first place. He did not think of this courtroom drama as a victory, "I think of it as one of the major failings in my life— it was a fight that could have been avoided." All in all, it was an enlightening ordeal and experience, a good lesson in life. One has to experience failure in order to succeed. One has to learn from previous failures.

K.J. demonstrated this ethos on a later occasion when a businessman who was a friend of many years suggested they buy a small medical office building as equal partners. The business colleague offered to supervise the renovation of the old building. As the bills came in for materials and labor, K.J. noted that they were unusually high for work on such a small building. His colleague owned other medical offices in another city and was charging 50 percent of those expenses to K.J. After much discussion, K.J. decided to 'buy him out' and communication between their families ceased for many years. One day, K.J. received a request to help this former acquaintance's son gain admittance to a prestigious Ivy League university. Without hesitation K.J. wrote to and called the Dean of Admissions. The young man was accepted by the university and went on to have a successful career. K.J. knew the importance of letting bygones be bygones.

Chapter 21

APPRECIATE STRENGTHS AND MANAGE WEAKNESSES

Coco Kejia Ruan

"Kindness is more important than wisdom, and the recognition of this is the beginning of wisdom."
— Theodore Isaac Rubin

Kindness can be described as the seed that bears beautiful flowers in the spring, the sunshine that melts snow in the winter, or the sugar added to a cupful of milk. K.J. always adds sugar to his milk; much to the surprise of his freshman classmates at Harvard. At their 25th reunion, some of his classmates remembered him only as the boy who put sugar in his milk. In K.J.'s experience, kindness can have another outcome— it can produce unfavorable results which we might call 'the lemons of life'.

K.J. has a special fondness for lemons, but he knows their bitterness all too well from his own childhood. Why bother 'growing lemons' by himself?

One of these bitter experiences began at midnight on a December evening in the 1980s. K.J. had flown into LaGuardia Airport having addressed a conference elsewhere. Despite being exhausted and cold, K.J. felt relieved. "Mr. Smith is picking me up from LaGuardia Airport and driving me home to Connecticut. At least I don't have to drive myself at this hour of the night," he thought. K.J. waited and waited. Half an hour passed, and nobody came. Mr. Smith was the night doorman at the medical office building where K.J. worked. K.J. had become acquainted with him soon after he started working there. No matter how tired K.J. was when he walked through the door, he always took time to speak to Mr. Smith, "How are you, Mr. Smith? It must be very tiring for you to be on the midnight to eight shift every day, or rather, every night."

In time, their conversations progressed from casual exchanges of greetings to discussions about Mr. Smith's personal life and financial struggles. One day, as K.J. routinely greeted him, Mr. Smith stopped K.J. and self-consciously inquired, "Dr. Lee, you know that my family is not that well-off. I need an additional job. If you ever need a driver or something, can I drive you?"

"Of course, you can! That will be wonderful!" K.J. concurred without a second thought. K.J. always feels an intangible sense of unease about driving long distances. Not because he is not a good, responsible driver, but because he is so careful and circumspect that he can't think of anything else when driving; he gets bored. For this reason, K.J. has always hired drivers for long-distance trips. However, his main motivation in concurring so readily with Mr. Smith's suggestion was that K.J. had always sympathized with him. With his limited technical abilities and verbal skills, the jobs available to him were poorly paid yet sometimes hard to secure. As a result, K.J. had long wanted to assist him without directly giving him money. By letting Mr. Smith be his driver occasionally, K.J. could kill two birds with one stone. What a brilliant idea!

K.J. never thought he would come to regret this seemingly perfect deal at the most unexpected moment. An hour had passed, and still there was no trace of Mr. Smith as the airport grew increasingly quiet. K.J. started to worry, "Had something happened to Mr. Smith? Was there a traffic accident? Had he suddenly fallen ill?"

"Dr. Lee!" in semi-darkness, a man shouted through the car window, "Dr. Lee, I am so sorry to be this late. I got lost in LaGuardia, and I had no idea how to locate you." There were no cell phones in those days. Looking into the man's sincere eyes, K.J. smiled and relented, "It's alright. You will get more used to it. Now, please drive me home safely, would you? I don't want my wife to worry about me." "Yes, sir," Mr. Smith said with determination.

K.J. closed his eyes to take a nap as he leaned back in the backseat. When he opened his eyes, he realized that this was not the way home. He looked at Mr. Smith in the rear-view mirror and saw how distressed he seemed— with his forehead furrowed and his hands tightly grasping the steering wheel. "Mr. Smith?" K.J. inquired. Mr. Smith was so occupied by driving that he didn't hear or reply. "Mr. Smith?" K.J. tried again, "where are we right now?" A look of guilt crossed Mr. Smith's face as he hesitated, "I am sorry, I have no idea where we are or where I am going."

Looking out of the car window into the immense darkness of the chilly December night, K.J. didn't know what he should feel. Disappointment? Rage? Helplessness? His reaction was unexpected, "Please pull over, Mr. Smith." Confused, Mr. Smith turned back to look at K.J. "Let me drive," K.J. explained.

Thus said, K.J. drove Mr. Smith back home and still paid him the service fee previously agreed upon. Sweet intention grew into lemons. When K.J.'s friends heard the story, they laughed and secretly thought that K.J. would have learned his 'lesson' from this experience and would not repeat it. How can you continue to employ someone whose capability is so far below the requirements of the job?

However, "never make the same mistake twice" didn't seem to apply in this case. In the early 1990s, K.J. acquired a piece of land by the ocean. It was close to Halloween, so K.J. was concerned that some neighborhood children might accidentally go into the house, which was under construction. He needed someone to stay there that night and fend off kids or burglars.

K.J. thought of Mr. Smith again, "This job doesn't require him to drive, nor does he need to know the directions well. The only thing that he needs to do is physically stay there and stay awake, just like he always does as the night doorman for the medical office building. Of course he can handle this!" Mr. Smith didn't hesitate to take on the task, "Dr. Lee, thank you so much for putting your trust in me once again. I promise I won't mess up this time!"

Concerned about Mr. Smith's driving ability, K.J. drove him to the house by the ocean himself and then drove back. His phone rang later that evening. It was almost 10 p.m. "Who could this be?" K.J. thought.

"Dr. ... Dr. Lee ... I am, I am ...," the voice on the other side of the telephone was trembling, "I am so scared. It's so dark here, I'm so scared. I don't want to stay here any longer." It was Mr. Smith. He had walked to the neighbor's house to borrow a phone. K.J. could visualize him squatting down and shrinking into a ball. The only thing to be done was drive back to the house to pick up Mr. Smith.

When Linda heard what had happened, she couldn't contain her laughter. K.J. laughed too, despite his disappointment. He thought he had hired someone so that he could have peace of mind on this night of 'trick or treat'. As it turned out, he was not only 'tricked', but he had to provide Mr. Smith with the 'treat': payment for two hours' 'work'.

This wasn't the last time K.J.'s kind nature got him into a ridiculous situation. He somehow had a fondness for nice people, or rather nice people always found their way to him. When K.J.'s eldest son, Kenneth, was getting married in New York, he asked to use the Bentley as the bridal car. Good things come in pairs, K.J. pondered, "If I let him borrow my car, I might as well find him a presentable driver."

Having learned about Mr. Smith's driving ability, he obviously wasn't an option. This time, K.J. found Mr. Richards, a handsome, tall, muscular man in his early fifties who would surely make a suitable driver for a bridal car. Mr. Richards had driven K.J. before, but not in the Bentley, and he was a very nice guy, as well as a professional driver. Mr. Richards arrived early at K.J.'s house that morning in a dark suit and tie, with a beaming smile on his face. "This man has such a good attitude," K.J. quietly observed. However, things went awry when Mr. Richards got in the car and tried to familiarize himself with the turn signal lever. It wasn't that he couldn't tell left from right, nor did he mistake the windshield wiper for the signal lights. Mr. Richards, on his first try, pulled the turn signal lever completely off the side of the steering wheel. Aghast, K.J. stood in complete astonishment for a long minute or two. He had thought of all the things that could potentially go wrong and come up with Plan Bs to fix them, but a bridal car without a turn signal lever? He didn't even think it was possible. Inside the car, Mr. Richards was equally in shock. He had never driven a car as 'delicate' as a Bentley, so he never considered his driving style would be too aggressive for the car.

With only an hour until the wedding there was no time for panic. "What would Kenneth and his bride think when they heard this news? It would surely ruin the mood for their special day." Putting aside his worries and anxiety, K.J. acted calmly and asked his wife Linda to reinstall the turn signal lever so that it at least *appeared* intact. Linda can fix anything! She has fixed broken TVs, radios, even the flat roof and gutters. She managed to fix the broken lever. When it was time to pull out and pick up the bride, K.J. looked at Mr. Richards imploringly and told him, "Please use your hands when you take turns instead of the signal lights." Fortunately, Mr. Richards didn't mess up again on Kenneth and Susan's big day.

Per usual, even though Mr. Richards had fumbled on an important task, K.J. didn't pass judgment on his overall ability and work ethic based on a single mistake. "Maybe he was bad at handling car gadgets, but there must be something that he is good at. I just haven't found it yet," was K.J.'s rationale. Maybe you can't use lemons to decorate birthday cakes because they aren't sweet enough, but you can make lemonade out of lemons, a popular drink, especially in the summer.

K.J. discovered Mr. Richards's real 'ability' when his middle son Lloyd went for a second interview with a less than reputable restaurant chain owner. Lloyd had already passed the first round of interviews, and according to him, his future boss had some eccentric habits. During the first interview, the restaurant owner had to use the restroom, and from there he continued the interview with the door propped open. Upon hearing this, K.J. was concerned about Lloyd's upcoming summer job, although Lloyd himself was not overly worried. Who knew what other eccentricities a person without basic manners might have? He considered talking Lloyd out of going for the second interview, but this didn't seem fair to the young man keen to gain experience in the hospitality industry during the summer between his two years of business school.

Stuck between a rock and a hard place, Mr. Richards came into K.J.'s mind. "Listen, Lloyd. I am going to have Mr. Richards drive you to your second interview and have him stay outside of the interview room waiting for you the whole time," K.J. instructed Lloyd. "What? Dad, this is ridiculous. Did you forget that Mr. Richards almost broke your Bentley? If I ever need a driver, I won't ask *him*," Lloyd refuted, "Besides. I am just going to an interview." "Just let him drive you," K.J. said calmly and earnestly. Seeing the sincerity in his father's eyes, Lloyd eventually acquiesced. In fact, K.J. had got it right this time. Upon arriving at the interview location, Mr. Richards walked in with Lloyd and loudly pronounced, "Mr. Lee, I will be waiting for you outside. Call my name if you need anything," and retreated. This was precisely what K.J. wanted— the tall and muscular Mr. Richards would act as Lloyd's 'bodyguard' so that the restaurant owner wouldn't dare to do any harm to his son. Mr. Richards was not the best driver, but he made a perfect bodyguard. K.J. was able to appreciate him for who he was and work around his weaknesses to make full use of his strengths. Lloyd did not accept the offer from the eccentric restaurant owner and moved on in his career. He is now the managing partner of a substantial real estate enterprise in London, UK, developing hotels, restaurants, sports arenas, theaters, offices and residences.

Even in his professional life, K.J. has collaborated with people with unconventional talents and equally unconventional personalities. Imagine a person who, when given four things to do, couldn't help himself but forget three of them and at times all four. A person who, during an intense meeting, opens three bottles of water and leaves all three bottles half empty at the end of the meeting. A person who, when he dines out at a restaurant, leaves the waiter and waitress to clean up not only the table, but also the floor. A person who forgets to turn off the light when he leaves the bathroom. Perhaps an aging, forgetful grandpa? One would never guess that this member of K.J.'s team graduated from MIT and is a genius at software engineering. Like his other habits, his intelligence comes in patches, which others have to help him piece together. He is fondly known by K.J. and his team as the absentminded 'Professor Einstein'.

Working with this man is usually too big a risk for any company to take, but K.J. is different. When he forgets the three things out of four, K.J. routinely sends him reminders. When he opens three bottles of water consecutively and does not finish drinking any of them, K.J. quietly picks up the water bottles and labels them for him. When he displays his messy table manners again at a restaurant or in a meeting room, K.J. gives apologetic glances to the waiters and waitresses and if possible, cleans up after he leaves. When he walks out of a restroom unaware of his surroundings, K.J. turns off the lights for him. K.J. never dreams of disrupting the mind of this genius engineer or improving his lack of orderliness, but rather helps him facilitate small things in life, so that he can focus his intelligence on the work he is best at. To his surprise, not only does Mr. Genius get his work done under K.J.'s brotherly guidance, his self-awareness increases drastically. One day towards the end of their collaboration, unlike his usual, whimsical self, Mr. Genius confesses to K.J., "You are the bird that sits on my shoulder. You are the best business partner and friend who has helped me overcome my shortcomings." From the outside, one can never change a person's lifestyle or alter his or her plans; but with loving concern and by appreciating the good in a person, we can turn them around for the better. It is this kind of genuine transformation that K.J.'s kindness helps to fuel.

K.J. has also tried to help another colleague, Mr. Carlson, in many ways. When the latter volunteered to help K.J. move to a new house, K.J. didn't assign him any difficult tasks. He only had to dump paper boxes and garbage. Weeks after the seemingly successful move, K.J. was looking for the brand-new garbage pail they had bought a few weeks before the move. When he called Mr. Carlson to inquire about its whereabouts, the latter replied, "I am sorry, Dr. Lee. When you told me to dump the garbage, I thought you wanted me to throw away the garbage pail as well, so that was what I did."

Always see the positive in people, just as you would make lemonade out of lemons.

Chapter 22

UNTANGLING THE HEALTHCARE WEB

Clementine Xinyi Li

"Don't attribute to incompetency that which can be attributed to conspiracy.

Don't attribute to conspiracy that which can be attributed to incompetency."

A modern-day renaissance man, K.J. wears many different hats. A surgeon's cap, when he performs otolaryngological surgery on his patients; a scholar's cap, as a student and then a university professor. Other hats are less literal, but far weightier: the hat of a son, husband, father; the many roles in his life that he has taken on and grown into, either by choice or by fate.

In balancing two of his most important hats, those of a doctor and an entrepreneur, K.J. developed two slogans that he shared during a lecture on healthcare, a hybrid industry where medicine and business intersect: "There are two ways of looking at it. First, 'I practice medicine, and I have to run a business.' Second, 'I run a business through the practice of medicine.' Do you know which one is correct?"

In his view, only the first is. Business and medicine may take on equal, parallel importance, but K.J. would never wear a businessman's hat without putting on a doctor's hat first. As he welcomes a patient into his office, what distinguishes his approach is not only phenomenal accuracy in diagnosis and treatment, but a personal touch, an aura of warmth and sincerity that comes from the knowledge that suffering patients waiting eagerly for attention and compassion should not be handled like a commodity. Though it is an industry, healthcare cannot be equated with the cold-hearted, impartial business of moneymaking, and K.J. has been an advocate for putting the 'care' into 'healthcare' throughout his medical career.

"A good doctor takes care of the disease, whereas a *great* doctor takes care of the patient. You have to treat patients as if they are you. When you have that in mind, you know how to behave as a medical practitioner." Whichever hat he may be wearing, there is a core quality that K.J. upholds constantly in medicine, in business, and in life— looking out for the interest of the other party. That value encompasses the one man under the innumerable hats.

That is exactly why his interest in his patients expands beyond the field of otolaryngology, to encompass the entire healthcare experience, and the system that provides it. Over the years, K.J. has worked with both the Clintons and Obama in multiple attempts to untangle the mess that is the American healthcare system. He was also interviewed by President George W. Bush's administration to head Medicare during the period when Medicare Part D was being considered. Ideologically, he is neither a strict Democrat nor a Republican. He believes there are good elements and people in each party. Of course, each party also has its negative aspects.

Back in 1993, when Hillary Clinton was the First Lady, she was appointed by her husband to solve the healthcare problem. This move sparked a great wave of censure and backlash, as the public protested against the appointment of Hillary as a non-elected official to take on such a momentous task. Amidst such an environment of controversy and uncertainty, K.J. and Hillary's first collaboration took place, more than two decades ago.

"I was introduced to Hillary, and we tried to come up with a solution in the form of a health savings account," K.J. recounted. Working on the proposal during his stay in Singapore, K.J. vividly remembers the day it was completed. All members of the delegation to Singapore signed it, and there was a sense of conclusion, achievement, and relief. K.J. personally examined and packaged the weighty proposal, carrying the wisdom and effort of some of the greatest minds in healthcare, and FedExed it to the United States, into the hands of Hillary Clinton, with high hopes of all the good this document could do for countless Americans.

However, Hillary turned it down. K.J. recounted her words, "She told me, 'K.J., this would work well only in Singapore. Singapore is composed of a homogenous group of people. They think alike, they esteem work ethics, and they share the habit of saving. It is not easy to have health savings accounts in the U.S."

Indeed, America has a population of over 300 million, almost 60 times that of Singapore's five million. Besides which, the American population was far from homogenous. The scalability and feasibility of the plan were placed under scrutiny, and subsequently rejected. Thus, K.J.'s first plan did not come to fruition. However, the health savings account idea has actually become quite popular in 2019.

Hillary and K.J.'s second encounter took place in 2008 during her first attempt at re-entering the White House, this time not as First Lady, but as Commander in Chief in her own right. During this collaboration, a fundamental problem as old as human society itself surfaced at the root of the healthcare fiasco: the clash between political needs— the need to make big profits and the greater good. K.J. explains, "Bill is the one who first proposed that 32% of each healthcare dollar is wasted, and the problem is not with insufficient funding but *wasted* funding."

The healthcare industry is a mammoth, complicated spider web of bureaucracy and paperwork benefitting stakeholders rather than patients. For each dollar spent, a good amount is squandered in the process of navigating that web, getting caught in its twists and turns, before reaching the spider crouching at the center. It is a political, institutional problem of budget allocation and system organization that can only be solved— if it is even possible— with the aid of political means. "What we need is to actually *reduce* healthcare spending, but no politician would do that because it's political suicide!" It was a simple enough problem but greatly complicated by politics and money, becoming virtually impossible to solve. Unbent as an arrow and unwilling to lose sight of the real goal, K.J.'s refusal to succumb to political forces repeatedly hindered his attempts to fix the system.

The interview by the Bush administration for the Administrator of Medicare position went smoothly, until the very last question, "Can you unequivocally support Medicare part D?" K.J. hesitated for a moment: he completely agreed with the plan that senior citizens should receive help to pay for costly medication, but he could not decipher the fact that Medicare would be prohibited from bargaining with the private pharmaceutical sector, as they would very likely hike pharmaceutical prices higher. Rather than indulging in the subtleties of politics and side-stepping the question in some manner, K.J. tried to brainstorm the pluses and minuses of Medicare Part D. Instead of being an interviewee trying to get the job, he only thought of getting his point across, and advising the White House on what he believed was right. The outcome was obvious; he did not get the job!

This was not the end of K.J.s involvement in politics. After his experiences in the White House, in Connecticut he was appointed by the Speaker of the House as a consultant on the state's healthcare policies. However, no one would listen to a man proposing to actually *cut* healthcare costs by reducing waste. Indeed, the politicians had something to gain from increased spending, whether it be securing their own political agenda through healthcare advocacy, or simply having the numbers look good on paper— an unfortunate illustration of how quantity works against quality.

Having learned this lesson, K.J. redirected his efforts to find another path. During the latter part of the 2008 presidential campaign and during Obama's presidency, K.J. made his third significant attempt at tackling the healthcare problem this time with a new idea.

"Electronic Health Records (EHR) was the idea I gave to Obama." K.J. said, terming the digitization of patient medical records as "the silver bullet to initiate healthcare reform." Digitizing all health records would not only reduce paperwork and minimize bureaucracy, it would also provide an overall smoother, more convenient experience for patients. If EHRs could be commercialized in an economical way that was user friendly and uniform throughout the healthcare industry, it would not only be a catalyst for positive change, but a huge leap towards a final answer to the healthcare problem.

However, it was another great idea badly executed. After billions of dollars' worth of funding from the federal government, EHR has actually created more problems for healthcare providers and consumers alike. To illustrate where we currently are with EHR technology, K.J. used an analogy of a decade-old faulty car. Every time you want to drive the car, it requires two hours of cleaning, fixing, and polishing, before you can drive it for a mere 10 minutes. The amount of resources, time, and energy devoted to EHR development and implementation is not yielding much benefit, at least not yet. In fact, it increases cost and reduces efficiency, causing stress to healthcare providers and patients alike. Worst of all, it is unreliable, introducing errors and inaccurate information into the system.

"We're trying to fix that car, find out how to eliminate the errors and inefficiencies, and make it run as good as new." K.J. explained. Such was the mission of his current enterprise, which recently developed a product, an app, going by the very appropriate and graceful name of Simplicity. Simplicity, as its name suggests, would function as a convenient interface used across all devices and EHR systems, eventually *simplifying* the entire healthcare experience.

K.J. continues to develop his vision for American healthcare. During the turmoil of the 2017 congressional attempt to repeal and replace Obamacare, he proposed a clear, concise, tangible nine-point strategy to reduce the current healthcare cost of 3.7 trillion dollars by 28% in the foreseeable future:

1) Streamline billing and claim processing.
2) Eliminate unnecessary 'facility fees'.
3) Utilize practice guidelines to reduce unnecessary, non-cosmetic, elective surgeries, as well as unnecessary procedures and tests.
4) Apply the 'favorite nation clause' to control pharmaceutical costs.
5) Deploy specialized mid-level providers.
6) Deploy appropriate usage of tele-medicine.

7) Doctors volunteering to care for the indigent, as was the case prior to the 1970s when doctors served the military, US Public Health Service or in hospital/medical school clinics.
8) Permit those under 65 years old to buy coverage from Medicare.
9) Deploy 2019 information technologies.

Based on his decades of experience as a doctor, K.J.'s plan comes from within the healthcare system and is in tune with medical workers' first-hand experiences to provide a comprehensive way of cutting costs while improving access and quality. It may seem like an oxymoron, but it is in fact very possible. K.J. firmly believes that until spiraling healthcare costs are appropriately reduced, all healthcare reforms will fail. He often exclaims, "Just imagine if a glass of milk cost $500, what kind of a situation would we end up in!"

Thus, at an age when most men seek retirement and a restful way of life, K.J. is working relentlessly to achieve a better healthcare delivery system for all. From the health savings account to his efforts to positively influence healthcare reform under President Obama; from EHRs and the advent of Simplicity, to the current nine-point proposal to reduce healthcare cost by 28%; after countless attempts and countless disappointments, K.J. seems to confirm Winston Churchill's definition of success, "Going from failure to failure without loss of enthusiasm."

Each person's reaction to perceived failure is a reflective and defining moment. Despite repeated failures and disappointments, K.J.'s response is to persist, choosing to let these experiences light his way and inform his future decisions, as he walks the arduous path towards the eventual fulfillment of a greater purpose.

"I'll make a plan, write it, edit it, submit it. Have it rejected or have it accepted partially without recognition. Write another one." To K.J., knowing and experiencing failure is part of an unavoidable human journey, but what is avoidable is accepting failure as final. Time after time, he moves on, learning lessons from defeat and re-orienting future endeavors so they have a better chance at success. From his failures he builds lighthouses.

Chapter 23

THE PATIENT IS U FOUNDATION, INC.

Sally Hyun Jung Jee

"Each of us has a unique part to play in the healing of the world."
– Marianne Williamson

Born into a devoutly Christian family, K.J. grew up with a faith that grounded him throughout his adult life. He took such Bible verses as Galatians 5:13 to heart, and the impulse to "serve [others] humbly in love" guided not only his personal life, but also his professional life. As a doctor, he was known to be exceptionally attentive, always putting his patients' needs above his own. K.J. worked to impart to a larger community the spirit behind his service.

K.J. established a lectureship at Harvard, Yale, and Columbia University College of Physicians and Surgeons. He called it the CT Lee Lectureship after his father. The program sponsored a dinner and a lecture once a year about the healing power of a Supreme Being. This Supreme Being is not necessarily Jesus; it refers to the equivalent entity in any religion. Knowing that his own faith reinforced his beliefs as a doctor, K.J. wanted to give future generations of healthcare providers an opportunity to explore their spirituality.

A few years ago, the dean of Columbia University College of Physicians and Surgeons asked K.J. if the school could repurpose the fellowship money to fund student scholarships. K.J. allowed the dean to do so, and his donations are now part of an effort to help Columbia's brightest medical students afford their tuition. At Harvard and Yale Medical Schools, however, the CT Lee Lectureship continues, in its original form, to this day.

From his days as an intern to his days as a professor at Yale Medical School, K.J. practiced medicine with compassion and respect for his patients. In the workplace, as well as in his many lectureships, he urged his colleagues to do the same. In fact, K.J.'s philosophy regarding patient care is to treat his patients as he would like to be treated. Three years ago, K.J. consolidated this philosophy into the not-for-profit The Patient Is U Foundation (TPIU), which he co-founded with a Chinese businessman and philanthropist[15].

TPIU works to ensure that all healthcare givers are compassionate and helpful to the sick— patients and potential patients. But how do we measure compassion? Compassion, like beauty, is in the eyes of the beholder. So, a crucial question to ask caregivers is, "How would you like to be treated if you were the patient?" This question reflects the central mission and motto of TPIU: "treat every step of the medical process— appointment making, parking, locating the doctor's office, registration, encounter with the doctor, receiving testing, treatment etc.— as if you are the patient."

For K.J., the medical process does not start at the hospital but at the patient's home, where the patient tries to make an appointment with the doctor over the phone. Often, when a patient calls the doctor's office, the call goes straight to voicemail. *If you are in a medical emergency, hang up and dial 911,* the voicemail instructs the caller. Then it goes into a complicated 'decision tree' for the patient to decipher— particularly challenging for an already anxious or elderly patient.

There are two definitions of an emergency. Most physicians, when talking about an emergency, refer to a life or death situation. But if you believe in TPIU, the emergency is whatever the patient considers an

---

[15] "The Patient is U Foundation" brochure. See page 200. Available at: http://kjlee.world/biography/uploads/TPIU.pdf.

emergency. A painful blocked ear after a flight can cause great discomfort including dizziness. To an otolaryngologist, it is not an uncommon situation. To the suffering patient, it can be very uncomfortable and frightening— not an emergency, but an urgent matter.

K.J. believes that a doctor's phone system has to be user-friendly. Instead of a voicemail, a "live human being who is smart, compassionate, and caring" should answer the call and make an appointment for the patient as soon as possible, respecting the patient's definition of urgency.

The next step in the process is for the patient to drive to the hospital or doctor's office and find a parking space. Clear instructions with photos should be sent to patients ahead of time. To streamline this experience, it is crucial to educate parking attendants as well. They should be polite and mindful of the fact that for most people, visiting a hospital causes much anxiety. They must, therefore, try to make the parking process as convenient and stress-free as possible, guiding patients to the areas closest to where they are seeing the doctor.

The next step is, of course, locating the doctor's office. With a small doctor's office this is usually easy, but finding a specialist's office in a large health system can be very stressful for a sick patient. Upon entering the huge building, a user-friendly, large print paper map should be handed to the patient with highlighter markings directing them to the correct office, just as a concierge at a hotel's front desk would do for hotel guests looking for a restaurant or sightseeing spot. Upon the patient's arrival, the secretary should be warm and inviting, and the patient should never have to wait an hour or more to see the doctor. Sometimes, when the patient finally enters the examining room, the doctor isn't there, and the patient has to wait even longer to be treated.

"If you'd made a reservation at a restaurant but had to wait for an hour to be seated, you'd walk right out. But in hospitals, the long waiting time is almost a culture," K.J. says. It is a dilemma; if the doctor is to accommodate 'emergencies', the schedule is overbooked and waiting on the day of the appointment could be inevitable. Sometimes it is not the actual waiting but the attitude of the staff and doctor that counts. A genuine apology showing concern, especially from the doctor, goes a long way.

Minimizing the patients' waiting time is not the only task at hand. Sometimes doctors neglect to follow up on medical test results, making patients anxious. Imagine that you just had a biopsy. A good doctor, of course, would notify you and send you a copy of the report, as well as keeping your report on file. However, some doctors think they "don't have the time" to notify each patient, and therefore say, "If you don't hear from me, it means the biopsy is normal."

"The report could have diagnosed cancer and been filed away without the doctor's knowledge. The specimen could be misplaced. There are other possible mishaps. Patients deserve for the doctor to call back, regardless of the result," K.J. says.

It is especially important for surgeons to reach out to their patients. Before a patient elects to have surgery, the doctor should explain to the patient and relatives (since the patient is likely to be emotionally distressed and might forget the information) the specifics of the surgical process, including the benefits, the risks, potential complications, and the ways in which these complications can be resolved. Alternative treatments should be covered in equal detail. Instead of using medical jargon that lay people have trouble understanding, the doctor should use simple, everyday vocabulary and draw diagrams if necessary. In the U.K. in June 2018, a useful acronym was coined which all doctors should practice: BRAN— Benefits, Risks, Alternatives, do Nothing may be the best choice.

Once the patient opts for surgery, the responsible surgeon, not an intern or resident, should meet with the patient just before the operation. In this meeting, the surgeon must confirm the site and the side of the body that will be operated on to prevent the disastrous, yet not entirely uncommon, mistake of operating on the wrong side or the wrong anatomical part. In the U.S.A, this practice is known as 'time out'.

However, all protocols, including 'time out', may fail if the responsible doctor is not present. The only protocol that doesn't fail is the doctor who will be performing the operation talking to the patient before being sedated, preferably in the presence of the nurse, anesthetist and family member.

During the 'time out' checks, K.J. recommends his colleagues use the words "correct side" rather than "right side" to avoid potential confusion.

For instance, if a surgeon is operating on the left ear of the patient, the surgeon should lightly touch this ear and ask, "Is this the correct ear to be operated on?" If the surgeon asks, "Is this the right ear?" the patient may construe the phrase "right ear" in two ways: the correct ear or the right— as opposed to the left— ear. "Correct ear," however, has only one possible interpretation.

After the surgery, the surgeon who operated on the patient or a knowledgeable, caring delegate should come out to the family and brief them on the patient's condition. When the patient has recovered from anesthesia, the responsible surgeon should discuss the surgery and its outcome with the patient. Who else could possibly know the patient's condition better than the surgeon? And when each patient has been discharged, the responsible healthcare provider or a knowledgeable, caring delegate should call the patient and ask if they have any questions. "Doctors whom I have operated on expected me to do this. Why should laymen deserve any less?" K.J. asks.

All this seems like common sense, but common sense is sometimes not so common. To K.J., being a doctor is never 'just a job'. It is a calling, a duty, and a way to serve others.

TPIU clearly strikes a chord with all those involved in healthcare, and its message continues to reach a growing audience. On October 15th, 2019 the foundation held its first Awards Gala Dinner, recognizing the achievements of physicians and healthcare administrators who embody the values of TPIU. The event was a huge success, with over 350 attendees from the healthcare profession, as well as patients, the president of a major university, dean of a prestigious medical school, the Attorney General of Connecticut, and other government officials; all showing their support for the organization. K.J. himself took to the lectern, quoting Hippocrates' teaching from 500 BC to "Cure sometimes, treat often, comfort always," and updating this for the 21st century to, "Cure as much as you can; go the extra mile; try harder, as if you are the patient. TPIU – treat often; comfort always."

The Patient Is U Foundation

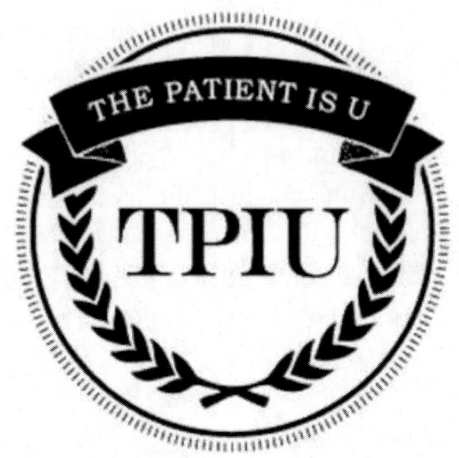

Mission Statement: To take care of patients as if you or your loved one is the patient.

To enhance humanism and offer solutions for the caregivers.

Objective: To encourage human communication in healthcare in this internet era

Action Items:

(1) To impart, empower and promote to all those who come into contact with the sick the importance of blending humanism with great outcome at a sensible cost. Knowledge to treat, heart to care.

(2) To educate the sick and their families to become better equipped to interact with the caregivers and navigate the complex system.

(3) To empower caregivers with tools to reduce the stress of practicing in the early twenty-first century – be the "wings of caregivers" to uplift them.

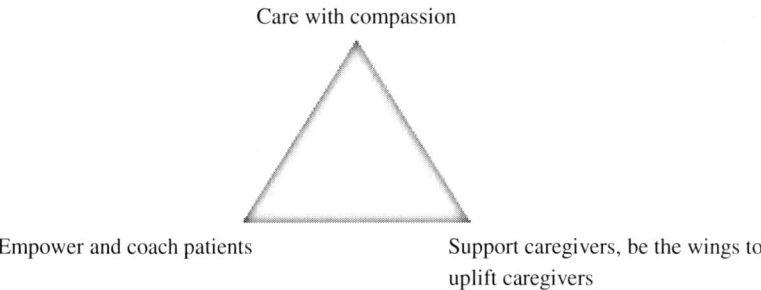

TPIU™ FOUNDATION

Providing excellent scientific medical care and achieving superb outcome are expected by every patient,

Humanistic, Compassionate Patient Care with unsurpassed "customer service" is paramount in any healthcare environment. We emphasize check and double check and the use of checklists.

TPIU Foundation's goals are to:

(1) Empower and share its philosophies to institutional healthcare providers such as hospitals, surgery centers, nursing homes as well as non-institutional providers such as doctors, nurses, medical secretaries and anyone who comes into contact with patients and their families. We will sponsor seminars, tutorials as well as mentorships. The process of caring for a patient starts with the initial phone call or visit to the web site. Phone calls to be answered promptly by a human and appointments given in a timely manner with easy, early access. The rest of the care to be equally accessible and rendered according to the principles of TPIU.

(2) Educate patients and potential patients on how to navigate a very complex healthcare system.

(3) Be the wings of caregivers to support them, to increase their morale. In this complex era when patients are asked to rate the practice and the physician, it behooves the Attending physician to communicate clearly about the care as well as introduce the team of caregivers including but not

limited to nurse practitioners, physician assistants, nurses, fellows, residents and medical students.

PART I. SAMPLES OF TOOLS FOR CAREGIVERS

Welcome, Getting to Know You

1) The first contact between a patient and the healthcare provider is when the patient calls for an appointment. The phone should be answered by a human being within three to five rings. If voicemail is absolutely necessary the voicemail should be easy to navigate to receive an appointment efficiently and assist the caller to reach the doctor when necessary. Doctors are advised to call into their patient phone lines periodically to experience what the patients' experience. Calling your "private" line will not get you the "patient experience."
2) Elective appointments to be given within ten working days unless the patient's schedule necessitates a later appointment. Urgent appointments to be given within 48 hours. Emergency appointments within the same day.
3) The registration and wait times in the general waiting area to be under 15 minutes.

Caring for You

1) The Attending doctor and his/her team of nurse practitioners, physician assistants, residents, fellows and medical students are familiar with the patient's available medical history and condition *before* meeting the patient, and maintains attentive eye contact while the patient is presenting his/her symptoms and past medical history, medications, previous tests etc.
2) The Attending doctor examines the patient personally in addition to that performed by the team.

3) Besides the team, the Attending doctor reviews tests, imaging results and other clinical data and discuss them and the physical findings directly and thoroughly with the patient/family as well as advises the next steps.
4) The Attending doctors and the team answer all the patient's questions and consider their wishes.
5) The scheduling of future tests or treatment is to be accomplished as efficiently as possible.
6) The Attending doctor reviews these new test results as soon as possible and discusses them with the patient/family. If the results are not ready when expected, the Attending doctor or his/her knowledgeable delegate is to call the patient to explain the delay and give an as accurate as possible, an estimate as to when the results will be ready.
7) The Attending doctor discusses treatment options (giving the pros and cons of each option as well as the risks for each option) and the post-operative care and expectations including but not limited to pain management. Following the UK acronym: BRAN – B=benefits, R=risks, A=alternatives, N=do nothing.

Treating You

1) On the day of surgery/treatment, the Attending doctor (NOT a delegate) meets with the patient (before induction of anesthesia if anesthesia is needed) to triple check and confirm the type of surgery/treatment, site and side of the surgery/treatment to be performed.
2) As soon as surgery/treatment is finished, the Attending doctor or a delegate who is fully knowledgeable about the patient and the details of the care as well as the specialty meets with the family to go over the surgery/treatment. As soon as the patient is awake, the Attending doctor repeats this process with the patient directly as well as covering the postoperative care.

3) The Attending doctor and/or the team makes rounds on the patient daily in a non-rushed fashion, answering all questions from the patient or family members. If he/she has to be out of town, a specific doctor can be delegated to care for the patient but he/she will have to be completely familiar with the patient's case and this doctor's credentials have to be commensurate with those of the original Attending doctor.

After You Leave

1) The evening of the discharge, the Attending doctor or a delegate who is knowledgeable about the patient's care and that specialty speaks to the patient or family member by phone to see how things are and to answer any further questions. The responsible caregiver or a fully knowledgeable delegate to call again in another 48 to 72 hours.

Always

1) Phone calls to be returned efficiently and promptly within hours, definitely within the same day.
2) A knowledgeable physician extender or delegate should be conversant in that specialty of medicine as well as familiar with that patient's condition.
3) In most instances, any bad news is to be delivered by the Attending doctor. A physician delegate knowledgeable in that specialty and the patient's care can deliver the good news or routine results.
4) "A good doctor takes care of the disease; a great doctor takes care of the patient."

Part II. 10 Suggested Questions for the Patient to Ask

Please be sure you ask all your questions to make certain that you understand what disease you have and what the treatment will be. The following sample of questions is to help you to get started. Make a list of questions ahead of time and bring the list to the appointment. You may have other questions you and your family need to ask. Please do not be shy about asking them and getting the answers. It may be necessary for you to ask the same question more than once to make sure you get and understand the complete answer.

1) What caused my problem?
2) Please list the reason for the treatment you are proposing. The pros and cons of this treatment and all the possible side effects or complications that may happen.
3) If there are any alternative ways to treat me, please describe them as well as their pros and cons, including "no treatment."
4) Could you give me an estimate of the length of hospital stay, and recuperation period. The amount of time it takes for the usual patient to recover enough to fly.
5) Please give me enough details on the postoperative care involved in terms that a layman can understand.
6) Please tell me the number of such cases the surgeon has performed, the good and the bad outcome/the results, the side effects and complications if any, the mortality rate if any, the re-admission rate, if any.
7) Could you kindly give me a copy of the curriculum vitae (CV) of the surgeon and/or the responsible physician?
8) Please give me a copy of all my medical reports including doctors' notes and all tests results. If imaging studies were done, please give me the typed written report as well as an electronic copy of the images; for example, a disc or a flash drive or e-mailed them to me.

9) If there are pathology reports, please give me a copy of the typed report.
10) Is there anything else you need or want to tell me and my family?

Ten Commandments of Patient Care

1) A patient is the most important person in any medical practice.
2) A patient is not dependent upon us ... we are dependent on him/her.
3) A patient is not an interruption of our work ... he/she is the purpose of it.
4) A patient does us a favor when he/she calls ... we are not doing him/her a favor by caring for him/her.
5) A patient is part of our business ... not an outsider.
6) A patient is not a cold statistic ... he/she is a flesh-and-blood human being with feelings and emotions like our own.
7) A patient is not someone with whom to argue or match wits.
8) A patient is one who brings us his/her wants ... it is our job to fill those wants to the best of our ability.
9) A patient is deserving of the most courteous and attentive treatment we can give him/her.
10) Caring for patients is the reason for our jobs.

~~~

The Patient Is U Foundation, Inc.

A 501(c)(3) nonprofit organization dedicated to promote

Skills to Treat and the Heart to Care at a Sensible Cost

"Excellent outcome is the main priority for both patients and caregivers"

TPIU encourages all those who come into contact with patients to interact as if they are, in fact, the patient.

Research has demonstrated that compassionate care and great patient experience lead to better outcome.

To enhance patient experience, we believe that patients very much appreciate:

- Being greeted by a user-friendly phone system including a helpful person with whom to speak;
- Not having to wait a long period of time to get an appointment for a visit, test or procedure;
- Receiving clear and understandable directions to the office building as well as directions to the office within the building;
- Having convenient and inexpensive parking with compassionate attendants;
- Having open and available lines of communication between the patient and all the caregivers, including the patient's Attending Doctor;
- All caregivers for any patient communicate with each other;
- Doctors' representatives or staff who are knowledgeable in their specialty and well versed in the patient's case;
- Obtaining test results and the Doctor's interpretation of those results promptly;
- Being informed of the pros and cons of the recommended tests, treatment(s), including the preoperative, operative and postoperative care and possible side effects thereof;
- Being informed of possible alternative tests or treatments and an explanation of the pros and cons of those tests and treatments;
- Making electronic health record user friendly and eliminate unnecessary government or insurance mandates so that the doctors can once again focus on patients.

It is helpful for the patients to prepare a written summary of their ailment and a list of questions before seeing the doctor.

TPIU will also outline steps to eliminate stress among caregivers in this day and age of a fast paced medical industry.

www.TPIU.org

Chapter 24

POSTSCRIPT

"I've learned that people will forget what you said, people will forget what you did, but people will never forget how you made them feel."
— Maya Angelou

In his twilight years, looking back at his life, K.J. feels privileged to have listened to his papa, becoming a doctor instead of a nuclear physicist, possibly developing new bombs. (His papa mentioned that an eminent nuclear physicist might get kidnapped or assassinated.) His clinical practice has helped thousands of patients in the United States and abroad. His books and lectures have educated otolaryngology-head and neck surgeons for five decades around the world.

In the last decade he has also been keenly aware of the caregiver's own well-being. The government and the business industry continue to impose more rules and regulations upon the practice of medicine. Many of these could have been implemented differently and in a less punitive manner. The current climate in healthcare has caused unnecessary stress among providers, to the point of causing many to retire early or switch careers. At this stage of his career K.J. has been called upon to give seminars on increasing physician morale and decreasing stress. K.J. firmly believes that the practice of medicine is a noble profession and a great career, and always will be. Even those who complain vociferously about the practice of medicine in this day and age are quick to 'brag' to friends and family when their children are admitted to medical school, start residency or become an attending doctor. K.J.'s seminars customarily start with recognizing increasing external 'interfering elements'. He calmly points out those elements that rightfully improve patient care and outcome, and he is quick to point out those elements that impede patient care. He then boosts morale by introducing strategies in workflow 'work around' for the mandates that interfere with patient care[16]. He then analyzes the business aspects of medicine, investment strategies and estate planning for the family. His PowerPoints include 'kumbaya philosophical' moments. He closes his seminars by teaching the participants techniques in negotiation. To him, negotiation is far from being confrontational.

At the time of writing, healthcare spending has reached over $3.3 trillion per annum in the US, which is 17.9% of GDP, equivalent to $10,348 per person per year[17]. In 2000, the healthcare premium for a single person was $2,500 and for a family was $6,400. In 2017, it was $6,700 for a single person and $18,800 for a family. K.J.'s analysis concluded that 20 to 28% of this can be saved without compromising care, but by eliminating waste and inefficiencies.

His healthcare policy emphasizes efficiency, outcome, quality of patient service and affordability. He specializes in using technology-based solutions to help hospitals and practitioners improve operational efficiency, reduce administration costs, and increase patients' access to quality healthcare services. He emphasizes that technology has to be simple, accurate, user-centric and reliable. He teaches that in spite of all the advances in technology, nothing beats the human touch. He has been recognized for his vision that practical clinical guidelines and the correct digitization of medical records are the backbone of successful healthcare reform. He has been awarded three Academy Presidential Citations by three Academy

---

[16] K.J. Lee, C. Lee, "Reduce Stress and Increase Morale In Your Practice." American Academy of Otolaryngology-Head & Neck Surgery/Foundation, Atlanta, Georgia, October 8, 2018. [PowerPoint presentation]. Available at: http://kjlee.world/biography/uploads/presentation-5bad363d6e3f5.pdf.

[17] National Center for Health Statistics. "Health Expenditures." Available at: https://www.cdc.gov/nchs/fastats/health-expenditures.htm.

presidents. The most recent 2017 citation was for his energetic diplomacy in the worldwide medical community and his expansive forward-thinking approach to finding solutions for problems. At the time of publication, K.J. estimates that about 28% of tests, procedures and non-cosmetic elective surgeries are not necessary. Besides raising the cost of healthcare, they cause pain and suffering as well as temporary disability for patients. To that end, he published *Healthcare Reform Through Practical Clinical Guidelines*[18], which was endorsed by Congresswoman Rosa DeLauro[19].

K.J.'s Step-Wise Solutions to Current Healthcare Problems

I. Introduction of a 'Pay For Value' Hybrid System Consisting of Both 'Pay for Outcome' and a Smaller Proportion of 'Pay for Each Service'

What Is the Problem?
- An inherent conflict of interest exists between generating more income through over booking, performing unnecessary tests, procedures, and surgeries on patients instead of using the most cost-effective treatments[20]. Lack of medical knowledge prevents patients from evaluating whether they have been treated with appropriate, cost effective treatment methods.
- Lack of preventive care.
- Lack of coordination of care and over utilization of emergency rooms.

---

[18] K.J. Lee, Y. Chan, "Healthcare Reform Through Practical Clinical Guidelines: Ear, Nose, Throat," Plural Publishing, 2015.
[19] "Healthcare Reform Through Practical Clinical Guidelines: Ear, Nose, Throat," endorsement by Congresswoman Rosa DeLauro. Available at: http://kjlee.world/biography/uploads/reforms-5ba927aebcb90.pdf.
[20] K.J. Lee, Y. Chan, "Healthcare Reform Through Practical Clinical Guidelines: Ear, Nose, Throat," Plural Publishing, 2015.

How Can We Solve It?

- K.J. cofounded The Patient Is U Foundation™ (TPIU), described in Chapter 23, to help laypeople navigate the complex healthcare system. He also published a book to help potential patients understand differential diagnoses and evaluate different treatment options[21].

- Deploy "evidence-based, practical, clinical guidelines for patients" to gradually empower patients to make informed decisions. These guidelines can also be seamlessly and unobtrusively embedded in an app linked to healthcare providers' electronic health records[22]. This will facilitate the clinician's workflow and thus decreases their stress.

- While following practical clinical guidelines could result in cost savings of over 20%, the guidelines would also address the incentive to prevent overutilization as well as underutilization, thus ensuring quality. Assigning part of the 'Pay for Value' compensation to 'Pay for Each Service' is wise[23,24,25]. Offer low cost, high yield, comprehensive preventative, checkups, (see Japanese example of a report showing the elements incorporated into an annual check-up[26]).

---

[21] K.J. Lee, "Differential Diagnosis: Otolaryngology," *Arco Diagnosis Series*, 1978.

[22] Pay for Performance, "P4P." Available at: http://kjlee.world/biography/uploads/reforms-5ba929ec5643e.pdf.

[23] "The Patient is U Foundation" brochure. Available at: http://kjlee.world/biography/uploads/TPIU.pdf.

[24] K.J. Lee, "From the Trenches," *Medical Economics*, November 25, 2013: 8. Available at: http://images2.advanstar.com/PixelMags/medical-economics/pdf/2013-11-25.pdf.

[25] K.J. Lee, "Hybrid Physician Payment System Can Ensure Quality, Customer Service," *ENT Today*, November 5, 2014. Available at: https://www.enttoday.org/article/hybrid-physician-payment-system-can-ensure-quality-customer-service/.

[26] Japanese check-up example. Available at: http://kjlee.world/biography/uploads/reforms-5baa2edf1e182.pdf.

- Invigorate the 'Home Room Doctor' concept, similar to the 'Home Room Teacher/Counsellor' in school[27,28]. This would benefit coordination of care services and decrease overutilization of the emergency room.

II. Streamline the Healthcare Billing Process and Increase Price Transparency

What Is the Problem?
- President Clinton once stated that 'paperwork made up as much as 32% of healthcare expenditure. On both the payers and payees' side, huge numbers of clerical and IT staff are hired just to complete paperwork and input data. The billing and collection process is burdened with inconsistent and conflicting rules and regulations.
- There is little transparency or rationale in listed prices, billed charges, maximum allowable fees, deductibles, and copays[29].
- There is no uniform way to identify a patient. Currently, one uses name, address, telephone number, date of birth, and social security number. There is no practical, efficient interoperability between different electronic health record products.

How Can We Solve It?
- Work with and learn from entities such as Amazon, Berkshire Hathaway and JPMorgan's healthcare company to devise a

---

[27] K.J. Lee, "Healthcare: Affordable quality coverage for all," *Otolaryngology-Head and Neck Surgery*, vol. 140, no. 6 (2009): 775-781. Available at: https://journals.sagepub.com/doi/abs/10.1016/j.otohns.2009.03.001.

[28] K.J. Lee, M. E. Lee, "Universal Healthcare: A Bold Proposal," *Connecticut Medicine*, vol. 64, no. 8 (2000): 485-491. Available at: http://kjlee.world/biography/uploads/article-5b8b08b7a6c12.pdf

[29] F. Schulte, D. Donald, "How doctors and hospitals have collected billions in questionable Medicare fees," *Center for Public Integrity*, September 15, 2012. Available at: https://publicintegrity.org/health/how-doctors-and-hospitals-have-collected-billions-in-questionable-medicare-fees/

streamlined 'billing and collection' process[30,31], which can be embraced by all providers and decrease operational costs for all parties[32,33].

- Amazon has proven that it can deliver goods and services at a low cost, coupled with quality and great customer experience. Solicit know-how of Amazon and similar companies to deliver cost-effective, unsurpassed healthcare outcomes along with superb patient experience.
- Significantly reduce the time spent on data entry and increase the transparency of billing and collection processes.
- Collaborate with provider communities and with the help of data analytics, discover the actual cost of care minus the 'red tape' involved for each service.
- Negotiate with provider communities to discover the most reasonable payment they will accept for each service.
- Identify each patient by a unique 13-digit healthcare number attached to their password-protected, patient-owned electronic health record. This would be entirely separate from the numerous 'patient portals' offered by hospitals and EHR companies ('Easy Patient Record').
- Offer practical user-centric interoperability. This technology is within reach.

---

[30] K.J. Lee, "Healthcare for 2019: A Dozen Steps." See page 219.
[31] K.J. Lee, "K.J. Lee & Associates' Proposal for the Amazon, Berkshire Hathaway and JP Morgan Healthcare Joint Venture, Executive Summary." http://kjlee.world/biography/uploads/article-5d9295672fb6c.pdf.
[32] K.J. Lee, "Super Management Service Organization – MSO." Available at: http://kjlee.world/biography/uploads/reforms-5ba92b1873fcd.
[33] K.J. Lee, "Here's how to reduce healthcare costs," *Medical Economics*, May 09, 2017. Available at: https://www.medicaleconomics.com/medical-economics-blog/heres-how-reduce-healthcare-costs

III. Enable, Expand, and Encourage the Use of Telemedicine

What Is the Problem?
- Time away from work or family, long waiting period for diagnosis and treatment of diseases.
- Current text/email exchanges between providers and patients often create slipshod record keeping and less than accurate or complete information.
- Telemedicine is currently insufficiently refined and appreciated by patients, providers and payers, preventing physicians and patients from taking full advantage of its potential benefits.

How Can We Solve It?
- Deploy telemedicine on a more widespread scale by standardizing appointment scheduling and patient record procedures. Compensate for the costs of telemedicine through the proposed hybrid payment system mentioned previously.
- Full and proper usage of telemedicine would bring significant healthcare cost savings for the patients, as well as making it more widely accepted by patients and providers.

IV. Facilitate the Use of Specialized Mid-Level Practitioners to Increase Access

What Is the Problem?
- Mid-level practitioners (advanced nurse practitioners and physician assistants) are qualified to treat certain patients but are underutilized.
- The predicted shortage of physicians can lead to longer waiting times and higher costs.
- Currently, a substantial amount of physicians' time involves treating basic symptoms that could be equally well cared for by *specialized* mid-level practitioners.

How Can We Solve It?

- Deploying the use of *specialized* mid-level practitioners paired with telemedicine will improve quality, increase access and decrease cost. To be successful, the mid-level practitioners need to receive specialty specific training.

V. Healthcare Technology

- Introduce a user-centric app customized to each practitioner's workflow, as the front interface of the provider's electronic health record (EHR). The metrics of practical clinical guidelines will be included within the app. This will further maintain and improve outcome and access, and reduce cost[34],[35],[36]. Simultaneously, it will solve the almost unanimous dissatisfaction of clinicians with the current EHRs available on the market[37,38,39,40,41,42].
- Enable patients to be more involved in their healthcare decisions. They will have easy 24/7 access and control of their password-protected healthcare records through 'Easy Patient Record'[43].

---

[34] "MACH III." Available at: http://kjlee.world/biography/uploads/reforms-5ba92b67691b9.

[35] K.J. Lee, "What to look for in an EMR," Talk Back, *Medical Economics*, February 5, 2010: 16. Available at: http://kjlee.world/biography/uploads/article-5b8b0768e7f24.pdf

[36] K.J. Lee, "Electronic Medical Records (EMR) – The Train Has Left the Station," *ENT & Audiology News*, vol. 16, no. 3 (2007): 2-3. Available at: http://kjlee.world/biography/uploads/article-5b8b0869d842a.pdf

[37] J. Bush, "Electronic health records 'inflict enormous pain' on doctors. It'll take more than stopwatches to learn why," *STAT*, September 06, 2016. Available at: https://www.statnews.com/2016/09/06/electronic-health-records-improve/

[38] J. K. Cohen, "Study: Physicians dissatisfied with EHRs more often want to leave jobs," *Health IT & CIO Report*, November 03, 2017. Available at: https://www.beckershospitalreview.com/ehrs/study-physicians-dissatisfied-with-ehrs-more-often-want-to-leave-jobs.html

[39] M. Miliard, "Docs 'stressed and unhappy' about EHRs," *Healthcare IT News*, October 09, 2013. Available at: https://www.healthcareitnews.com/news/docs-stressed-unhappy-about-ehrs.

[40] D. Gorn, "These doctors think electronic health records are hurting their relationships with patients," *Future of You*, July 21, 2017. Available at: https://www.pbs.org/newshour/health/doctors-think-electronic-health-records-hurting-relationships-patients.

[41] K. Loria, "Physicians leaving profession over EHRs," *Medical Economics*, January 24, 2018. Available at: https://www.medicaleconomics.com/modern-medicine-feature-articles/physicians-leaving-profession-over-ehrs

[42] HITC Staff, "peer60: Physicians are Extremely Unhappy with All Major HER Vendors," *HIT Consultant*, October 11, 2016. Available at: https://hitconsultant.net/2016/0/11/35967/#.XNk3zfZFyP8.

[43] "Easy Patient Record Version 2." Available at: http://kjlee.world/biography/uploads/reforms-5ba92bb52bdfb.

Unlike today, where patient records are scattered and uncoordinated, 'Easy Patient Record' will aggregate records and streamline the process. 'Easy Patient Record' solves the interoperability and interconnectivity issue.

Is U.S. Healthcare Broken?

K.J.'s vision is that it is not broken. With his fundamental common-sense proposals for clinical and business solutions to eliminate bureaucracy, waste, over- and under-utilization and excessive profits, he believes the U.S. healthcare system can thrive, and indeed act as a beacon for others to emulate.

K.J. believes that through the grace of God and serendipity he has been fortunate to learn from and be encouraged by his family, including his children, friends, colleagues, teachers and even adversaries. As a toddler, he played at business by 'selling rice' in the jungle to his maternal grandmother and two sisters. He values his mother's teaching that "good accounting and arithmetic makes good friends," and her warning that forwarding or lending money to friends and family can ruin relationships. His father taught him to be careful and hardworking. He particularly values his parents teaching him not only to make a daily 'to do list', but also to look at it many times a day and act on it. Checking and double checking can prevent many ills. It is always better to appreciate others and yet not be blind to their deficiencies. His children taught him that 'less is more', along with diplomacy and management of people. Since early childhood he has learned to be persistent but not stubborn. At times it is wise to compromise. At times it is smarter for oneself to change, rather than expect others to change. When coming to an impasse, he learned to think outside the box, be ingenious. Honesty and keeping one's word are important to him. In his life he has witnessed the relief and at times even rewards of not holding grudges. He has cured, treated and comforted thousands of patients and their families. Through his publications he has educated five decades of otolaryngology-head and neck surgeons around the world. Together with Linda, his beloved and capable, loving wife of 53 years, a wise counselor, and a "cannily accurate diagnostician," he has raised three boys— Harvard graduates and decent human beings, all with a great work ethic and a passion for their work. They are married to three beautiful, accomplished, caring women. K.J. and his wife are also enjoying their five grandchildren, who are well brought up by their parents. He hopes his offspring will learn a little bit more about him through reading this book[44,45,46].

He counts himself fortunate to have met serendipitously four talented writers from Columbia University to pen this biography. He also wants it to be known that he is fortunate to have a very able editorial consultant, a very efficient publishing consultant and a very accurate editorial assistant.

To him, this memoir is not about a famous man but an ordinary soul. He is no Nobel Laureate, Einstein, Warren Buffett, Bill Gates, Jeff Bezos or Steve Jobs, although he did his Harvard senior paper under Nobel Laureate George Wald, had lectures with Novel Laureate James Watson and is a personal friend of Nobel Laureate Eric Kandel. He believes that his hybrid provider compensation model[47] though simple is the ultimate formula that will solve healthcare economics. What he has experienced in his life can be shared and achieved by ordinary hard- working young people. He is humbled that you are reading *Leeway*.

HEALTHCARE FOR 2019; A DOZEN STEPS

Healthcare reform is not difficult when we put the patient and the patient's family front and center. In light of our capitalistic economy and our

---

[44] K. Liu, "Dr KJ Lee: From Penang to Presidency of the AAO-HNS... and beyond!" *ENT & Audiology News*, vol. 27, no. 1 (2018): 48-50. Available at: https://www.entandaudiology news.com/features/ent-features/post/dr-kj-lee-from-penang-to-presidency-of-the-aao-hns-and-beyond.

[45] *Connecticut State Medical Society, Action News*, Winter, 2018: 7. Available at: https://csms.org/wp-content/uploads/2018/03/Winter-2018-Action.pdf.

[46] "Abbreviated Curriculum Vitae of K.J. Lee." Available at: http://kjlee.world/biography/uploads/reforms-5ba92c33ef6df.

[47] K.J. Lee, "From the Trenches," *Medical Economics*, November 25, 2013: 8. Available at: http://images2.advanstar.com/PixelMags/medical-economics/pdf/2013-11-25.pdf.

political ideologies, to achieve successful reform we have to address these issues as well. Healthcare reform is about collaborating among all stakeholders, not winning or losing by a stakeholder. It is a joint private-public system offering choices of providers and insurance carriers. We should avoid terms like universal healthcare which can be misconstrued as socialized medicine.

We can start with practical steps to eliminate waste and inefficiencies in the system.

1) From the providers' corner, a significant percentage of tests, procedures and surgeries can be avoided without compromising care. Besides raising costs, redundant care causes harm, pain and suffering and absenteeism from work. Each specialty of medicine has already or will develop practice guidelines to guide providers to practice quality medicine that is cost effective. As a matter of fact, these lessons are taught in medical schools and residencies.

2) Providers' compensation: Change the "pay for volume" system to "pay for value." To start with we can develop a hybrid payment system, pay X% of the compensation based on volume and the Y% of the compensation is based on value.

3) Reorganize the emergency rooms to treat emergencies. To successfully achieve that, two steps need to be done.

   a) To avoid missing a true emergency, the triage medical officer should be the most experienced doctor in the emergency room and not the least experienced doctor, physician assistant or nurses. An experienced doctor can quickly and accurately discern the true emergency cases from those that are not, without having to order a host of unnecessary tests. Unnecessary tests cost money and reduce efficiency. An experienced doctor is less likely to misdiagnose.

   b) Physician groups to organize for their patients to be evaluated and treated outside the costly emergency room setting until an emergency case has been established by the physician on call.

4) Develop and deploy more reliable telemedicine.
5) Develop more "price and outcome" transparency through the application of "blockchain" and MDMI health information technology.
6) Develop more preventive care. Examples can be borrowed from other countries such as Japan.
7) Allow those over 50 to be able to "buy into Medicare" as well as Medicare Advantage or Medicare supplement.
8) Increase compensation to primary care physicians especially those that do "care coordination." This will increase morale among primary care physicians. This will solve the shortage of primary care doctors. In large companies, the Chief Executive Officer (CEO) may not be an expert on all aspects that a Chief Financial Officer (CFO), Chief Technology Officer (CTO), or Chief Operating Officer (COO) may know, but the CEO coordinates and manages all aspects of the company, at times through his executive team. Similarly, the primary care doctor is the CEO of the patient's health, the whole body. The primary care doctor may diagnose and treat the patient with the help of the specialists. As CEO, primary care doctors to have compensation commensurate to a CEO. Looking at it through this lens, let us develop reimbursement policies to better reimburse primary care doctors. For example, the reimbursement for a particular E/M code submitted by a primary care doctor could be 135% of the reimbursement of the same E/M code when submitted by a specialist.
9) Train and deploy more midlevel providers (physician assistants, nurse practitioners) in primary care and in each specialty.
10) Eliminate preexisting disease exclusion.
11) Incorporate elements of the Federal Employee Health Benefit Program for the general population.
12) Since it is so expensive to administer the Medicaid system for the indigent and providers consider the Medicaid reimbursement does not cover their cost, let us take a page from the 1950s to 1960s.

a) Every licensed provider is to donate ½ day a week to care for the indigent at the local hospital or local health clinic.
b) The local hospitals donate the clinic space and the clinic staff. We can also use the school based health clinics for providers to render their care.

K. J. Lee, M.D., F.A.C.S.
Email: kjleemd@aol.com
Phone: 203-645-4758

APPENDIX 1. A SELECTION OF THE LEE FAMILY'S CHRISTMAS CARDS (1966-PRESENT)

Cards designed by Linda Lee

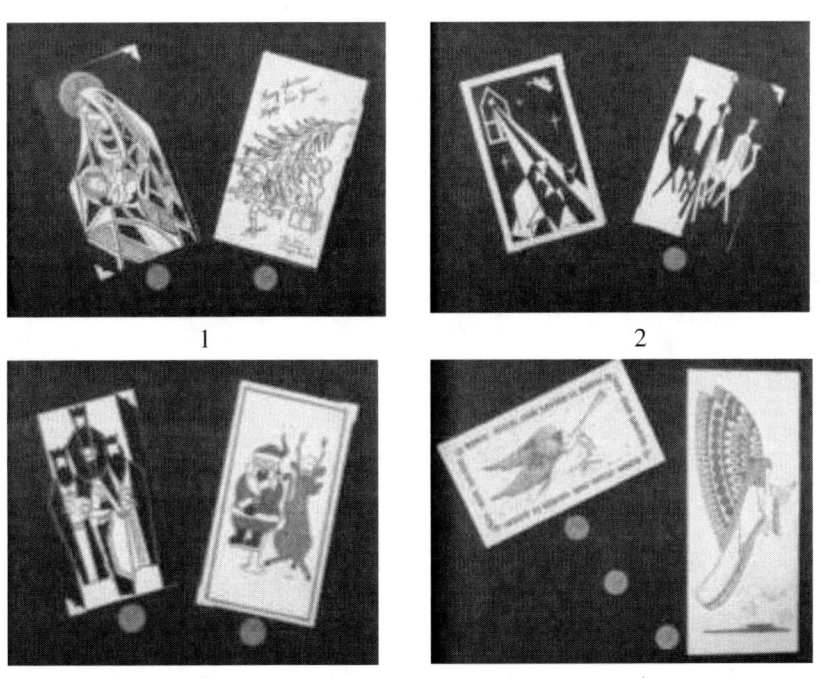

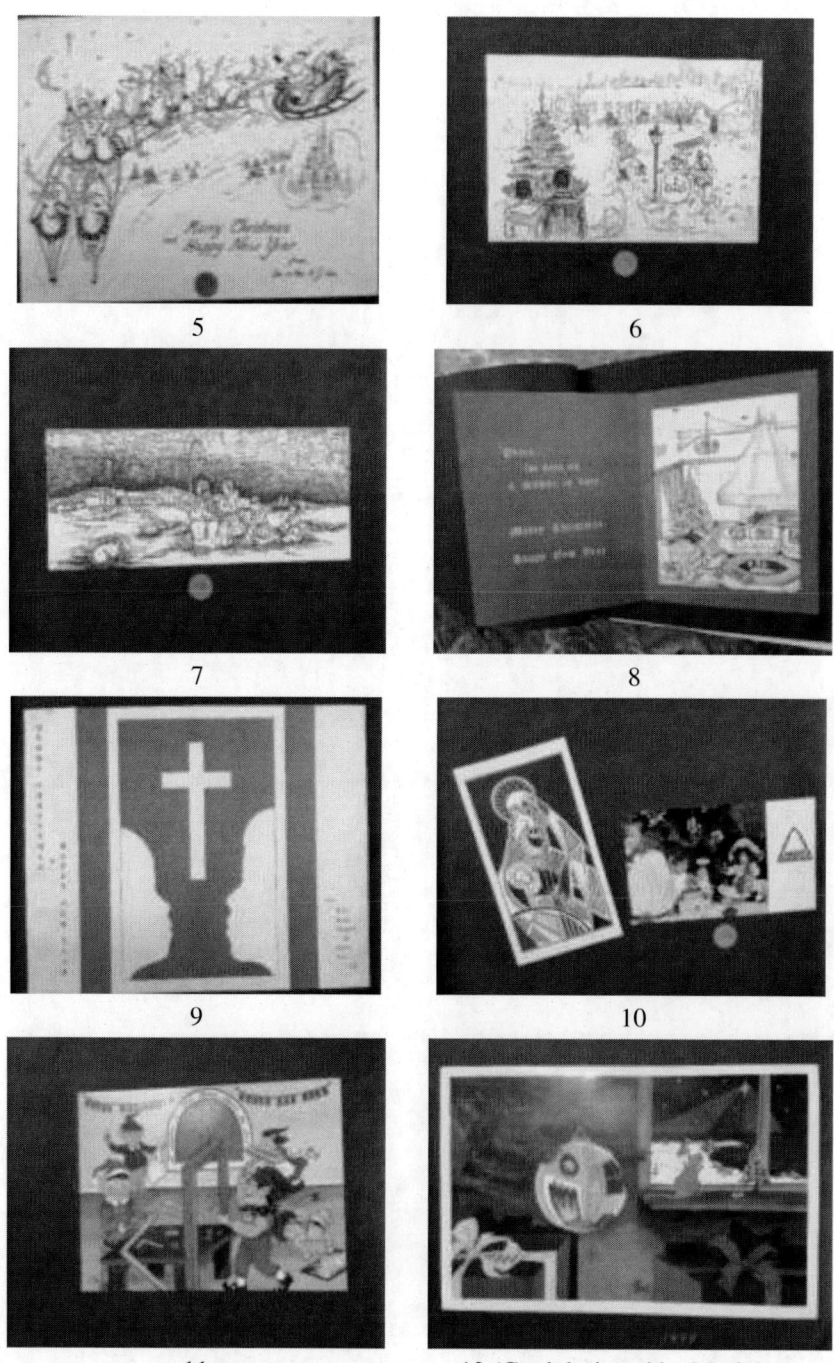

12 (Card designed by Mark Lee)

Appendix 1. A Selection of the Lee Family's Christmas Cards ... 225

FAMILY PHOTO CHRISTMAS CARDS

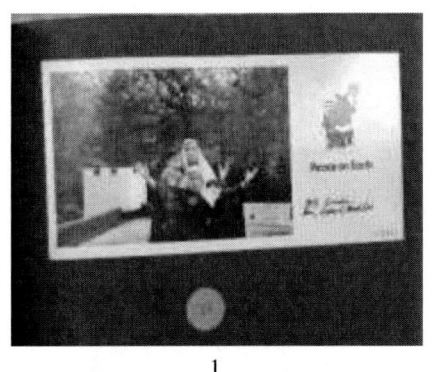

1

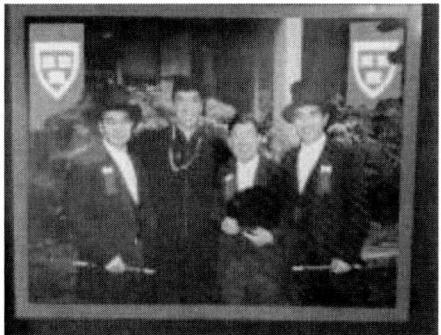

2

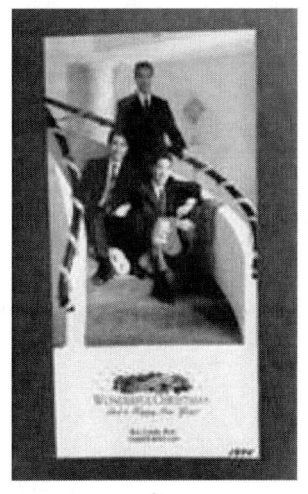

3

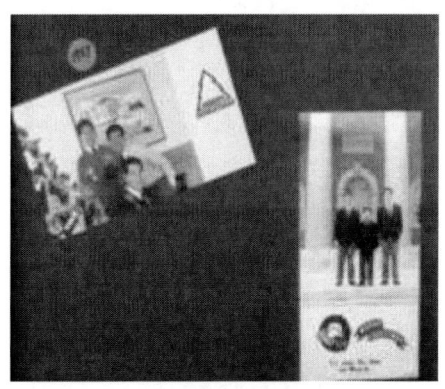

4

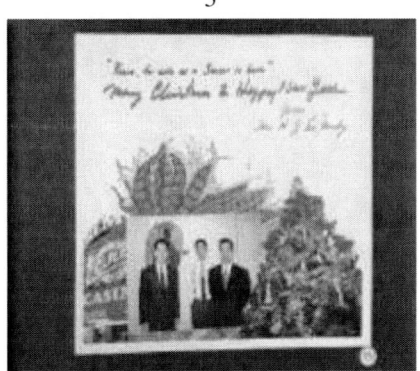

5

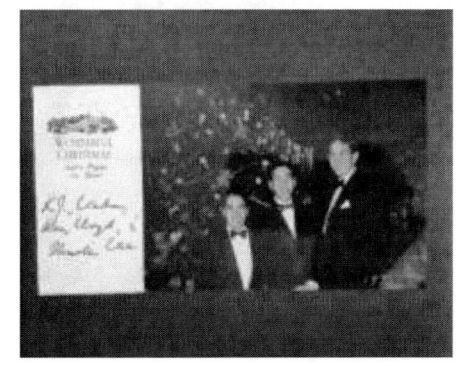

6

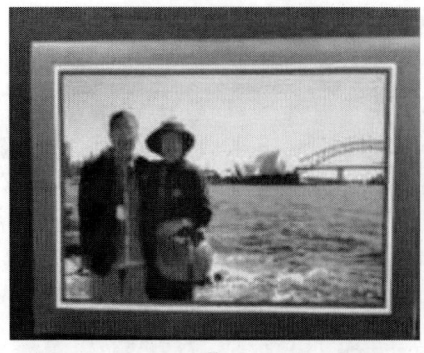

7

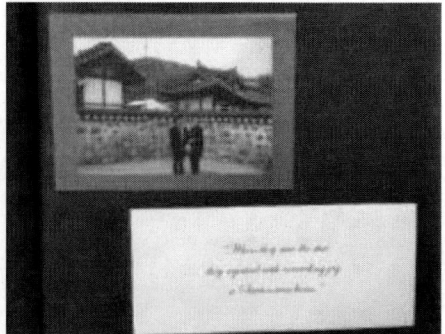

8

9

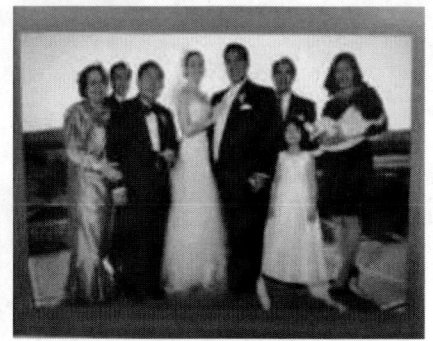

10

11

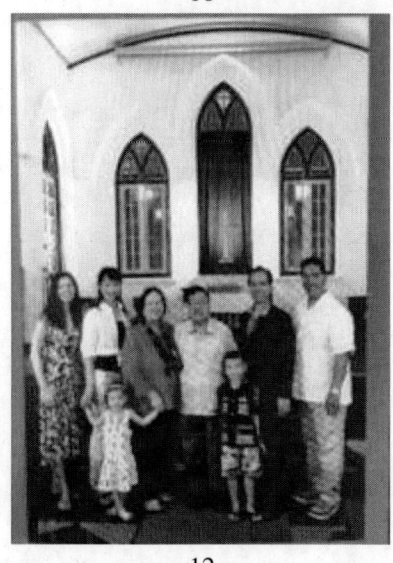

12

Appendix 1. A Selection of the Lee Family's Christmas Cards ...

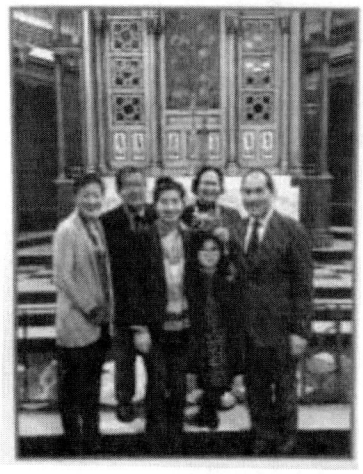

13

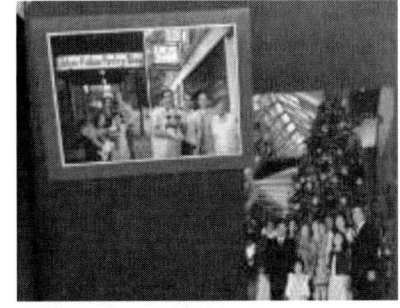

14

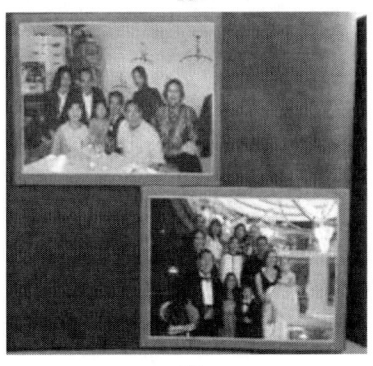

15

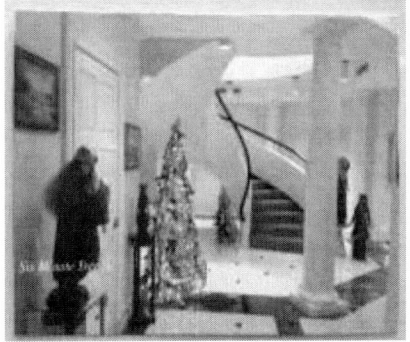

16

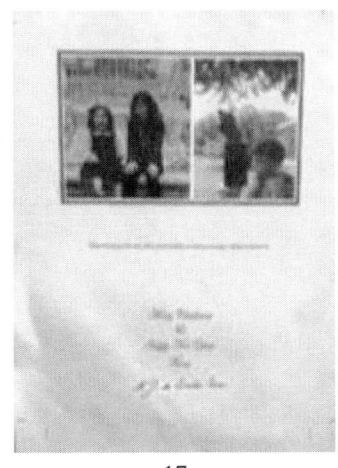

17

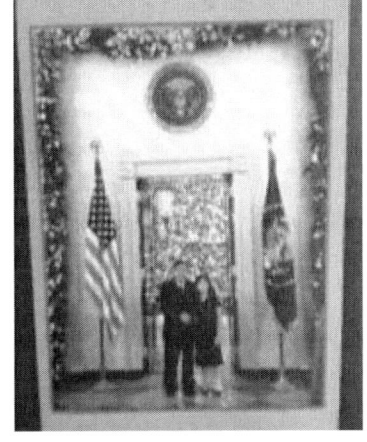

18

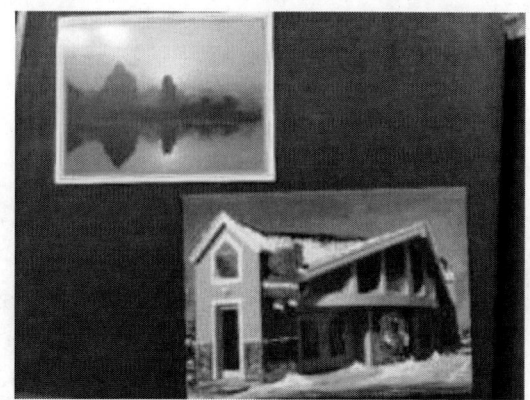

19

APPENDIX 2. ARTICLES BY DOCTOR LEE

RESULTS OF TYMPANOPLASTY AND MASTOIDECTOMY AT THE MASSACHUSETTS EYE AND EAR INFIRMARY.

KEATJIN LEE, M.D.,

and

HAROLD F. SCHUKNECHT, M.D.,

Boston, Mass.

The primary objectives of surgery for chronic suppurative disease of the ear are the elimination or arrest of disease and the preservation or improvement of auditory function. The concept is not new, for even the earliest otologists[1] performed temporal bone surgery with the hope of preserving the sound transmitting mechanism of the middle ear. Before the availability of antibiotic drugs for the control of bacterial infection, it was not always prudent to compromise the removal of diseased tissues for the sake of preserving function. It was observed, however, that good thresholds of hearing sometimes occurred even though the ossicles and tympanic membrane were partly or completely destroyed by disease or surgery. These cases were the result of fortuitous patterns of healing in which the function of the ossicular system or the phase difference at the oval and round windows was preserved. Tympanoplasty tries to achieve these goals without compromising the desired end result of a safe, dry, and asymptomatic ear.

Following the leadership of Wüllstein[2,3,4,5] and Zollner[6,7,8] many otologic surgeons[9,20,11,12,13,14,15,16,17,18] contributed importantly to the development of effective surgical procedures. The early enthusiasm for tympanoplasty diminished somewhat when longer periods of postoperative observation revealed a high incidence of recurring disease and deterioration of the tissues utilized for reconstruction. Among the reasons for failure were: 1. eustachian tube dysfunction; 2. deficient middle ear mucosa; 3. tympanosclerosis; 4. incomplete removal of diseased tissues; 5. necrosis or resorption of tissues used in reconstruction; 6. postoperative fibrosis; and 7. inadequate postoperative care. Through clinical experience and laboratory research the results have improved. Improvement can be attributed to the more careful selection of candidates for surgery, a better understanding of the behavior of tissues in tympanoplasty procedures and the application of greater surgical skill.

In 1961, the Board of Surgeons of the Department of Otolaryngology of the Massachusetts Eye and Ear Infirmary established a Tympanoplasty

Service for the purpose of providing a more uniform and effective training experience for the residents; thus, the responsibility for the care of clinic patients requiring middle ear and mastoid surgery because of chronic suppurative disease was concentrated in the hands of eight members of the staff. At that time there were 39 members of the active staff and 14 residents. Based on their accumulated experience, these surgeons established a set of guidelines which would be followed in the management of all patients; furthermore, the members of the Tympanoplasty Service provided an instructional course in temporal bone dissection for the residents. In actual practice, some variations in procedure were necessary to meet the exigencies of the particular case; however, major changes in methodology were made only by mutual agreement.

The procedural guidelines developed to govern the Tympanoplasty Service were as follows.[19]

1. The selection of patients for surgery is to be the responsibility of a member of the Tympanoplasty Service.

2. Canalplasty, that is, enlargement of the cartilaginous and bony external auditory canal, is to be performed on all operations except simple myringoplasty.

3. The post-auricular incision is to be used for all operations requiring mastoidectomy.

4. Complete and thorough radical mastoidectomy is to be performed for all patients having active chronic suppurative disease or cholesteatoma of the mastoid.

5. The mastoid cavity is to be obliterated with pedicled or free fascial-muscle grafts except when there is uncertainty that disease has been completely eradicated. Both superiorly and inferiorly based pedicled grafts are to be used for most cases and, usually, a free graft of connective tissue is to be placed in the epitympanic space.

6. In Type III tympanoplasty, the posterior bony canal wall is removed to the level of the facial nerve and the tympanic graft (or tympanic membrane) is to be placed on the head of the stapes.

7. In Type IV tympanoplasty, the tympanic graft, or tympanic membrane, is to be placed on the promontory to create a hypotympanic air pocket incorporating the round window. The oval window niche is to be exteriorized and skin grafting performed to prevent fibrous obliteration of the niche.

8. The skin of the posterior canal wall is to be prepared as a laterally based pedicled flap (Koerner flap) and replaced on the anterior surface of the pedicled grafts used for mastoid obliteration.

9. Packing is to consist of strips of rayon cloth placed on all surfaces in

the form of a rosette, and cotton soaked in cortisporin. The packing is to remain in position for two weeks.

10. Three weeks following surgery, all unepithelized surfaces are to be covered with thin split thickness skin grafts (0.003-0.005 inches) as an out-patient procedure.

MATERIAL.

Following these general principles, operative procedures were performed on 1,074 ears over a five-year period (January 1, 1962, to December 31, 1966) with follow-up periods of two to seven years. The case material represents all clinic patients and all private patients of the full-time staff, without exception. The authors have located and personally examined all the patients totalling 936 cases (87 percent), 282 (30 percent) of which were private. One hundred thirty-eight cases were lost to follow-up study. In 97 (9 percent) of these cases, the patients have moved from the New England area and were not available for study, while 41 (4 percent) were lost despite an intensive search.

Of the 936 operations studied, there were 172 revisions (18.4 percent), 97 of which were performed on patients having the first procedure at the Massachusetts Eye and Ear Infirmary, and 75 on patients first operated upon elsewhere. Of the 172 revisions, 68 were tympanoplasties, 77 tympanoplasties with mastoidectomies, 25 radical mastoidectomies, and two total obliterative procedures. The principal reasons for revision were continued suppuration, perforation of the graft, and recurring cholesteatoma. The procedural guide lines used were the same as for the first operation. The statistics reported include all revisions which were treated as primary operations.

The final follow-up study consisted of a historical review, an otological examination with the aid of magnification, an audiometric evaluation and measurement of size of the meatus and volume of the cavity. The volume of the cavity was obtained by determining the quantity of warm polymyxin solution (50 mcg per ml) required to fill the cavity to the margin of the concha.

The data were processed through an IBM No. 7094 Computer at the Harvard Computer Center.

The Wüllstein[4] method of classification of tympanoplasty procedures was followed.

Type I. Repair of the tympanic membrane, usually with exploration of the middle ear and often with canalplasty. Synonym: myringoplasty.

Type II. Repair of the tympanic membrane and reconstructive procedure to restore the ossicular lever mechanism of the middle ear.

TABLE I.
Distribution of Cases.

Types of Operation	N	Totals
Tympanoplasty alone:		
Type I	218	
Type II	8	
Type III	82	
Type IV	23	
		331
Tympanoplasty with mastoidectomy:		
Type I	2	
Type II	0	
Type III	16	
Type IV	3	
		21
Tympanoplasty with mastoidectomy and obliteration:		
Type I	8	
Type II	0	
Type III	254	
Type IV	126	
		388
Tympanoplasty with attico-antrostomy:		
Type I	7	
Type II	5	
Type III	6	
Type IV	11	
		29
Other procedures:		
Radical mastoidectomy alone	83	
Radical mastoidectomy with obliteration	45	
Modified radical mastoidectomy alone	19	
Modified radical mastoidectomy with obliteration	11	
Total obliteration ("Rambo")	9	
		167
Total number of cases studied		936 (87%)
Lost to follow-up study		138 (13%)
		1074

Type III. Reconstructive procedure with placement of graft or tympanic membrane on the capitulum of the stapes, possibly with interposition of autogenous tissue graft, usually with radical mastoidectomy.

Type IV. Reconstructive procedure with placement of graft or tympanic membrane on the promontory and exteriorization of the oval window, usually with radical mastoidectomy.

A listing of the total case material by type of operative procedure appears in Table I. Unless otherwise stated, the data include service and private patients. Several operative procedures were performed in inadequate numbers to constitute significant statistical analysis; they are listed in Table I, but not discussed further.

RESULTS.

Tympanic grafting or use of the remaining tympanic membrane to establish the desired end result was performed in 769 tympanoplasty operations. The incidence of graft success is shown in Table II. In this table, as in several others, we have presented the statistics for the more experienced (M. E.) and the less experienced (L. E.) surgeons, or to be more specific, the difference between service patients, who were the prime responsibility of the residents operating under supervision, and the private patients of

TABLE II.
Incidence of Graft Success.

			N	Success	(%)
Tympanoplasty alone:					
	Type I	L.E.	154	105	68
		M.E.	64	57	89
	Type III, IV	L.E.	57	42	74
		M.E.	48	39	81
Tympanoplasty with mastoidectomy and obliteration:					
	Type III	L.E.	162	135	83
		M.E.	92	76	83
	Type IV	L.E.	88	75	85
		M.E.	38	32	84

L.E. — Less experienced surgeons, service cases.
M.E. — More experienced surgeons, full-time staff cases.

TABLE III.
Causes of Tympanic Graft Failure.

Perforation	139
Graft Cholesteatoma	6
Lateral Displacement of Graft	12
Total	157

(Six of the 12 with lateral displacement of graft occurred in Type I procedures.)

the full-time staff. The causes for the 157 (20.4 percent) graft failures appear in Table III. All of the six graft cholesteatomas appeared in ears having tympanic split thickness skin grafts, a procedure which was eventually discontinued. It is probable that many of the perforations occurring prior to 1963 were also due to graft cholesteatoma. There were 12 ears in which failure was due to lateral displacement of the graft. The cause for this probably was improper packing or postoperative fibrous retraction.

Age was found to have no significant effect on the success of grafting (Table IV). Age also had no effect on the postoperative hearing results, nor did it influence the success of achieving a dry ear. The youngest patient was five and the oldest was 67.

All patients who had active suppuration prior to surgery were treated with parenterally administered antibiotic drugs and frequent local treatment by aspiration, removal of granulations and insufflation with 5 percent chloromycetin powder for six weeks prior to surgery. Despite this treatment, suppuration persisted in 262 of 769 ears (34 percent) undergoing tympanoplasty.

TABLE IV.
Age and Graft Success.

Age	N	Success	(%)
1-10	94	77	82
11-20	222	173	78
21-50	366	293	80
51-60	71	54	76
Over 61	16	15	94
Total	769	612	80

TABLE V.
Pre-Operative Suppuration and Graft Success.

	N	Success	(%)
Tympanoplasty:			
Suppuration	39	24	62
Without suppuration	292	226	78
Tympanoplasty with mastoidectomy:			
Suppuration	223	185	83
Without suppuration	166	140	84

TABLE VI.
Pre-Operative Suppuration and "Dry" Ear Success (Tympanoplasty with Mastoidectomy).

	N	Dry	(%)
Suppuration	223	194	87
Without suppuration	166	143	86

The statistics in Table V show that, for tympanoplasty alone, the presence of suppuration adversely affected the success of grafting, whereas for tympanoplasty with mastoidectomy, the presence of suppuration had no significant effect.

In ears subjected to tympanoplasty with mastoidectomy, the presence or absence of pre-operative suppuration did not affect the percentage of dry ears following surgery (Table VI).

Of the 31 traumatic perforations, eight were caused by the slap of a hand to the ear, eight by objects introduced into the canal by the patient to clean the ear, four by industrial accidents, three by automobile accidents, and the remainder by miscellaneous injuries. Simple myringoplasty was performed in 21, whereas more extensive surgery was required in 10. Results of tympanic grafting in these cases were similar to those of post-infectious cases.

The location and the size of the perforation had no effect on the success rate of tympanic grafting.

TABLE VII.
Tubal Patency and Postoperative Rinne Test (512).

		N	Positive	(%)
Type I	Patent	135	124	92
	Not patent	17	12	71
Type III	Patent	122	65	53
	Not patent	74	19	26
Type IV	Patent	42	14	33
	Not patent	39	9	23

TABLE VIII.
Type of Graft and Success Rate.

	N	Success	(%)
Fascia + skin	72	63	88
Fascia	227	194	85
Skin	324	247	76
Vein	37	29	78
Total	660	533	81

Multiple perforations were present in 22 ears, but no patients had evidence of tuberculosis on roentgen films of the chest or positive cultures for acidfast organisms from the middle ear.

In 429 patients undergoing tympanoplasty an attempt was made, preoperatively, to determine whether air passed through the eustachian tube on forced inflation by the techniques of auto-inflation, politzerization, and the use of the Senturia calibrated inflating device. Patency was detected in 299, with successful grafting occurring in 79 percent; non-patency in 130, and successful grafting in 81 percent, thus showing no statistical difference. A study of tubal patency on hearing, on the other hand, showed that postoperative hearing as manifested by the Rinne test is adversely influenced by lack of tubal patency (Table VII).

Of the 769 tympanoplasty procedures listed in Table I, 660 (86 percent) procedures utilized the tympanic grafts listed in Table VIII. The tympanic membrane was adequate to complete the tympanoplasty in 51 ears (6.6 percent); other types of grafts were used in 41 (5.4 percent) and in 17 (2 percent), the operative description failed to specify the type of graft used. Fascial grafts were used in 299, of which 72 also had split thickness skin grafts (the so-called composite graft) with a success rate of 86 percent. Split thickness skin alone was used in 324 ears and was successful in 76 percent. Vein was used alone in 37 cases with success in 78 percent (Tables VIII and IX).

TABLE IX.
Graft Failure and Type of Graft.

	N	Perforation	Graft Cholesteatoma	Lateral Displacement
Fascia + skin	9	6	1	2
Fascia	33	26	0	7
Skin	77	71	5	1
Vein	8	8	0	0
Total	127	111	6	10

TABLE X.
Postoperative "Dry" Ear.

	N	"Dry"	(%)
Radical mastoidectomy	83	60	72
Radical mastoidectomy with obliteration	45	35	78
Tympanoplasty with mastoidectomy and obliteration	388	338	87

The data show that for the successful grafts the type of tissues used did not affect the final hearing levels.

An analysis of the number of dry ears following surgery shows 72 percent for radical mastoidectomy alone, 78 percent for radical mastoidectomy with obliteration, and 87 percent for tympanoplasty with mastoidectomy and obliteration (Table X). The incidence of postoperative crusting and ulceration was correspondingly less for tympanoplasty with mastoidectomy and obliteration (Table XI). The difference may reflect a selectivity factor in that tympanoplasty with the obliterative procedure was performed only when it was determined that all disease had been removed; thus, the non-obliterated mastoids may have had more extensive disease. There were 10 patients with bilateral chronic suppurative otitis media. In each of these 10 patients, tympanoplasty with mastoidectomy and obliteration was performed on one ear, and radical mastoidectomy was performed on the opposite ear. Pre-operatively, both ears had about the same extent of disease.

Postoperatively, all of the 10 ears in which tympanoplasty with mastoidectomy and obliteration was done were dry and asymptomatic. Five out of the 10 ears in which radical mastoidectomy was done remained wet postoperatively.

Operative procedures were performed on 226 ears for severe disease consisting of either gross infection, extensive cholesteatoma, labyrinthine fistula, facial nerve involvement, or CNS complications. In these ears, postoperative suppuration was controlled more often by tympanoplasty with mastoidectomy and obliteration (Table XII). It is of interest to note that

TABLE XI.
Postoperative Condition of Cavity.

	Radical Mastoidectomy	Radical Mastoidectomy with Obliteration	Tympanoplasty with Mastoidectomy and Obliteration
N	83	45	388
Suppuration or Crusting	22 (26%)	9 (20%)	42 (11%)
Ulceration	16 (19%)	5 (11%)	27 (7%)
Cavity	3.1 cc	2.4 cc.	2.3 cc
Meatus	10 mm	10 mm	10.6 mm

TABLE XII.
Procedures Performed for More Severe Disease States.

	Radical Mastoidectomy	Radical Mastoidectomy with Obliteration	Tympanoplasty with Mastoidectomy and Obliteration
N	76	32	118
Postoperative Suppuration	21 (27.6%)	7 (22%)	17 (14.4%)

the cavity size for radical mastoidectomy (83 ears) was 3.1 cc whereas it was 2.3 cc for radical mastoidectomy with obliteration (433 ears) (Table XI).

Auditory thresholds were determined immediately before surgery and from two to seven years following surgery. Pure tone measurements were made with three Beltone 14A and one Beltone 15A audiometers. Air conduction stimuli were measured with a Brüel and Kjaer Model 158 Audiometer Calibrator. Bone conduction was calibrated at monthly intervals utilizing subjects with mild sensori-neural hearing loss according to the techniques of Roach and Carhart.[20] Masking of the non-test ear was accomplished with Beltone narrow-band masking instruments, Model No. 102. Speech reception thresholds were routinely measured with live voice stimuli with Grason-Stadler speech audiometer, Model 162. All tests were administered in IAC rooms (series 1400 ACT, 400 ACT, 400 A). The ISO stand-

TABLE XIII.
Postoperative Bone-Air Gap (Averaging 500, 1,000, 2,000 Hertz).

	N	Criteria	Success N	(%)
Type I	235	Less than 10 db Gap	184	(78%)
Type III	358	Less than 20 db Gap	143	(40%)
Type IV	163	Less than 30 db Gap	75	(46%)
Radical Mastoidectomy	128	Less than 30 db Gap	44	(34%)
Modified Radical Mastoidectomy	30	Less than 20 db Gap	14	(47%)

TABLE XIV.
Postoperative Thresholds (Shown in Percentage).

	N	0-15 db	16-25 db	26-35 db	36-45 db	46-60 db	Over 60 db
Type I	235	72	14	10	3	1	0
Type III	358	6	13	28	30	15	8
Type IV	163	0	7	17	25	33	18
Radical Mastoidectomy	128	3	2	10	30	25	30
Modified Radical Mastoidectomy	30	13.3	13.3	20	13.3	26.7	13.3

TABLE XV.
Gain of Bone Conduction Thresholds.

	N	n	%	Average Gain
Type I	235	47	20	9 db
Type III	358	80	22	8 db
Type IV	163	40	24	11 db
Radical Mastoidectomy	128	31	24	14 db
Modified Radical Mastoidectomy	30	13	43	13 db

ard calibration was adopted in 1963 and audiograms made before that date were corrected to match the ISO standard using the following values: 250 - 15 db, 500 - 15 db, 1,000 - 10 db, 2,000 - 10 db, 4,000 - 5 db, 8,000 - 10 db.

The pure tone thresholds are evaluated by averaging the three speech frequencies (500, 1,000, and 2,000 Hertz). The bone-air gap values show the difference in decibels between the averaged postoperative bone and air conduction thresholds. The bone-air gaps for several success criteria are shown in Table XIII.

The postoperative average pure tone thresholds for several success criteria are shown in Table XIV.

The number of patients experiencing gain or loss in bone conduction thresholds are shown in Tables XV and XVI. Table XVI does not include the two patients who had surgical injury to the horizontal canal and sustained profound hearing loss.

The results of the Rinne tests are shown in Table XVII.

Interpositioning procedures were performed on 72 ears of which 44 consisted of bone or cartilage graft on the capitulum of the stapes; 25 of bone or cartilage graft to the footplate of the stapes and three of malleus to the capitulum of the stapes. These techniques did not improve postoperative hearing results as compared to non-interposition procedures and were eventually discontinued.

TABLE XVI.
Loss of Bone Conduction Thresholds.

	N	n	%	Average Loss
Type I	235	48	20	7 db
Type III	358	83	23	10 db
Type IV	163	38	23	10 db
Radical Mastoidectomy	128	32	25	14 db
Modified Radical Mastoidectomy	30	5	17	9 db

TABLE XVII.
Postoperative Rinne Test (512 Hertz).

	N	Positive
Type I	235	83%
Type III	358	43%
Type IV	163	28%
Radical Mastoidectomy	128	18%
Modified Radical Mastoidectomy	30	50%

Surgical injury to the facial nerve occurred in two patients. One was crushed in its intratympanic region by a less experienced surgeon, and one was totally transected near the stylomastoid foramen by an experienced surgeon. The latter nerve was surrounded by cholesteatoma and granulation tissue. Both patients sustained permanent mild paresis and dissociated movement. Eleven patients had pre-operative facial paresis, of which six recovered in two weeks, three within six months, and two sustained permanent paresis. Three had total pre-operative paralysis, of which one recovered within two weeks, one within six months, and one recovered partially and has permanent paresis.

Labyrinthine fistulae were found in 27 ears, 23 in the horizontal canal, one in the posterior canal, two in both the horizontal and posterior canals and one in both the horizontal and superior canals. Five of the 27 patients with fistulas had no pre-operative vertigo.

Of 103 patients who complained of vertigo pre-operatively, 22 had labyrinthine fistulas. Seventy-six reported great relief of vertigo following surgery.

The horizontal canals of two ears were opened inadvertently at the time of surgery, and both sustained profound loss of hearing.

Fourteen ears were profoundly deaf pre-operatively. Nine received labyrinthectomy because of pre-operative vertigo or because of invasion of the inner ear by granulation tissue or cholesteatoma. The total obliterative procedure of Rambo[21] was performed on five of these 14 ears.

A severe hearing loss for frequencies above 1,000 cps, not present before surgery, was sustained by eight patients, seven of which occurred in Type

TABLE XVIII.
Incidence of Cholesteatoma.

	N	Pre-Operative Cholesteatoma	Postoperative Cholesteatoma			
			Graft	Middle Ear	Mastoid	Total
Tympanoplasty	331	18 (5.4%)	2	3	1	6
Tympanoplasty and Mastoidectomy	409	213 (52%)	4	9	2	15
Tympanoplasty and Attico-Antrostomy	29	14 (48%)	0	0	0	0
Mastoidectomy only	158	101 (64%)	0	1	3	4
"Rambo"	9	1 (11%)	0	0	0	0
	936	347 (37%)	6	13	6	25 (2.7%)

III tympanoplasty and one in Type I tympanoplasty. The cause for this loss is assumed to be acoustic stimulation type injury due to surgical manipulation of the ossicles. The principal cause probably is contact of the rotating burr with the ossicles.

An unsatisfactory external auditory meatus occurred postoperatively in 48 ears. Severe stenosis occurred in 25, partial stenosis in nine, and collapsing meatus in 14. Surgical correction was performed for 20.

Some degree of medial displacement of the auricle occurred in 179 (31 percent) patients having radical mastoidectomy procedures and 14 patients registered dissatisfaction with the cosmetic appearance of this flattened auricle.

Otosclerosis was found to co-exist with chronic suppurative disease in seven ears, of which two had Type III and five had Type IV tympanoplasty. Care was used in differentiating otosclerosis from tympanosclerosis. Removal of the stapes footplate and introduction of a fatty connective tissue graft was performed at a subsequent surgical procedure in four. The average hearing gain from this second procedure was 20 db. These procedures are not included in the statistical studies.

Cholesteatoma was found at the time of tympanoplasty and mastoidectomy in 347 (37 percent) of 936 ears. Cholesteatoma occurred postoperatively in 25 ears (2.7 percent) of which six were located in the tympanic graft, 13 in the middle ear and six in the mastoid (Table XVIII). Postoperative cholesteatoma occurred in 11 (2.5 percent) of 444 ears with mastoidectomy and mastoid obliteration and eight (6.5 percent) of 123 ears with mastoidectomy without obliteration.

A summary showing the incidence of complications of all types is shown in Table XIX.

TABLE XIX.

Complications of Tympanoplasty and Mastoid Surgery.

	N
1. Facial Nerve Injury	2
2. Surgical Injury to the Labyrinth	2
3. Acoustic Trauma	8
4. Meatal Stenosis	34
5. Postoperative Cholesteatoma	25
6. Tympanic Graft Failure	157

SUMMARY AND CONCLUSIONS.

A study was made of the findings and results of 936 tympanoplasty and mastoidectomy procedures performed at the Massachusetts Eye and Ear Infirmary between January 1, 1962, and December 31, 1966. Of this group 654 were service cases on whom surgery was performed by the residents under supervision, and 282 were private patients. All surgeons followed a set of guidelines for the surgical procedure and postoperative management.

The data were compiled and processed through an IBM No. 7094 Computer at the Harvard Computer Center.

Tympanoplasty alone was performed in 331 ears; tympanoplasty with mastoidectomy in 21; tympanoplasty with mastoidectomy and obliteration in 388; and tympanoplasty with attico-antrostomy in 29. Radical mastoidectomy alone was performed in 83; radical mastoidectomy with obliteration in 45; modified radical mastoidectomy in 19; modified radical mastoidectomy with obliteration in 11; and the total obliterative procedure (Rambo)[21] in nine.

The presence of suppuration was found to affect adversely the results of tympanoplasty alone but had no effect when mastoidectomy was combined with tympanoplasty. Age, on the other hand, had no effect on the results of tympanoplasty.

An assessment of patency of the eustachian tube was made pre-operatively in 429 cases, and it was demonstrated that lack of patency had an adverse effect on the hearing results but had no effect on the grafting results.

For tympanic grafting, temporalis fascia proved superior to split-thickness skin grafts, the success rates being 86 percent for the former and 76 percent for the latter.

An analysis of the number of dry ears following surgery shows 72 percent for radical mastoidectomy alone, 78 percent for radical mastoidectomy with obliteration, and 87 percent for tympanoplasty with mastoidectomy and obliteration.

Obliteration of the mastoid with fascial-muscle pedicled grafts reduced the final cavity size from 3.1 cc (radical mastoidectomy) to 2.3 cc (radical mastoidectomy with obliteration) and resulted in fewer symptomatic cavities.

Of 235 Type I tympanoplasties (Wüllstein classification), 78 percent achieved a bone-air gap of 10 db or less. Type III tympanoplasties (358 cases) showed 40 percent with a bone-air gap of 20 db or less. Of 163 Type IV tympanoplasties, 46 percent had a final bone-air gap of 30 db or less. For modified radical mastoidectomy a 20 db or less bone-air gap was achieved in 47 percent and for radical mastoidectomy a 30 db gap was achieved in 34 percent.

Among the 936 cases studied, 347 (37 percent) had pre-operative cholesteatoma and 25 (2.7 percent) developed postoperative cholesteatoma. Of the 444 ears with mastoidectomy and mastoid obliteration, 11 (2.5 percent) developed recurrent or had residual cholesteatoma.

Major complications include two facial nerve injuries and two surgical injuries to horizontal semicircular canals. Minor complications include eight stimulation injuries to the cochlea, 179 displaced auricles, and 34 meatal stenosis.

These are the experiences in a large clinic with a strong teaching responsibility. The establishment of a set of procedural guide lines, incorporating particularly the wide-field approach, aided the young surgeons in developing surgical skills with minimal risk of injury to the ear or facial nerve. The study shows that tympanoplasty has added a dimension of improvement in results over radical and modified radical mastoidectomy, both in terms of the number of dry ears and the hearing improvement; nonetheless, tympanoplasty, at least as we practiced it, is not a panacea for the management of the chronic suppurating ear. There is much room for improvement. We doubt that the glowing short-term results reported by numerous surgeons will stand the test of time.

ACKNOWLEDGMENT.

The authors thank Miss Rhoda Kimmel and the Audiology Staff for performing the audiometric tests.

BIBLIOGRAPHY.

1. BERTHOLD, E.: Ueber Myringoplastik. *Wien. med. Bl.*, 1:1627, 1878.

2. WÜLLSTEIN, H.: Funktionelle Operationen im Mittelohr mit Hilfe des freien Spaltlappen-Transplantates. *Arch. Ohren-Nasen-Kehlkopfheilk.*, 161:422, 1952.

3. WÜLLSTEIN, H.: Die Tympanoplastik als gehörverbessernde Operation bei Otitis Media chronica und ihr Resultate. *Proc. Fifth Internat. Cong. Otol., Rhinol. and Laryngol.*, p. 104, 1953.

4. WÜLLSTEIN, H.: The Restoration of the Function of the Middle Ear in Chronic Otitis Media. *Ann. Otol., Rhinol. and Laryngol.*, 65:1020, 1956.

5. WÜLLSTEIN, H.: Tympanoplasty Today. *Arch. Otolaryngol.*, 76:295, 1962.

6. ZÖLLNER, F.: Die Schalleitungsplastiken. *Acta Otolaryngol.*, 44:370, 1954; 45:168, 1955.

7. ZÖLLNER, F.: The Principles of Plastic Surgery of the Sound-Conducting Apparatus. *Jour. Laryngol. and Otol.*, 69:637, 1955.

8. ZÖLLNER, F.: Present-Day Status of Surgical Treatment of Chronic Otitis Media. *Deutsche Med. Wschr.*, 86:2309, 1961.

9. GOODHILL, V.: Some Crucial Problems in Case Selection and Surgical Technique in Tympanoplasty. *Ann. Otol., Rhinol. and Laryngol.*, 76:587, 1967.

10. GUILFORD, F. R., and WRIGHT, W. K.: Basic Techniques in Myringoplasty and Tympanoplasty. *The Laryngoscope*, 68:525, 1958.

11. JANSEN, C.: Cartilage-Tympanoplasty. *The Laryngoscope*, 73:1288, 1963.

12. MORITZ, W.: Hörverbessernde Operationen bei chronischentzündlichen Prozessen beider Mittelohren. *Ztschr. Laryngol., Rhinol., Otol.*, 29:578, 1950.

13. PORTMANN, M.: "Open" or "Closed" Technique in Surgery of the Middle Ear. *Ann. Otol., Rhinol. and Laryngol.*, 77:927, 1968.

14. PROCTOR, B.: Type IV Tympanoplasty. *Arch. Otolaryngol.*, 79:176, 1964.

15. SHEEHY, J. L., and PATTERSON, M. E.: Intact Canal Wall Tympanoplasty with Mastoidectomy. *The Laryngoscope*, 77:1502, 1967.

16. SHEEHY, J. L., and GLASSCOCK, M. E.: Tympanic Membrane Grafting with Temporalis Fascia. *Arch. Otolaryngol.*, 86:391, 1967.

17. WRIGHT, W. K.: Tissues for Tympanic Grafting. *Arch. Otolaryngol.*, 78:291, 1963.

18. Symposium on Tympanoplasty and Mastoidectomy. *Arch. Otolaryngol.*, 89:184-251, 1969.

19. SCHUKNECHT, H. F.; CHASIN, W. D., and KURKJIAN, J. M.: Stereoscopic Atlas of Mastoidotympanoplastic Surgery. C. V. Mosby Co., St. Louis, Mo., 1966.

20. ROACH, R. E., and CARHART, R.: A Clinical Method for Calibrating the Bone Conduction Audiometer. *Arch. Otolaryngol.*, 63:270, 1956.

21. RAMBO, J. H. T.: The Primary Closure of the Radical Mastoidectomy Wound: A Technique to Eliminate Postoperative Care. *The Laryngoscope*, 68:1216, 1958.

***

Universal Healthcare: A Bold Proposal

K.J. LEE, M.D. AND MARK E. LEE

Presented at Healthcare Solution Workshop/Conference,
8 April 2000, Foxwoods Resort.
Revised by the Healthcare Solution Task Force.

ABSTRACT—One problem with the American health-care system today is not that it's too expensive but that it's too wasteful. The amount spent on health-care in the United States is sufficient to take care of the medical needs of every citizen. The reason that it does not is that the money is far too often is misspent. America already is spending 14% of the gross domestic product and yet we have health-care chaos and 44 million uninsured. Another problem is the lack of trust between payors, insurance carriers, regulators, employers, employees, providers, and patients. Although the financing aspect of health-care is tremendously important, it is even more important to design a plan to spend the money wisely, align the incentives of insurers, payors, patients, and providers, and restore trust between parties. Otherwise we shall continue to be in chaos regardless of how much money we spend on health-care.

In this article, we outline our proposal for an ideal comprehensive national health-care plan that will guarantee that we spend our health-care dollars wisely.

K.J. LEE, M.D. Chair, Healthcare Solution Task Force, Associate Clinical Professor, Yale University School of Medicine, Chief of Otolaryngology, Hospital of St. Raphael, New Haven, Chairman and CEO, MedWin of Connecticut, LLC, New Haven, CEO, The Primary and Specialist Medical Center, Managing Partner, Southern New England Ear, Nose, Throat, and Facial Plastic Surgery Group, New Haven; MARK E. LEE, Summer administrative intern, MedWin of Connecticut, LLC, New Haven.

Our plan would cover all Americans, including the 44 million uninsured, and it would do so at less than the cost of the current system.

Because insurance companies are not equipped to oversee medical practice, our plan would place the day-to-day management of the health-care system in the hands of physicians and local physician-run, physician-owned "provider groups." The physicians in these provider groups would be charged with two primary responsibilities: 1) clinically, they would be responsible for providing total quality cradle-to-grave health-care for every patient in their group and 2) economically, they would be responsible for the budget and to spend it wisely. Physicians will be compensated fee-for-service plus an incentive for efficiency, patient satisfaction, and outcome in a broad sense. Physicians would enjoy wide latitude in clinical decision-making without being second-guessed by distant third parties. Our plan places the fiscal responsibility on physicians while at the same time establishing a system of checks and balances to ensure that patients are protected and well cared for. Unlike outwardly similar plans, under this proposal the physicians are owners of the provider groups and the incentives between payors, insurers, providers, and patients are better aligned. It will eliminate the debate about giving patients the right to sue health plans and employers. It would empower large legally organized physician groups to negotiate with insurers.

Our plan is a model for spending money wisely. We believe it would benefit, and therefore be embraced, by all parties—physicians, other healthcare providers, employers, insurance companies, the government, and above all the American public.

Appendix 2. Articles by Doctor Lee

Introduction

THERE is little dispute that the quality of medical care available in the United States is the best in the world. Yet despite all of our technologic advances and successes, today's American health-care delivery system is in a state of chaos. Providers, patients, insurers, employers, and regulators are all dissatisfied. One problem with the American health-care system is not that it's too expensive, but that it's too wasteful. The amount of money spent on health-care in the United States today is sufficient to take care of all the medical needs of every citizen. The reason that it does not is that the money too often is misspent. America is already spending 14% of the gross domestic product and yet we have health-care chaos and 44 million uninsured. Another problem is the lack of trust between payors, providers, patients, insurers, employers, and regulators. This is evident from the debates in Congress, litigation, draconian precertification processes mandated by insurance companies, and a maze of complicated regulations imposed by Medicare. Although the financing aspect of health-care is tremendously important, it is even more important to design a plan to spend the money wisely, align the incentives of insurers, payors, patients, and providers, and restore trust between parties. otherwise we shall continue to be in chaos regardless of how much money we spend in the health-care industry. In this article we submit for consideration our proposal for a new universal health-care delivery program.

Our plan would significantly reduce, if not virtually eliminate, wasteful spending. As a result, health-care insurance would become affordable for every American, including the 44 million who are now uninsured. It realigns incentives thus restoring trust among all parties.

The framework of this proposal is the establishment of local, comprehensive, integrated, physician-run "provider groups." The health-care services rendered by these groups would be paid for from a budget paid by employers, consortiums of patients, or the government, either directly or through an insurance company.

Physicians would be responsible for keeping costs in check by eliminating waste while still rendering necessary medical care in a timely fashion. Moreover, clinical decision-making authority, much of which has been usurped by third parties, would be returned to the physician who is in the ideal position to recognize and avoid wasteful spending.

Cutting waste would account for only part of the savings. Free-market competition would provide more. Physicians would compete in the open market for patients which would ensure that quality care would be rendered at a competitive price.

Background

In the days before health-care costs began escalating out of hand, the physician and patient interacted in a confidential, one-on-one encounter. They had the same goals. They discussed the mosaic of competing and complementary considerations that go into making a treatment decision-cost, convenience, risk, benefit, etc., and they generally agreed on how to proceed. If the patient had insurance, the company paid the bill and few questions were asked.

But as costs increased, insurers began to demand a greater say in how their money was being spent. Third parties are not interested in the mosaic of competing and complementary considerations. They are interested in only one piece of the mosaic: cost. One way they could control costs was to foster an environment that not only encouraged, but demanded underutilization. Therefore, they set up strict claims-review processes and began to deny coverage of services.

This led to a situation in which physicians were being second-guessed by the third parties. Doctors complained that untrained, uninformed strangers in distant cities were telling them how to treat patients. But the insurers controlled the purse strings, so they made the rules. And in doing so, they created an enormous bureaucracy and mountains of paperwork.

Eight Steps to Spending Wisely

Our plan would eliminate waste in eight ways: cutting paperwork, ensuring appropriate utilization, coordinating care, implementing a system of early intervention and disease management, avoiding unnecessary emergency room and hospital admissions, behavior modification, copayments, and promoting preventive medicine and wellness.

Paperwork reduction.—One of the benefits of our plan is that it would curtail the level of bureaucracy and significantly cut the amount of paperwork. Because the mechanics of our plan's financing are uncomplicated and the decision-making authority would not be shared by antagonists, we would no longer need an army of claims processors and claims reviewers in hundreds of thousands of physicians' and insurers' offices across the country. Microsoft chairman Bill Gates has estimated that 20% to 30% of the annual trillion-dollar cost of the U.S. health-care system is for paperwork.[1] Cutting paperwork under our plan would reduce the overall cost of health-care by 11%.

Appropriate utilization.—The long-standing point of bitter contention between third parties and physicians-utilization—would finally be settled. While insurers have a stake in *underutilization*, physicians today have an inherent financial (as well as clinical) interest in *overutilization*. From a financial standpoint, physicians today are pieceworkers—the more they do, the more they earn. The temptation exists to do more than is necessary.

Our plan seeks to bring these two diametrically opposed concepts into balance. Medical necessity would be defined by the physician and the patient, rather than by an uninvolved, distant insurance worker. Under our plan, the objectives of all parties concerned would be aligned.

Coordination of care.—Another expensive failing of the current system is that treatment is uncoordinated and communication among doctors is lacking. When patients today are referred through the system from one physician to the next, their charts and test results too often don't accompany them. As a result, specialists duplicate costly tests that have already been performed and they institute treatment protocols that are not synchronized with those of the primary-care physician.

Our plan takes steps to alleviate this problem by calling for the centralization and computerization of the medical records of each patient in the provider group. While maintaining confidentiality, all physicians in the group would have rapid access to complete and current information on each patient in the group, including the latest treatments and test results. Thanks to the revolutionary advances in information technology during the past decade, creating a computerized record system for each provider group can be achieved quite easily. Until recently the input of history and physical findings was not user-friendly; the refinement of scanning and voice recognition natural speech writer has put electronic medical records within reach. Having the testing results at hand will avoid unnecessarily repeating tests.

Early intervention and disease management.—In the current health-care delivery system, it is not possible for physicians to identify patients with serious chronic illnesses. Physicians can do nothing until such a patient takes the initiative and makes an appointment. By the time many of these patients do seek treatment, their diseases have progressed to the point that routine care is no longer sufficient and expensive measures must be taken.

Our proposed model would lower the cost of health-care by taking steps to minimize medical problems through early intervention and disease management. Whenever a group of patients signed on with a provider group, the physicians in the group, or the mid-level providers, would examine each patient assigned to him or her and flag the charts of those whose conditions warrant close observation. An advanced nurse practitioner would call these patients periodically, daily, if need be, depending on the seriousness of the condition, to monitor the patient's health, to remind the patient to take his or her medication, and to provide any other advice or instruction that is helpful. If the nurse suspected any trouble, a home or office visit could be arranged immediately. These patients would be considered "preferred clients," and they would receive "VIP treatment."

Unnecessary admissions.—Two of the biggest contributors to waste in the current system are unnecessary emergency room visits and hospital admissions. Emergency room visits can cost thousands of dollars, and hospital admissions can cost tens of thousands. Avoiding improper utilization would save the system millions of dollars.

Under our model, patients would be instructed to call one of the physicians in their provider group *before* going to the emergency room, whenever feasible. A clinician would see and examine the patient at a location near or adjacent to the emergency room and determine whether or not emergency care or hospitalization is actually necessary. If so, the patient would receive whatever care is required expeditiously. But when the situation is a false alarm—for example, simple indigestion rather than a heart attack—the patient would be reassured and treated appropriately without hospitalization. The patient would be spared the trouble of unnecessary hospital tests, which can be risky and painful, and the system would be spared the unnecessary expense.

Behavior modification.—One factor that could derail the best intentions of this model would be an insistent, implacable demand by patients for tests, treatments, and procedures that are not medically necessary. Physicians would need to educate patients at every opportunity that some services are not only unnecessary, but can do harm. Behavior modification could be achieved through ongoing public service campaigns, such as those that are changing attitudes about smoking, drunk driving, and other issues. The population would need to be educated, beginning in grammar school, through all of the media vehicles, including the internet. For example, credible spokespersons would explain that overuse of antibiotics causes drug resistance, that taking unneeded medications exposes patients to unnecessary side effects, that x-rays and MRIs are not risk-free, and that surgery should almost always be the last resort.

Copayments.—The patient's copayment for certain services would be another way to minimize overuse. Copayments would be high enough to discourage attention-seeking and unneeded care, but reasonable enough to be affordable.

Preventive medicine and promoting wellness.—Finally, perhaps the best way to avoid overuse is to keep patients healthy and satisfied. Each provider group will emphasize preventive medicine through screening and early detection of disease and promote wellness through nutrition, exercise, and life-style changes. This is what the population wants. It saves lives and money.

Avoiding both under- and overutilization, together with improving coordination obtaining accurate medical information, would reduce health-care expenditures by another 15%.

Local Provider Groups

The provider group model proposed here would make health-care affordable in two ways. First, health-care delivery would be subject to market-force competition. Second, each physician in the provider group would be encouraged to have ownership in the group and thus be personally responsible for keeping costs in check while rendering quality, compassionate, and courteous care.

Competition.—Provider groups would compete in a "market share area." The geographic size of each market share area would depend on its location but would be based on the size of its population and take into account a reasonable commuting distance.

Provider groups would be made up of a staff of primary-care physicians and specialists. Each provider group would be responsible for providing and paying for whatever health-care services their patients require, from influenza vaccinations to tertiary care. The group's income would derive from the premium or a percentage of the premium paid by employers, consortiums of patients, or the government. The money would be paid to the group either directly or through an insurance company. In addition to primary care, covered services would include specialty care, hospitalization, nursing care, physical and occupational therapy, home health care, etc. Provider groups would also pay for durable medical goods, acute care, subacute care, outpatient surgery, and diagnostic procedures, etc. The group would be able to hire ancillary personnel as full-time employees or contract for their services on an outsource basis.

To foster competition, each market share area would be serviced by at least three provider groups. Natural market-force competition would keep costs down and ensure value to payors and patients alike. Each group would compete on the basis of quality, service, and price.

Ownership and physician compensation.—Unlike outwardly similar models, each provider group would be owned by the providers who practice in it, although a few providers might not wish to participate in ownership, at least initially. The risks and rewards of ownership would provide ample incentive to see that the plan succeeds.

Patient satisfaction, the quality of care rendered, and appropriate and efficient management of resources are crucial to the success of a provider group that is held accountable for managing the health-care budget assigned to the group. The physicians' component of the budget will be divided between primary-care physicians and each of the specialty groups in accordance with actuarial data compiled by Milliman and Robertson, custom modified for each group. *Each physician's compensation would be paid in the following manner: part of the compensation could be a base amount, another portion could be related to productivity, another portion could be related to appropriate utilization of resources, and yet another portion could be related to patient satisfaction and outcome.* The portion related to productivity will be billed fee-for-service to the group, not to a distant insurance company or a complex governmental agency. The process is simple and cost effective. For the primary-care physicians, a portion of the dollars assigned to the primary-care department will be given to the primary-care physicians as a base compensation proportionate to the number of patients selecting him/her to be their primary-care physician. The rest of the dollars allocated to the primary care department will be divided into a pool to pay the physicians fee-for-service, a pool for appropriate utilization, and a pool for patient satisfaction and outcome. A similar arrangement can be made for the specialists except that the money allocated to a specialty will be divided into pools to pay fee-for-service, to pay for appropriate utilization, and to pay for patient satisfaction and outcome. There is no need for a base compensation among specialists as the patient will not be selecting a specialist until he or she has a need for one. At the end of a predetermined period, as decided by the individual group, all the money in the physician's component of the budget as well as surpluses in the rest of the budget will be distributed in such a manner as to encourage the rendering of quality care with excellent customer service and appropriate utilization of resources. The details on compensation, which are beyond the scope of this paper, are described in detail by Lee and Lee[2], and by Lee et al[3]; suffice it to state that the formula encourages the physicians to render quality, appropriate, affordable care efficiently, with excellent customer service while managing the health-care budget effectively.

Because practicing physicians are in the best position to understand when clinical services are needed and when they are not, they are able to make smart decisions regarding utilization. They would be able to provide quality care for all without contributing to the enormous waste of money and resources that plagues the system today. Furthermore, utilization review is more efficient when it is conducted locally by the medical director of each provider group rather than by uninvolved insurance company employees in distant locations. Local utilization review can be conducted personally and in a timely manner and physician education can take place on the spot.

There is more than a financial incentive for physicians to participate in such an arrangement. There are psychologic rewards as well. Physicians have been complaining for years about loss of autonomy, the mass confusion, and the "hassle factor." For example, in order to obtain prior authorization, physicians usually must call an 800 number. All too often, the party on the other end of the line has no idea what the physician is talking about. Moreover, a single phone call can take as long as 45 minutes and disconnections are a frequent occurrence.

Under our proposed model, physicians would regain right to make their own decisions and do so in a much-streamlined process. Physicians would not be micromanaged and they would earn a reasonable income. They would also enjoy the satisfaction of playing an important, if not historic, role in eliminating the enormous excesses and mismanagement inherent in the current system.

Funding of the Budget

The premium for each patient would be paid to the provider group by employers, consortiums of individuals, or the government, either directly or through an insurance company, as described by Lee in 1998.[4] The budget would cover the cost of complete cradle-to-grave healthcare for all patients in the group. Each patient would contribute a reasonable copayment for office visits and other routine services.

Our plan would provide access to equal care for workers and their dependents who are now covered by their employers, citizens and dependents who are now covered by government programs, and the 44 million uninsured.

The employed population.—To cover its employees and their dependents, a large employer would compare the quality, service, and prices offered by the three provider groups in its market area. By having a choice, the employer would be able to negotiate and obtain the best value for its health-care dollar.

Once the employer has chosen a provider group, it would pay the fixed amount—say, for example, $150 per month per patient. This payment would guarantee total care for each patient. All expenses incurred by the provider group would be paid out of the pool it receives. The physicians in the provider group would have control of the pool and would have an incentive to apportion the money wisely. Under the current chaotic system, the available pool is still limited but the physicians are not in control nor held accountable for spending the money wisely.

Medicare and Medicaid beneficiaries.—In the case of patients who have government-funded coverage, the government would pay an insurance company or the provider group a lump sum for each patient. The provider group would use these funds to cover the costs of service in the same manner as it uses employer-paid funds.

The uninsured.—Most of the 44 million Americans who do not have health insurance are either the working poor whose employers do not provide benefits, the owners of small businesses, or self-employed individuals. There are three ways to provide coverage for these workers. All three would be funded, or at least partially subsidized, by the money that would be saved by implementing other facets of this proposed plan.

One proposal is to improve the welfare system so that it would provide different levels of welfare coverage according to the recipient's financial status—in other words, two different means tests. Some of the working poor and their families would qualify for a complete welfare package, including Medicaid, food stamps, child support, housing support, etc. Others whose needs are not as great would receive only Medicaid coverage.

The second solution would be for single working people to join together and form a health-care purchasing consortium. Such a consortium could be organized according to the worker's neighborhood or town, his occupation, or on the basis of any other common ground shared. They could also obtain coverage through business coalitions such as the Council of Smaller Enterprises and the local chamber of commerce. Members of the consortium would contribute to its general fund, and the consortium would pay the premium to the provider group directly or through an insurance company the same way that the large employer and Medicare and Medicaid would. By banding together, members of the consortium would increase their bargaining power and obtain a lower price for coverage than they could as individuals. The consortium also would be able to keep costs down by comparing the quality, service, and price offered by the different provider groups in its market share area and choosing the one that offers the best value for its members.

A consortium might be unwilling to accept an uninsured person who has many illnesses for fear that this person would use a disproportionate share of the budget pool. In this case, such a patient would be assigned by lottery to one of the provider groups in that market share area at the same rate negotiated by the consortium.

The third method would be to mandate that *all* employers provide health-care coverage for their workers. This could be accomplished without placing an undue burden on small businesses or penalizing them for their size. First, government would be encouraged to provide these small businesses with a tax break and/or other benefits, such as a loosening of the minimum wage requirements. Second, just like individuals, small businesses could keep their costs down by forming or joining a consortium.

Of course, there will always be people who decline to purchase coverage, preferring to take the risk and pay for healthcare out pocket as needed. These people might actuary be the wisest shoppers of all. In any case, they would be free to make their own choices.

Adoption of this plan would finally provide good health-care coverage for the 44 million uninsured working people

Appendix 2. Articles by Doctor Lee

in this country whose situation has for so long been an unsolvable dilemma.

Quality Assurance

In most walks of life, supervisors reprimand workers for *under*performance. In medicine, physicians are chastised for overperformance that is, *over*utilization. It does not matter to an HMO whether the provider is simply conscientious, unaware of the cost-benefit ratio, or is out for economic gain. Under our plan, physicians would be encouraged to use resources wisely because they would have a personal financial incentive to render the appropriate level of care. Overutilization wastes resources, while underutilization results in poor outcomes and patient dissatisfaction, which can lead to a loss of patient volume and perhaps a lawsuit. Moreover, underutilization leads to a higher severity of illness which leads to greater cost.

Naturally, fears would arise that with such a system the physician might be tempted to underutilize, that is to forgo a test or treatment in order to save money. Our proposal would counter any such inclinations by tying compensation to measures of patient satisfaction and outcomes, as discussed earlier. The medical director of each provider group would concentrate on monitoring *under*performance rather than *over*performance. Hence, a group or an individual provider who cut corners, had consistently poor outcomes, and/or received poor patient satisfaction reports would be disciplined and, if necessary, terminated from the program.

In addition, our proposal calls for three "patient's rights" safeguards:

1. All patients would have the right to file a complaint with the provider group as well as with outside agencies and the government. Groups that receive a large number of substantiated complaints could either be fined or have a contract revoked.
2. All patients would be able to complain to their employer or to their consortium's representative. Any employer or representative who received an excessive number of complaints about a particular provider group would most likely drop its arrangement with that group and purchase its coverage from a competing group at the first opportunity. Again, quality care would be assured by this market-driven element of the plan.
3. All patients would retain the right to sue their physicians and any other provider in the group.

These patients rights would be a powerful inducement not to cut corners. Physicians fear lawsuits, and with good reason. When a large corporation is served a lawsuit, it generally does not suffer an institutional emotional crisis. Large companies have staffs of in-house counsel and in most cases the wherewithal to defend themselves if they choose to do so. But when an individual doctor is sued, he or she finds it frightening and traumatic. Physicians do not have teams of lawyers in-house to defend them and their reputations. Hence, physicians are less likely than HMOs to cut corners in order to make a profit. Physicians are more averse to risk and more fearful of lawsuits than large corporations.

Staffing Underserved Areas

Certain remote rural areas and certain pockets in urban areas might find themselves lacking an adequate number of health-care providers. A volunteer system could be established—call it "HealthCorps"—wherein qualified generalists and specialists who have just completed their training would be recruited to help out in these underserved areas for two years. This system would not lower the standard of care because these same physicians would otherwise be practicing elsewhere.

As an inducement to join HealthCorps, participating physicians would receive some form of relief from the debt they incurred with student loans. Many physicians begin their professional careers with a debt load in the six figures. HealthCorps would be an attractive option for many young doctors. This program might also encourage low-income students to pursue a career in medicine.

Role of the Insurance Industry

Under our model, the insurance industry would play a significant role. It would underwrite coverage, handle actuarial calculations and other administrative functions, as well as provide stop-loss insurance, reinsurance, catastrophic insurance, liability insurance, and "wraparound insurance" for out-of-network and out-of-area coverage.

Other Alternatives

Congressman "Pete" Stark proposes for anyone to be able to buy into Medicare coverage by paying HCFA a certain premium per month, thus receiving the same care as Medicare beneficiaries. The "working poor" will receive subsidies from the government to buy into Medicare. This solution creates a single payor system which will simplify claims processing to a certain degree.

Another proposal is to have insurance coverage only for the expensive diagnostic procedures and hospitalizations, leaving patients to pay for office visits and consultations. However, these alternatives do not answer waste resulting from teams of claims processors within the system, inappropriate utilization, poor coordination of care, inadequate early intervention/disease management, and unnecessary admissions to hospitals and emergency room visits.

Implementation

It is not necessary for the whole nation to convert to this system overnight. It can coexist with other plans and be phased in slowly. The government can grant tax credits or other incentives to encourage large local provider groups to organize legally with proper infrastructure and personnel. In certain circumstances, insurance companies or large employers may be willing to sponsor or joint venture with large provider groups to adopt and develop this proposed plan. Without external stimulation, it is not easy to get large numbers of physicians working together ... like herding cats. Under this proposal there will be no need to debate in Congress regarding patients' ability to sue the health plans or employers. Medical decisions are made between patient and providers. We would have given physicians the ability to organize legally into large groups for certain economy of scale/negotiation and yet not violate antitrust statutes. That is free-market competition. It takes the need out of debating the Campbell Bill. Perhaps the Campbell Bill can be modified to promote this proposed plan.

Conclusion

There are many other health-care plans throughout the country. We believe none is as comprehensive as the plan we propose here, none designed the detailed steps to align incentives between regulators, insurers, payors, providers, and patients as well as minimize wasteful spending and restore trust among parties. Our plan ensures universal coverage and it would save an abundance of money that could be used to lower premiums and provide coverage for the 44 million uninsured Americans. Our goals and incentives are concordant with the desires of all parties concerned. Our plan places trust in and reliance on the free-market system which has benefited our country like no other. It eliminates the antagonism that exists between parties in the health-care industry. It can be phased in and it needs the support from government, insurers, and large employers. We estimate that under our model, the percentage of the gross domestic product consumed by health-care would fall below the current figure of 14%. No matter how health-care is financed or how much money is allocated to healthcare, until America develops a coherent delivery system that eliminates wasteful spending, restores trust, and aligns incentives between all parties, the chaos will not end.

REFERENCES

1. Gates W, Hemingway C. Business @ the Speed of Thought. Ch. 19. New York: Warner Books, 1999;333-55.
2. Lee KT, Lee MM: In-house data. MedWin of Connecticut, LLC.
3. Lee KJ, Colbert-Alvarez J, Lee ME: Survival in the era of managed care. In: Myers EN, ed. Advances in Otolaryngology–Head and Neck Surgery. Vol. 13. St. Louis: Mosby-Year Book, 1999: 353-68.
4. Lee KJ: How global capitation can calm chaos in healthcare markets. Am J Integrated Healthcare 1998; 1:101-3.

NOTE: Reader comments and opinions invited.—Ed.

Otolaryngology–Head and Neck Surgery (2009) 140, 775-781

INVITED ARTICLE

Healthcare: Affordable quality coverage for all

Keat Jin Lee, MD, New Haven, CT

No sponsorships or competing interests have been disclosed for this article.

ABSTRACT

The quality of medical care available in the United States is the best in the world. However, today's American healthcare delivery system is unacceptable. It is too expensive, disjointed, and wasteful. The amount spent on healthcare in the United States is sufficient to meet everyone's needs; the reason it does not is that the money is misspent. Healthcare makes up 16 percent of the gross domestic product, or $2.3 trillion, yet 46 million people are uninsured, the majority of people are underinsured, and even those with insurance suffer significant hassles in receiving healthcare. Medical errors occur at alarming rates. The lack of quality measures to define best practices leads to a wide variation of practices and costs. Fragmented healthcare leads to errors. The goal of this paper is to explore a set of 20 comprehensive steps to begin reform of healthcare in this country.

© 2009 American Academy of Otolaryngology–Head and Neck Surgery Foundation. All rights reserved.

Before healthcare costs began soaring, the physician and patient interacted in a confidential encounter. They discussed various treatment alternatives, including cost, convenience, risk, and benefit—and decisions were made.

The primacy of the doctor-patient relationship has been eroded over the past two decades, as insurers have demanded more power in determining how and what services are performed, as a way to control cost. While there is no question that insurers have succeeded in reducing fees paid per service, the level of success they have achieved in reducing over-utilization of healthcare services is in question. But the resulting substantial increase in costs for administration and paperwork is not. Between 20 percent and 30 percent of the healthcare dollar is currently spent on overhead, and if healthcare insurance profits are included, that percentage is even higher.[1] While payers have achieved success in reducing the fees paid per service, that savings has been eclipsed by the significantly higher costs of administering an extraordinarily complex payment system, and by profit margins causing rapidly increasing insurance premiums.

Unfortunately, the rise in influence of for-profit, third-party payers has also created an antagonistic relationship between payers and providers, as well as between payers and patients, with providers and patients resenting the power of individuals without sufficient medical training or familiarity with the cases to make decisions.

Simply putting more money into the healthcare system will not solve the problem, nor will shifting the economic burdens from one party to another (eg, state to federal, employers to employees). In 2004 we spent $1.7 trillion; in 2008 we spent $2.3 trillion, and we are worse off. Without comprehensive reform that seeks to change the manner in which healthcare services are paid for and to dramatically eliminate the waste brought on by obsolete paperwork, a bloated bureaucracy, and corporate overhead, the roots of the problem will never be solved. The cost of health care hinders America from competing in the world economy. Healthcare is intertwined with the economy, and we are afraid that if the situation is not remedied, the healthcare industry can implode in a way similar to the mortgage-financial industry. Fixing healthcare is investing in human capital. No single stakeholder is to be blamed for all the ills; there is plenty of blame to go around. We need the leadership to step in and step up for the patients. We present below 20 steps to positively reform healthcare. They include the following principles:

- Healthcare is a right, a commodity, and a service. We have to balance these three concepts.
- Coverage for all; no pre-existing disease exclusion. (Avoid the term "universal healthcare." It has been misconstrued as socialized medicine, big government.)
- Healthcare reform is about collaborating among stakeholders, not winning by a stakeholder.
- It should be a private system offering choices of doctors, hospitals, and insurance carriers.
- Decisions are made between the providers and the patients and not in the halls of Congress or the corporate offices of insurance companies.
- It is a private system with government oversight to control cost, improve quality and efficiency, and decrease abuse and excessive profits.
- No healthcare reform can be successful unless it also addresses the fee-for-service compensation system for providers, which rewards volume of services (utilization),

Received February 10, 2009; revised February 23, 2009; accepted March 3, 2009.

as opposed to a system that rewards good outcomes and being a good steward of the healthcare dollar.

20 STEPS TO SPENDING WISELY, WITH COMMON SENSE

1. Improve Transparency at All Levels for All Stakeholders

Transparency should be improved at all levels for all stakeholders so that consumers know the percentage of their healthcare dollar that is spent on patient care, administration, and profits. Just as in the case of the Federal Employee Health Benefit Program (FEHBP), and similar to public utility regulation or the Federal Reserve Board, there should be governmental oversight regulating the rate of increase of insurance premiums, copayments, and profit margins. The free market has not worked well in controlling the rate of increase of health insurance premiums. (Transparency about providers is discussed in Step 4.)

2. Simplify and Standardize Administration/Paperwork

There are currently countless incompatible and inconsistent forms and protocols to obtain approval for tests and treatment and to receive reimbursement from third-party payers. This requires each provider to have a staff team who do nothing but process paperwork to get permission to order a test or do a procedure and for reimbursement, not to mention the payers themselves who have large staffs solely for these administrative functions. A national standard is needed to simplify and standardize the administrative process for all government and commercial health plans. Simply creating a national standard and a streamlined, efficient system will result in substantial cost savings. Bill Gates estimated that 20 percent to 30 percent of the annual trillion-dollar cost of the U.S. healthcare system is for paperwork alone.[2]

3. Expand Medicare

Although in theory there is free market competition among insurance companies to help consumers, in reality there is such an unlevel playing field between insurance companies and consumers that consumers are helpless and frustrated. It is like the story of David and Goliath.

Allowing people under 65 years old to buy into Medicare by paying the premiums is a step forward. When there is healthcare insecurity and massive unhappiness, it is the government's responsibility to step in and offer a solution. This is not big government or socialized medicine. The patients continue to have their choice of doctors, hospitals, and other providers as well as having the choice to choose other commercial insurance over Medicare.

Besides, seniors and the disabled make up the current Medicare pool of patients, considered as "adverse risk pool." By adding younger, healthier working people, it will create a better-balanced risk pool.

4. Implement a New Compensation Formula for Providers That Ensures Quality and Appropriate Levels of Utilization, Outcome, and Patient Satisfaction

Quality assurance is pursued, measured, and ranked in almost every industry except medicine. The current "fee-for-service" system, which rewards over-utilization without regard to quality assurance, should be reformed. Any reform should link compensation to measures of quality, be it patient satisfaction or outcomes. It would be better to monitor quality than over-utilization. Utilization—the longstanding point of bitter contention between payers and providers—would be resolved. While insurers have a stake in under-utilization, providers have an inherent financial and clinical interest in over-utilization.

Reforming the traditional 100 percent "fee-for-service" model can resolve utilization issues, by calculating a portion of a provider's compensation based on methods other than fee-for-service. Currently, 100 percent of a provider's compensation is typically derived from the standard fee-for-service model. What if only 55 percent of a provider's compensation were based on a fee-for-service structure, but the remaining 45 percent were calculated differently? For example, 15 percent could be based on appropriate utilization, being a good steward of the healthcare dollar. The quantity and types of tests requested and procedures performed by a provider would then be reviewed to determine which doctors are prescribing appropriate levels of utilization and which ones are ordering unnecessary tests and procedures, with rewards going to providers who achieve appropriate standards of utilization. Another 15 percent of a provider's compensation could be based on patient satisfaction, as determined by validated surveys filled out by patients. Another 15 percent of total compensation could be based on outcomes achieved, as determined by a review of the health of the patient based on the provider's treatment plan, as well as comparing the provider's practice to evidence-based protocols. It is critical that outcome and utilization standards are based on science, not based on reducing the amounts the insurance companies have to pay for medical care.

Quality and evidenced-based medicine are like the "holy grail." One of the most pressing health policy concerns hinges on identifying what is effective and not effective clinical service.[3] Certain conditions are treated by primary care providers as well as by many different specialties, making it even harder to standardize diagnosis and treatment. The process outlined in Table 1 constitutes one methodology to arrive at evidence-based medicine or best practice. The new technology described in Step 6 can facilitate the implementation of best practices and evidence-based medicine. Table 2 illustrates five examples of quality indicators.

Appendix 2. Articles by Doctor Lee

Table 1
One method to arrive at "best practice"

Step 1	Identify the common ailments.
Step 2	Identify which type of providers diagnose and treat this ailment.
Step 3	Assemble a task force of no more than 15 and no fewer than 10 to represent each provider specialty to define the best, most cost-effective practice. The Cochrane Studies, etc, will be reviewed and debated.
Step 4	After a consensus is made, publish an Opinion Letter to be distributed to each group for comments, to be received within one month.
Step 5	Implement this as evidence-based medicine until amended in one or two years, or as new medical knowledge makes this Opinion Letter invalid.

At a glance, this method of compensation may appear to be labor-intensive. To facilitate this new compensation formula for providers, a web-based, secured, affordable electronic medical record system (EMR) described in Steps 5 and 6 is needed. With this technical tool, a reviewer can remotely study a statistically valid sample of a provider's patients periodically, instead of adjudicating every claim under today's 100 percent fee-for-service model. This will simplify the compensation process and decrease the 20 percent to 30 percent administrative costs. The provider can validate through the EMR that the analysis is accurate. Currently, analyzing pay-for-performance uses "claims and reimbursement data," not the clinical medical data through an electronic medical record system. Using claims data rather than clinical data from electronic medical records is an inaccurate method to study utilization.

The 55 percent fee-for-service component needs to be in place to avoid the mistake some payers made when providers were paid 100 percent on a "per capita, per patient, per month basis," which resulted in patients having difficulty getting a face-to-face appointment with the provider.

In *addition* to the formula mentioned above, to align financial incentives with patients' health would be to pay certain providers an *additional* compensation to serve as a primary care or "homeroom/quarterback" coordinating provider for the patient—to perform disease management for chronic illnesses, practice preventive medicine, and serve as a "gateway" to coordinate all of that patient's care with specialists as necessary. (This is not to be confused with the concept of a "gatekeeper," employed by some payers, which requires a patient with a broken leg, for example, to see a primary care physician to get a referral in order to be able to see a specialist. That "gatekeeper" system has proven to be costly and unwieldy for the patient and the system.) The coordinating provider would be paid to help patients make intelligent decisions about obtaining healthcare services without having a financial incentive to over-utilize. This additional compensation and its significant role would also help to encourage medical students to become primary care physicians, of which there is an acute shortage.

The simple goal of those proposals is to explore new ways in which providers can be paid that leads to appropriate levels of utilization and improved patient health. We may evolve into another model that uses large multispecialty provider groups. However, it would be difficult to implement that model for the whole nation at this time.

There is more than a financial incentive for physicians to participate in this new compensation formula. Physicians have been complaining for years about loss of autonomy, the mass confusion, and the "hassle factor." For example, in order to obtain prior authorization, physicians usually must call an 800 number. All too often, the party on the other end of the line has no idea what the physician is talking about. A single phone call can take as long as 45 minutes to precertify a single diagnostic test or treatment, and getting disconnected is a frequent problem.

Under our model, physicians and patients would regain the right to make their own decisions. There will be no "precertification" or having someone second-guessing decisions made between patients and providers. Providers will be compensated in a more progressive and much-stream-

Table 2
Examples of quality indicators

A. Surgery
1. Did the responsible surgeon meet with the unsedated patient, or if the patient is sedated, with a member of the family to reconfirm the type, the site, and the side of the operation in the presence of the operating room nurse and anesthesiologist/anesthetist?
2. In an elective procedure, did the responsible surgeon have a preop visit with the patient before the day of surgery, going over the indications for surgery, the alternative treatments, the risks of surgery, and the potential complications?

B. Laboratory medicine
1. Did the technician drawing blood from a patient label the blood tubes first and then draw the blood from that patient? Alternatively, did the technician draw the blood and label the tubes right in front of the patient before moving on to other duties?
2. When a specimen is passed on from the doctor's office or operating room to a courier to take the specimen to the laboratory, is there a "receipt system" acknowledging accountability for the specimen?
3. Does the doctor ordering a diagnostic test have a "tracking system" to make sure he/she receives the result in a timely manner and inform the patient in a timely manner?

lined process, eliminating the labor-intensive chore of debating individual claims. This will reduce the 20 percent to 30 percent administrative costs.[1,2]

We can bring more accountability into the Medicare reimbursement system. Currently the Medicare (CMS) payment formula for providers, Sustainable Growth Rate (SGR), is budget neutral, which means that if the payment for a particular service is increased or if the frequency for that particularly service increases, the payment for services in all specialties and primary care are decreased to keep the Medicare budget neutral. To make primary care and each specialty more accountable, we can alter the formula to have the budget neutrality principle apply to primary care's bucket and each specialty's bucket.

5. Establish "Homeroom/Quarterback" Provider to Coordinate Care

An expensive failing of the current system is that treatment among providers is fragmented and uncoordinated, and communication is lacking. Implementing the "homeroom/quarterback" coordinating provider mentioned above will help alleviate the problem. Further, when a patient today is referred by one physician to another, typically the patient's chart and test results will not accompany them, leading to either extensive clerical time spent calling, obtaining, photocopying and sending the chart, or simply duplication of costly tests that have already been performed. Without all of the patient's data readily accessible, treatment protocols are instituted that are not synchronized with those of other physicians. To decrease fragmentation and increase efficiency, the development of a secured, user-friendly, and confidential EMR system, accessible to all providers, can lead to coordinated care and reduce medical errors caused by a lack of up-to-date patient information.

6. Deploy Affordable, Secured, Confidential, Web-Based, User-Friendly Electronic Medical Records (EMR) with Interconnectivity

Bringing the health information system into the 21st century is essential to achieving healthcare reform. Levinson pointed out the shortcomings of the EMR being deployed today.[5] Later technology is able to centralize and catalog medical records for all patients in an affordable, secured, confidential, web-based data warehouse, utilizing user-friendly interfaces for input and retrieval of information. To assure its ease of use, it needs to be a hybrid of digitization and image preservation (the use of scanners). In a 2007 article, Lee described the user interface as intuitive, utilizing cyberspace filing cabinets and cyberspace gateways to other providers' medical records.[6,7] In medicine, unlike accounting, not all data should be digitized. While maintaining confidentiality through encryption, screen names, patient numbers, and passwords controlled by the patient (or perhaps iris/retina scan, or finger/palm print), all authorized providers would have immediate access to the complete information on each patient. Until the public feels comfortable with the security and privacy issues, psychiatric, addiction, and HIV data will not be stored in this EMR. Health information technology is needed to improve quality through the practice of evidence-based medicine, preventive medicine, and disease management. Automatic "test tracking" will coordinate all the tests that have been ordered by any provider, ensuring that no tests are overlooked or abnormal results ignored. Artificial intelligence is to be incorporated to facilitate practice guidelines. EMR can increase transparency by enabling utilization and outcomes to be tracked and analyzed—making it easier for evidence-based or utilization-based compensation and other alternative methods of compensating providers (see Step 4). A RAND Corporation study estimated that the savings from an EMR system could be as much as $77 billion annually. Bringing the health information system into the 21st century is the cornerstone to reform healthcare, reduce cost and errors, and increase quality.

7. Create a Unique Healthcare Identifier Number

Creating a unique healthcare identifier number for each person will increase efficiency, accuracy, and the security of exchanging vital medical information among authorized caregivers, without requiring patients to reveal their social security numbers, currently used as identifiers.

8. Deploy More Specialized Advanced Nurse Practitioners and Specialized Physician Assistants (Mid-Level Providers)

A substantial portion of a physician's time involves treating patients who can be equally well cared for by mid-level providers, if they are appropriately linked to physicians through telemedicine embedded in the EMR system. Increased use of mid-level providers who work closely with physicians can increase the efficiency of patient care while reducing costs. However, if these mid-level providers are not linked to doctors physically in the same office or through real-time telemedicine, errors can happen. Funding for the training of nurse practitioners and physician assistants should be increased, which will in turn create new job opportunities.

We believe a properly organized network of physician supervising through telemedicine embedded in an EMR system can make the so-called WalMart pharmacies' "Retail Health Clinics" staffed by mid-level providers work with high quality and reduce costs.

We emphasize "specialized" mid-level provider, because to maintain quality, a mid-level provider needs to have additional training (six months) in a specialty in which he or she is going to practice.

9. Implement a System of Early Intervention and Disease Management

Healthcare costs can be further reduced by minimizing medical problems through early intervention and disease management. Patients with serious chronic illnesses should be flagged early by providers and receive follow-up care from an advanced nurse practitioner, such as by calling these patients periodically to monitor their health, reminding them to take their medication, and providing further instruction. If the nurse suspects any trouble, a home or office visit should be arranged immediately. Early intervention can be very helpful in preventing diseases from progressing to the point that routine care is no longer sufficient, requiring expensive measures as well as causing further pain and suffering. To be successful, we need a real time, secured web-based, user-friendly electronic medical record system.

10. Improve Costly, Inefficient Emergency Rooms

One of the biggest contributors to waste in the current system is unnecessary emergency room visits. Having a "homeroom/quarterback" coordinating provider (mentioned above) will decrease unnecessary emergency room (ER) visits. An EMR system will enable the ER provider to understand the patient's health better and potentially avoid repeating unnecessary tests. In addition, emergency procedures could be improved and cost reduced by better organization of patient flow into 1) trauma/real emergencies; 2) non-emergencies; and 3) triage, for patients who are in between trauma and non-emergency, conducted by an experienced doctor who can make an accurate diagnosis without ordering unnecessary tests, and who would not miss an emergency condition. Under the current system, the triage function is often performed by a less experienced doctor.

11. Promote Public Health Education and Establish a Wellness Corps

Preventive medicine, emphasizing screening for early detection of disease and promoting wellness, nutrition, exercise, and lifestyle changes, saves lives and saves costs. We should implement a Wellness Corps, similar to JFK's Peace Corps, in which young graduates can serve in all communities promoting healthy lifestyles, to reduce obesity and other chronic diseases. The public should be educated that some medical services, tests, and procedures are not only unnecessary but have the potential to cause harm. Ongoing public service campaigns would be helpful to educate and change attitudes about medical services, as such campaigns have done with attitudes about smoking and drunk driving. For example, the public should learn that overuse of antibiotics leads to drug resistance, that taking unneeded medications exposes patients to unnecessary side effects, that x-rays and MRIs are not risk-free, and that surgery should almost always be the last resort.

12. Reduce the Cost of Pharmaceuticals

Pharmaceutical costs can be reduced by 1) increasing the availability of safe generic drugs; 2) allowing safe reimportation of drugs made in the United States and sold at lower prices in other countries; 3) working with the World Trade Organization (WTO) so that other developed countries help shoulder the cost of research and development by paying the same price for drugs as in the United States; 4) allowing Medicare to negotiate with pharmaceutical companies; 5) reducing media advertisements to consumers; 6) reducing the marketing costs of gifts and perks to providers; and 7) increasing translational research, thus bringing new drugs more quickly from the laboratories to the bedside.

13. Eliminate Pre-existing Disease Exclusions

There will be no pre-existing disease exclusion under our proposal. In order to make this economically viable, everyone needs to pay for insurance, be covered by a government program, or pay into a pool. (See Step 14, below.)

14. Expand Coverage Through a Purchasing Consortium, Insurance Exchange, Federal Employees Health Benefit Program, School-Based Clinics, and Making Coverage Portable

Coverage needs to be expanded to those who are uninsured, and there are many ways to accomplish this goal. Every baby should leave the hospital not only with a birth certificate and a name, but with health insurance as well.

One step is to modify the welfare system so that it would provide different levels of welfare coverage according to the recipient's financial status; some would qualify for a complete welfare package; others would receive only health coverage. This model is practiced in some states.

Our possibility is to help single working persons and small employers join together and form a healthcare purchasing consortium/exchange, or to buy into a program like the FEHBP. Such a consortium could be organized according to neighborhoods, towns, occupation, or any other common denominator. Coverage might also be obtained through business coalitions such as the Council of Smaller Enterprises and the local Chamber of Commerce. Another suggestion was that persons under 65 be allowed to buy into Medicare. All employers should be required to provide healthcare coverage for their workers. The burden on small businesses could be alleviated by tax breaks and/or other benefits. Everyone insists that health insurance should be portable without penalty when changing jobs. Those who refuse to purchase coverage, preferring to take the risk and pay for healthcare out of pocket as needed, would be required to pay an amount into a pool.

The use of school-based health clinics to treat certain ailments and to immunize schoolchildren could prove to be convenient and save costs. The human resources and the physical spaces are already here and part of the education budget. The nurse practitioners at the school-based clinic can be linked through telemedicine embedded in the EMR record to obtain consultations with physicians.

It is suggested that providers giving humanitarian, uncompensated care in indigent/rural/disaster-stricken communities be granted license reciprocity between the home state of the provider and the state needing humanitarian care. They also requested the same professional liability protection similar to providers caring for the armed forces. Currently, many providers give humanitarian uncompensated care abroad because they are unable to do so within our country because of the two aforementioned issues.

15. Establish Parity for All—Rich and Poor, Young and Old, Working and Unemployed, Different Ethnicity; and Parity for Mental Health Services

Any reform plan should strive to achieve parity for all, regardless of income, age, race, or working status.[6,9] We have to pay more attention to mental health. It is not only a healthcare issue, it impacts greatly on the workforce and families.

When Medicare and Medicaid reimbursements are reasonable, all licensed providers will be obligated to accept Medicare and Medicaid patients.

16. Establish Sensible Tort Reform

Frivolous and costly litigation raises the cost of healthcare for everyone. Ways need to be explored to reduce this component of healthcare costs by limiting meritless lawsuits, as has been done, for example, in the area of securities litigation reform. The Fair & Reliable Medical Justice Account mentioned by Senator Baucus in his "Call to Action, Health Reform 2009"[d] should be considered. We need to explore avenues to grant immunity to someone who steps forward and admits his or her mistake. Learning from our errors can prevent future errors, estimated to save billions of dollars and save lives. Similarly, once we have established evidence-based quality guidelines, when a patient has a poor outcome although the provider has followed the established guidelines, the provider should not be sued. The fear of being sued costs the healthcare system billions of dollar in unnecessary tests and second opinions.

17. Establish Health Corps to Staff Underserved Areas

Areas that are lacking in adequate numbers of healthcare providers (some rural and inner-city areas) should be addressed by establishing a volunteer system such as the "HealthCorps," wherein qualified generalists and specialists who have completed their training would serve in these underserved areas for two years. This system would not lower the standard of care because these same physicians would otherwise be practicing in better-served areas. Besides salaries and benefits, as an inducement to joining the HealthCorps, participating physicians would receive relief from student loan debt, thus also encouraging individuals from less affluent backgrounds to go into medicine.

Medical schools are partially funded by the government. Medicare, through its reimbursements to hospitals, pays for postgraduate education of doctors. Hence, it could be argued that residents should be required to serve (with compensation) in underserved areas for two years, or perform translational or evidence-based research at the National Institutes of Health (NIH). They would also have their student loans forgiven. In the 1960s and 1970s, all doctors were required to serve in the armed forces or in the U.S. Public Health Services, or to do research at NIH for two years.

18. Deploy Appropriate Use of Copayments

Patient copayments are not a new idea, but another method to minimize over-utilization; they should be high enough to discourage unnecessary care, but reasonable enough to be affordable. It has also been pointed out that copayments punish the sick who can least afford the copay.

19. Establish Sensible End-of-Life Care and Living Wills

It has been said that 80 percent of one's healthcare expenditure could be spent in the weeks before life ends. As a nation, we need to deliberate on how to handle end-of-life care, not to ration, but to spend the healthcare dollar wisely. Everyone should be strongly encouraged or required to have a living will stored in his or her electronic medical record.

20. Establish Teaching Ethics to Medical and Paramedical Personnel

Teaching ethics early and reinforcing such teachings later to medical and paramedical personnel would promote a culture that discourages over-utilization and promotes an emphasis on quality healthcare that achieves good medical outcomes for patients.

CONCLUSION

No matter how healthcare is financed or how much money is allocated to it, the problem will not be solved until America develops a coherent delivery system that eliminates wasteful spending, restores trust, and aligns incentives between all parties through a compensation formula for providers, based not solely on volume but also on quality (outcome, customer service) and stewardship of the healthcare dollar. Lasting reform will require presidential leadership to step in and step up to make some significant, innovative changes, and to bring together all stakeholders for the benefit of the nation. We need common sense for uncommon times.

Besides creating the Federal Health Board,[9] perhaps the President can appoint two dependable, detail-oriented people to help: 1) a Healthcare Reform Coordinator who can work with all the stakeholders, and who understands the ins and outs of how the best (not perfect) system can function and who pays attention to the details of implementation to have as smooth a transition as possible; and 2) a Health Information Technology Coordinator to supervise the refinement and implementation of a secured, confidential, user-friendly, low-cost, web-based electronic medical record system that offers real-time connectivity to other systems. It should be a system with artificial intelligence that can also incorporate evidence-based medicine and be used to mine the data for analysis (again, in a secured manner) protecting the privacy of patients.

Having a great vision and policy is important; however, "the devil is in the details." We need to have knowledgeable, common-sense people to implement it. As a country, we have strayed from common sense and become overcome with greed. Just as fire can cook our food and keep us warm, but can also destroy our homes, proper implementation of reform can help us, but improper implementation can destroy the system.

AUTHOR INFORMATION

From the Yale University School of Medicine and the Hospital of St. Raphael.

Corresponding author: K. J. Lee, MD. Chief of Otolaryngology, Yale University School of Medicine, 98 York Street, New Haven, CT 06511.

E-mail address: kjleemd@aol.com

AUTHOR CONTRIBUTION

Kwai Jin Lee, sole author.

DISCLOSURE

Competing interests: None.

Sponsorships: None.

REFERENCES

1. Woolhandler S, Campbell T, Hermulstein D. Costs of healthcare administration in the US and Canada. N Engl J Med 2003;349(8):768-74.
2. Gates W, Hemingway C. Business @ the speed of thought. New York: Warner Books; 1999. p. 333-55.
3. Eden J, Wheatley B, McNeil B, et al. Knowing what works in healthcare. Washington, DC: National Academic Press; 2008. p. 33-56.
4. Lee KJ, Lee M. Universal healthcare, a bold proposal. Conn Med 2000 Aug;64(8):485-91.
5. Levinson SR. Practical EHR. Electronic record solutions for compliance and quality care. Chicago: AMA Press; June 30, 2008.
6. Lee KJ. Electronic medical records (EMR)—The train has left the station. ENT News July-Aug 2007. Vol. 16 No. 3.
7. Lee KJ. Helpful practical points on electronic medical records from the patient's point of view. The Tide Lines July 2008; Vol 10, #1.
8. Baucus M, U.S. Senator (D) (Montana) Chair, Senate Finance Committee. Call for Action, Health Reform 2009. US Congress White Paper. November 12, 2008.
9. Daschle T. Critical: What we can do about the health-care crisis. New York: St. Martin's Press; 2008.

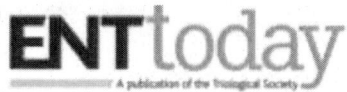

Hybrid Physician Payment System Can Ensure Quality, Customer Service

November 5, 2014

I read with great interest the front page article by Thomas R. Collins ("Medicare Payment Data Release Concerns Some Otolaryngologists") published in the August 2014 issue of *ENTtoday*, as well as the article by Win Whitcomb, MD, MHM, ("Physician Pay Shifts from Volume to Value") published in the same issue. Both discussed physician compensation.

It appears that two initiatives are going to happen: pay for performance and the application of clinical guidelines. In most walks of life, people are evaluated for their performance and, oftentimes, compensation is linked to such evaluation. In most industries, there are standardized, acceptable ways, or a range of ways, to perform a job well. Clinical guidelines are being developed at a steady rate by academic institutions and organized medicine. If we do not craft these guidelines, nonmedical entities will impose their guidelines upon us. Much as we prefer not to have cookbook medicine, we can embrace well-crafted guidelines that allow for legitimate deviation. Current software is available to track the data.

It is the consensus that a "fee for service" or "pay for volume" model is not sustainable in the U.S. Capitation, ACO, and similar formulas being proposed do not solve the problem; in fact, they can create new problems.

The closest model is the so-called hybrid payment system (HPS). HPS takes into account human nature. It incentivizes the providers to be accessible on one hand and good stewards of the healthcare dollar on the other hand. As consumers, we all want quality, customer service, and "bang for our buck." The HPS comes the closest to fulfilling the consumer's wish. Besides, we are patients, or, someday, we will be patients, consumers of healthcare. The HPS incorporates the use of good clinical guidelines. As a collateral benefit, we can slowly affect tort reform. If the provider follows the guideline and an untoward event happens, the filing of a suit should not be permitted, or it should at least be a powerful aid in the defense.

The HPS keeps the fee-for-service payment system; however, instead of paying 100% of the claims, X% of the claims, which can range from 70% to 99%, is paid within one week from the date of claim, with no denial and no hassles. This will decrease unnecessary administrative costs on the payers' side and on the providers' side. Every quarter, the payer and the provider will review online the electronic medical records of a small but statistically significant number of the provider's patients to measure the provider's performance based on how he/she follows the practice guidelines. It is not cookbook medicine. Current technology allows physicians to deviate from the guidelines, documenting good reasons for the deviation to avoid a bad score. Depending on the results of this evaluation, the provider will get Y% of the claims or part of Y%.

Once we decide what X% is, we can decide what Y% of the claims will be. If X% is 70%, Y% can range from 40% to 0%. X% + Y% can be equal to 110% or less.

A quality, cost-effective doctor who does not underutilize or overutilize will get paid 110% of the maximum allowable fee. He/she will not only get the full value of the claims, but a 10% bonus can be added. Those who score lower will get paid between 70% and 100% of the claims.

HPS also borrows but modifies the principle of "HMOs withholding" of a prior era. In the eighties, the return of the "withhold" depended on the total performance of all the providers in the network and the financial health of the HMO. In this new HPS, each provider is measured according to his/her own performance. Hence, we are holding each provider accountable for his/her actions according to the criteria set by pay for performance. His or her compensation is thus not dependent on other physician performances.

The old "capitation model" or putting providers on salary without incentive will lead to less "access" for the patients, encouraging underutilization as well as making the provider want to pass the patient on to another provider (or refer to another specialty) to take care of and incurring unnecessary extra medical visits.

This HPS methodology will decrease cost without compromising quality and access. Once rational payment systems are adopted, providers will have no conflict with their conscience to overutilize and upcode, or underutilize or limit patient access. HPS is not going to be perfect at the beginning, but once we work with it, we can amend and improve it.

K.J. Lee, MD
Associate Clinical Professor
Yale Medical School
New Haven, Conn.

Medical Economics AHCA

Here's how to reduce healthcare costs

May 09, 2017
By KJ Lee MD FACS

The recent White House-Congressional fiasco epitomizes the lack of basic understanding regarding healthcare and healthcare reform.

Further reading: Cost, not access, is underlying problem facing American healthcare

Obamacare (ACA) and the Republicans' AHCA, each with its pros and cons, are more like "health insurance coverage reform" or "healthcare payers reform" rather than healthcare reform for patients. Offering "coverage" is different than offering "real access" to receive efficient, quality, compassionate healthcare in a timely manner.

Just because someone has an insurance, Medicare or Medicaid card, does not necessarily help him or her get an appointment for treatment in an efficient, timely manner. In addition, it does not guarantee the patient can afford the co-pay or deductible required before he or she is examined. The goal of our healthcare solution is to offer access at a sensible price.

> "Just because someone has an insurance, Medicare or Medicaid card, does not necessarily help him or her get an appointment for treatment in an efficient, timely manner."

In 2004, the United States spent $1.7 trillion on healthcare.[1] In 2008, we spent $2.3 trillion, or 16% of Gross Domestic Product (GDP). In 2016, we spent more than $3 trillion. It is not that we are not spending enough money on healthcare, the problem is that we are not spending the money wisely. There is wastage, redundancy, inefficiency, bureaucracy, and perhaps, even charging more than necessary in some sectors. We have to align the long-term incentives of insurers, payers, providers and patients. We need to restore trust between parties. Otherwise, we shall continue to be in chaos regardless of how much money we spend in healthcare. We are reshuffling the deck chairs on the sinking Titanic.

Hot topic: House Obamacare bill won't fix healthcare system, doctors say

As Warren Buffett once told me at a dinner meeting, "each person comes to Washington to look for more money in healthcare; no one comes to Washington to reduce the unsustainable skyrocketing cost of healthcare." This skyrocketing cost has already made us less competitive in the world economy. It is not necessary for finger pointing. If we all collaborate, it can be achieved without too much sacrifice from each sector of the healthcare industry.

The following is a plan to reduce healthcare cost by 28%, making it much more affordable. This will make "healthcare insurance coverage reform" and "healthcare payers reform" easier. Thus, a "replacement" or "improvement" of ACA can be achieved less acrimoniously.

Next: Streamlining and expanding Medicare

I. Streamline the current manner in which providers bill insurance companies, Medicare, Medicaid or patients. It is a very convoluted and expensive system. To illustrate simply: A $100 item is billed out between $1,500 and $2,000 or sometimes more. After months of back and forth and mountains of paperwork, consuming millions of hours of computer time, the bill is settled for $125.32, part of which is paid by the insurance carrier or Medicare and part of it by the patient's co-pay or deductible. There is a simpler way.

President Bill Clinton once said that eliminating this mountain of paperwork could save 30% of the healthcare dollar. To be conservative, simplifying the medical billing system would save at least 20% of the healthcare dollar, bringing relief to both the payers and the providers...a win-win situation. The poor patients would be relieved.

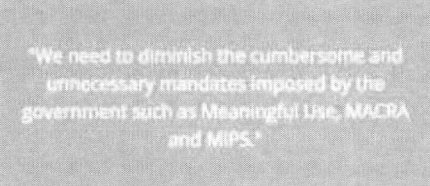

"We need to diminish the cumbersome and unnecessary mandates imposed by the government such as Meaningful Use, MACRA and MIPS."

II. The surge of hospitals charging very high "facility fees" has exacerbated the skyrocketing cost of healthcare. It is not uncommon that the facility fee is 5 to 10 times the fee charged by the doctor for an office visit, which does not require the use of an operating room, emergency room, intensive care unit or an admission for an overnight stay in the hospital.

Further reading: Medicaid expansion must remain safe in healthcare reform

III. A certain percentage of non-cosmetic elective surgeries, not tests, may be unnecessary. This amount is considered enough not only to raise the cost of healthcare, but also causes pain and suffering, potential complications and absenteeism from work. I realize each surgeon believes that she or he does not perform such unnecessary surgery, it is the other guy. Medical Societies have started to produce evidence-based clinical guidelines to decrease unnecessary surgeries. Introducing appropriate common sense, non-draconian "pay for value" instead of "pay for volume" reimbursement could be the first step to decrease healthcare costs, or perhaps, a hybrid of the two methods. At the same time, we need to diminish the cumbersome and unnecessary mandates imposed by the government such as Meaningful Use, MACRA and MIPS. As one national leader advocates, too much regulation stifles productivity. There is a simple way to achieve value.

IV. A pill produced by the same company is sold in the U.S. at a cost multiple times of the same pill sold in other countries. We understand fully that the cost of developing a new drug is prohibitive. Is there a solution for all parties if we all work together? We should take a good look at the arduous process of developing a new drug. Will the application of a modified "favorite nation clause" help? We need Solomon's wisdom to create a win-win for industry and patients.

In case you missed it: Fight not over to preserve ideal patient care, says ACP

V. Expanding Medicare for younger and healthier people to buy into it will help to sustain and stabilize Medicare. We are not proposing free healthcare for all. As it is, Medicare has an adverse selection actuarially of its members. Insurance companies, expert on actuarial science, are needed at the table to decrease healthcare costs.

VI. Rather than allocating different budgets for Medicaid, block grants, debating whether it is federally or state funded, could we explore the mechanism for all licensed providers to donate a percentage of their time and resources to take care of the less privileged, the way it was done in the '50s and '60s?

Next: We are all patients, whether in the past, present or in the future

We could expand the system to encourage more recently qualified doctors to serve in the U.S. HealthCorps for two years, caring for the less privileged and in areas having insufficient doctors. In return, these doctors could get their student loan forgiven. Besides, it gives these doctors great satisfaction and experience like those who served in the armed forces or U.S. public health services prior to the 1970s.

Further reading: Uncertainty in healthcare driving DPC growth

VII. Deploy telemedicine. The current sporadic practice of medicine through e-mails and text messages can create slipshod medicine leading to errors. Both patients and providers can be distracted while e-mailing or texting and there is no opportunity to dialogue properly. Instead, introduce a new method, deploying virtual visits via Skype or FaceTime at an appointed time so that both patients and providers are concentrating. This also creates the appropriate medical record keeping. The provider should be compensated but at a more cost-effective rate, as overhead may be lower. This will decrease healthcare cost and make it more convenient for both providers and patients. Furthermore, the patients do not have to miss work.

VIII. We should also deploy more nurse practitioners and physician assistants who are well trained in the specialty in which they practice. It has been pointed out that a generalized nurse practitioner or physician assistant can lower the quality of healthcare. A well supervised specialty trained nurse practitioner or physician assistant can lower the total healthcare cost for the country and at the same time maintain quality of care as well as improve access. Another win-win.

Hot topic: Why are women leaving medicine?

IX. The modern health information technology with "machine learning," artificial intelligence, more user friendly interface and enhanced connectivity between providers, e.g. the Department of Defense and the Veterans Administration can facilitate aspects of the above to cut costs and increase efficiency.

The above is not a panacea to completely cure our healthcare chaos. It took us decades to get here, but if we all chip in, we can reduce healthcare costs by at least 28% of over $3 trillion without significantly compromising, and instead, increasing the quality of healthcare.

Simplifying the medical billing alone can save 20% of healthcare cost, helping payers and providers achieve a win-win. The above could be a first step to bring parties together in a round table to improve healthcare for the patients. We are all patients, whether in the past, present or in the future. Once Democrats and Republicans, conservatives and liberals, work together on the above nine points for the common good, the debate on ACA and AHCA will hopefully be more cordial.

Reference:

1. Otolarygology-Head and Neck Surgery (2009) 140, 775

* * *

IDEAS FOR THE ADMINISTRATION AND CONGRESS TO LOOK AT HEALTHCARE REFORM FROM ANOTHER PERSPECTIVE

The recent White House-Congressional fiasco epitomizes the lack of basic understanding regarding healthcare and healthcare reform. The so-called Obama Care (ACA) or the Republicans' AHCA, each with its pros and cons, is more of a "health insurance coverage reform" or "healthcare payors reform" rather than healthcare reform to take care of the patients. Offering "coverage" is different than offering "real access" to receive efficient, quality, compassionate, healthcare in a timely manner. Just because someone has an insurance, Medicare or Medicaid card, does not necessarily help him/her get an appointment for treatment in an efficient, timely manner. In addition, it does not guarantee the patient can afford the co-pay or deductible required before he/she is examined. The goal is to offer access at a sensible price.

In 2004, the United States spent 1.7 trillion dollars in healthcare. In 2008, we spent 2.3 trillion dollars or 16% of Gross Domestic Product (GDP). In 2016, we spent over 3 trillion dollars. Hence, it is not that we are not spending enough money on healthcare, the problem is that we are not spending the money wisely. There is wastage, redundancy, inefficiency, bureaucracy, and perhaps, even charging more than necessary in some sectors. We have to align the long-term incentives of insurers, payors, providers and patients. We need to restore trust between parties. Otherwise, we shall continue to be in chaos regardless of how much money we spend in healthcare. We are reshuffling the deck chairs on the sinking Titanic. As Warren Buffet once told me at a dinner meeting, "Each person comes to Washington to look for more money in healthcare, no one comes to Washington to reduce the unsustainable sky rocketing cost of healthcare." This skyrocketing cost has already made us less competitive in the world economy. If unchecked, it will get worse unless all segments of the healthcare industry work collaboratively, to reduce inefficiency and waste. It is not necessary for finger pointing. It can be achieved without too much sacrifice from each sector of the healthcare industry.

The following will outline a plan to reduce healthcare cost by 28%, making it much more affordable. This will make "healthcare insurance coverage reform" and "healthcare payors reform" easier. Thus, a "replacement" or "improvement" of ACA can be achieved less acrimoniously.

I. We can start by streamlining the current manner in which providers bill insurance companies, Medicare, Medicaid or patients. It is a very convoluted expensive system. To illustrate simply: A $100 item is billed out between $1,500 and $2,000 or sometimes more. After months of back and forth and mountains of paperwork, consuming millions of hours of computer time, and after many months, the bill is settled for $125.32, part of which is paid by the insurance carrier or Medicare and part of it by the patient's co-pay or deductible. As in most other industries, there is a simpler way. President Clinton once said that eliminating this mountain of paperwork could save 30% of the healthcare dollar. To be conservative, simplifying the medical billing system would save at least 20% of the healthcare dollar, bringing relief to both the payors and the providers.....a win-win situation. The poor patients would be relieved.

II. The surge of hospitals charging very high so called "facility fees" has exacerbated the sky rocketing cost of healthcare. It is not uncommon that the "facility fee" is 5 to 10 times the fee charged by the doctor for an office visit which does not require the use of an operating room, emergency room, intensive care unit, or an admission for an overnight stay in the hospital.

III. It has been estimated that a certain percentage of non-cosmetic elective surgeries, not tests, may be unnecessary. This amount is considered enough not only to raise the cost of healthcare, but also causes pain and suffering, potential complications and absenteeism from work. I realize, each surgeon believes that she/he does not perform such unnecessary surgery, it is the other guy. This article is not to point fingers but to bring us together "to heal" the system. Medical Societies have started to produce evidence based clinical guidelines to decrease so called unnecessary surgeries. Introducing appropriate common sense, non draconian "pay for value" instead of "pay for volume" reimbursement could be the first step to decrease healthcare costs, or perhaps, a hybrid of the two methods. At the same time, we need to diminish the cumbersome and unnecessary mandates imposed by the government such as Meaningful Use, MACRA, MIPS. As one national leader advocates, too much regulations stifle productivity. There is a simple way to achieve value.

IV. How do we deal with the cost of pharmaceutical products? A pill produced by the same company is sold in the US multiple times the cost of the same pill sold in other countries. The common drugs like the epi pen, have skyrocketed in price. We understand fully that the cost of developing a new drug is prohibitive. Is there a solution for all parties if we all, as US citizens, as human beings, work together? We should take a good look at the arduous process of developing a new drug. Will the application of a modified "favorite nation clause" help? We need Solomon's wisdom to create a win-win for industry and patients.

V. Expanding Medicare for younger and healthier people to buy into it will help to sustain and stabilize Medicare. As it is, Medicare has an adverse selection of its members. Insurance companies, expert on actuarial science, are needed at the table to decrease healthcare costs.

VI. Rather than different budgets for Medicaid, block grants, debating whether it is federally or state funded, could we explore the mechanism for all licensed providers to donate X% of their time and resources to take care of the less privileged the way it was done in the 50's and 60's? Perhaps we could expand the system to encourage more recently qualified doctors to serve in the US HealthCorp for 2 years caring for the less privileged and in areas having insufficient doctors. In return, these doctors will get their student loan forgiven. Besides, it gives these doctors great satisfaction and experience like those who served in the Armed Forces or US Public Health Services prior to the 1970's.

VII. Deploy tele-medicine. The current sporadic practice of medicine through e-mails and text messages can create "slip shot" medicine leading to errors. Both patients and providers can be distracted while e-mailing or texting and there is no opportunity to dialogue properly. Instead, introduce a new method, deploying virtual visits like skype or face time at an appointed time so that both patients and providers are concentrating. This also creates the appropriate medical record keeping. The provider should be compensated but at a more cost effective rate, as overhead may be lower. This will decrease healthcare cost and make it more convenient for both providers and patients. Furthermore, the patients do not have to miss work.

VIII. We should also deploy more nurse practitioners and physician assistants who are well trained in the specialty in which they practice. It has been pointed out that a generalized nurse practitioner or physician assistant can lower the quality of healthcare. A well supervised specialty trained nurse practitioner or physician assistant can lower the total healthcare cost for the country and at the same time maintain quality of care as well as improve access. Another win-win.

IX. The modern health information technology with "machine learning", "artificial intelligence", more user friendly interface (UX) and enhanced connectivity between providers, e.g. the Department of Defense and the VA can facilitate aspects of the above to cut costs and increase efficiency.

The above is not a panacea to completely cure our healthcare chaos. It took us decades to get here. If we all chip in, it will reduce healthcare costs by at least 28% of over 3 trillion dollars without compromising, but in fact, increasing the quality of healthcare. Simplifying the medical billing alone can save 20% of healthcare cost, helping payors and providers, a win-win. The above could be a first step to bring parties together in a round table to improve healthcare for the patients. We are all patients, in the past, now, or will be in the future. Once Democrats and Republicans, conservatives and liberals, work together on the above nine points for the common good, because it is the right thing to do, the debate on ACA and AHCA will hopefully be more cordial.

The Sublabial Transseptal Transsphenoidal Approach to the Hypophysis.

KEAT-JIN LEE, M.D., F.A.C.S.,

New Haven, Conn.

PUBLISHED BY

THE LARYNGOSCOPE

EDITORIAL OFFICE:
517 South Euclid Avenue
St. Louis, Mo. 63110, U.S.A.

BUSINESS OFFICE:
9216 Clayton Road, Suite 18
St. Louis, Mo. 63124, U.S.A.

THE SUBLABIAL TRANSSEPTAL TRANSSPHENOIDAL APPROACH TO THE HYPOPHYSIS.*

KEAT-JIN LEE, M.D., F.A.C.S.,
New Haven, Conn.

ABSTRACT.

A simple and safe technique for the sublabial transseptal transsphenoidal approach to the hypophysis and parasellar region is described. A review of the literature reveals that this technique and other transsphenoidal routes to the hypophysis were performed more than half a century ago. These procedures fell into disfavor because of low magnification and insufficient illumination of the operative field, infection and inadequate postoperative endocrine replacement therapy. With today's antibiotic therapy and hormonal replacement, plus the use of the operating microscope, the transsphenoidal route to the hypophysis has gained renewed interest among neurosurgeons and otolaryngologists.

Each of the transsphenoidal routes and the advantages of the "from below" approach are described. The applications of the transsphenoidal approach and the nonsurgical modalities for hypophysectomy are reviewed.

The simplicity and safety of the sublabial transseptal transsphenoidal approach depend on a thorough familiarity with the surgical anatomy, proper positioning of the patient, and the availability of appropriate instrumentation. Photographs of specially prepared whole head anatomical specimens plus skull dissections with radiographic correlation illustrate the pertinent anatomy. Some of the vital structures to be identified and avoided are the optic canals, carotid arteries, circular sinuses, cavernous sinuses, III, IV, V, VI cranial nerves, foramen rotundum, medial walls of the orbits, medial walls of maxillary sinuses, medial pterygoid plates and pterygoid canals. A method for preoperative determination of key distances within the patient's skull is described along with other preoperative tests. This paper discusses the self-retaining speculum and other new instruments for this procedure. A gauge mounted on the front end of the speculum is calibrated to measure the size of the opening at the tip of the speculum.

Thirty cases are included in this report, six of which are presented in detail. No operative mortality, CSF rhinorrhea, visual damage, carotid or cavernous sinus hemorrhage, fracture of the medial pterygoid plates or maxilla were encountered in this series. Three patients developed diabetes insipidus and two patients had meningitis which responded to antibiotic therapy.

———— O ————

INTRODUCTION.

The goal of this dissertation is to illustrate the simplicity and safety of the sublabial transseptal transsphenoidal approach to the hypophysis and parasellar region. Various extracranial routes will be discussed as well as other modalities of selective destruction of the hypophysis. The simplicity and safety of this approach depend on a thorough familiarity with the surgical anatomy from the anterior nasal spine to the dorsum sellae, on proper positioning of the patient as well as on the availability of appropriate instrumentation. To illustrate the surgical anatomy, the author has prepared whole head anatomical specimens and skull dissections with radiographic correlations. A method for preoperatively determining key distances within the patient's skull will be described. Working with toolmakers, the author has designed a self-retaining speculum, modified an air drill and other dissecting instruments for this procedure.

*Presented as a Candidate's Thesis to the American Laryngological, Rhinological and Otological Society, Inc., 1978, receiving Honorable Mention.
Send Reprint Requests to K. J. Lee, M.D., University Towers, 95 York St., New Haven, Conn. 06511.

REVIEW OF THE LITERATURE.

Chiari,[1] Cushing,[2,3] and Hirsch[4] performed the transsphenoidal approach more than half a century ago. They lacked neither surgical skill nor imagination but were hampered as much by infection, poor magnification and illumination of the operative field as by inadequate postoperative endocrine replacement therapy. With current availability of antibiotics and hormonal replacement therapy plus the use of the operating microscope, the transsphenoidal route to the hypophysis has gained renewed interest among neurosurgeons and otolaryngologists.

The advantages of the "from below" approach compared to the transcranial removal of the hypophysis or stalk section have been amply discussed by Burian,[5] Montgomery,[6] Hardy,[7] James,[8,9] and Hamberger.[10] These advantages include:

1. A more direct and rapid access to the pituitary fossa in general and to the anterior lobe in particular. (Tumors of the hypophysis primarily originate in the anterior lobe.)

2. An adequate view of the total hypophyseal bed which is not possible through the transcranial route. This view enables a more accurate dissection of the tumor from the normal gland. In cases where hypophysectomy is used as a means of manipulating endocrine function, as in patients with breast carcinoma, this view allows an increased certainty of complete extracapsular enucleation of the gland under magnified vision.

3. Less probability of injury to the optic chiasm, optic and olfactory nerves.

4. The ability to remove a pituitary tumor which has herniated into the sphenoid sinus. This is not possible via the transcranial route without injuring or sacrificing the optic nerve.

5. A decrease in mortality and morbidity. Angell James[9] presented a transfrontal mortality rate of 12% compared to less than 2% via the transsphenoidal route. Postoperative seizures, hematomas, brain damage, and cerebral edema are rare in the cases utilizing the "from below" approach. Craniotomy is particularly hazardous in diabetic patients where postoperative cerebral edema and hemorrhages from the diffusely abnormal vessels are frequent causes of death. Therefore the transcranial approach is not suitable for controlling diabetic retinopathy. In certain acromegalic patients, frontal bossing increases the technical difficulty in the transfrontal approach.

6. Metastatic involvement of the calvarium is another contraindication to the transfrontal approach.[11]

It is well agreed that tumors with suprasellar extensions as evidenced by displacement of the third ventricle or cerebral vessels may have to be approached transcranially as a primary or secondary procedure following decompression and partial resection "from below." In some instances a prefixed chiasma impedes access to the tumor, causing some neurosurgeons who use the transcranial route to sacrifice part or all of one optic nerve. Others prefer to sacrifice part of the frontal lobe.[12] In such an instance, a two-stage approach — transsphenoidally to resect the inferior portion of the tumor and transcranially to remove the suprasellar extension — should be utilized to avoid damage to either the optic nerve or the frontal lobe.

Extracranial Routes.

All extracranial routes to the sella turcica take advantage of the proximity of the sphenoid sinus to the sella. Hence all "from below" routes are transsphenoidal. However, there are numerous means of access to the sphenoid sinus.

In 1904, Horsley[13] attempted to resect pituitary tumors through the middle cranial fossa, while in 1905 Krause[12] performed the anterior craniotomy approach. Schloffer[12] in 1907 worked through a lateral rhinotomy incision and dislocated the septum. He was the first to perform the transsphenoidal approach. The mortality rate at that time was reported as 25%. Minor technique modifications were subsequently made by various surgeons including Proust[14] in 1908, Kanavel[15] in 1909, and Kanavel and Grinker[16] in 1910. In 1910, Halstead[17] introduced the sublabial incision. In the same year, Hirsch[12] performed the transsphenoidal operation endonasally under local anesthesia. Following a submucous resection of the septum through the nares, Hirsch approached the sphenoid sinus within the envelope of mucoperichondrial and mucoperiosteal flaps. The anterior wall of the sphenoid sinus was opened with rongeurs. The intersphenoidal septum was removed and the sella opened with chisels and rongeurs. The size of his opening was approximately 1.5 x 1.75 cm. To supplement surgical removal of the tumor, Hirsch implanted radium after the sixth postoperative day. He further stated that should there be recurrence of visual changes suggestive of tumor regrowth, he could either implant additional radium in the office or resect the recurrence through the same route. He reported only two cases of cerebrospinal fluid leak which were repaired with a septal mucosal flap. In his series of 277 pituitary adenoma patients covering a 4 to 19 year follow-up, Hirsch[15] reported an operative mortality of 5.4% with 65% obtaining a lasting good result. He compared his series to Olivecrona's[18] transfrontal series of 291 pituitary adenoma patients followed for 14 to 18 years showing an 11.7% operative mortality with 54.5% obtaining a lasting good result.

In 1912, Cushing[2] combined Halstead's sublabial incision with Hirsch's submucosal resection approach to the sphenoid sinus. The sublabial incision provided a wider entrance to the operative field. The overall mortality rate of Cushing's series as reported by German and Flanigan[19] was 6.3%. However, the mortality rate for the last 10 years of the series was markedly reduced to 2.4%. They noted that hematoma was the greatest hazard following the frontal approach, whereas meningitis was the greatest hazard in the transsphenoidal approach. One case of fatal hemorrhage secondary to an adjacent carotid aneurysm was reported.

Chiari[1] in 1912, Kirchner and Van Gilder[20] in 1975 described the external ethmoidectomy approach to the sphenoid sinus for transsphenoidal hypophysectomy. In 1963, Montgomery[6] described a transethmoido-sphenoidal hypophysectomy procedure coupled with a septal mucosal flap for closure of the surgical defect. Angell James[8,9] used a combined transethmoidosphenoidal and transnasal technique. He viewed through the ethmoidal incision and introduced the instruments through the nose. Through the ethmoidal incision, he fenestrated the posterior third of the septum from the cribriform plate to the palate.

Bateman[21] used the endonasal approach of Hirsch to open the sphenoid sinus combined with a separate right external ethmoidectomy approach for illumination of the field and inspection through the operating microscope. The suction tip was introduced through the external ethmoidal incision with his left hand while the punch forceps, diathermy or dissectors were used with his right hand through the septal incision. This technique is similar to that described by Angell James.

The disadvantages of the external ethmoidectomy approach are the 1) external scar, and 2) the obliquity which diminishes the safe distance between the operative field and the vital structures (internal carotid artery, cavernous sinus and II, III, IV, VI, 1st division of V cranial nerves). The oblique approach also makes it more difficult to cope with the different degrees of pneumatization and anatomical variations of the sphenoid sinus.

Hirsch[12] mentioned that Fein and Denker described a transantrosphenoidal route in 1910 which was repopularized by Hamberger[10] in 1961. The maxillary sinus was entered through a buccal mucosal incision. After the transantral ethmoidectomy was performed, the sphenoid sinus was readily exposed. In certain cases, Hamberger resected the superior-posterior part of the nasal septum to optimize exposure. The distance from the anterior wall of the maxillary sinus to the pituitary is about 9 cm. After the anterior wall of the sphenoid sinus was removed, the anterior wall of the sella was entered with a thin chisel. The disadvantage of this approach is obliquity as experienced in the external ethmoidectomy approach.

Preysing in 1913 and Tiefenthal in 1920 described a transpalatal approach as reported by Hirsch.[12] Through their interest in the repair of choanal atresia, Trible and Morse[22] approached the hypophysis through a transpalatal-transsphenoidal route.

The advantages of this approach are: *1*. The route is short and direct. *2*. The operative field is wide. *3*. It is a midline procedure. *4*. It does not leave an external scar.

The disadvantages are: *1*. It involves a moving functioning organ, the soft palate. In order to avoid functional impairment, this route cannot be easily used again should postoperative bleeding or CSF rhinorrhea occur. *2*. It is not suitable in a patient with trismus or macroglossia as occasionally encountered in acromegaly. *3*. It involves working through a contaminated field. *4*. It does not lend itself well to the use of an operating microscope.

Macbeth[23] indicated that the transseptal route offered a narrow operating field and hence found it undesirable for removal of the pituitary gland. However, with the instruments and the technique to be discussed later in this dissertation, this operative field is quite adequate for bimanual manipulation. Macbeth disliked the transethmoidal route because of its oblique approach and also objected to working through a contaminated field in the transpalatal technique. In his opinion, the transantroethmoidal route neither lent itself well to the use of the operating microscope nor was its oblique approach desirable. Therefore, Macbeth introduced the nasal osteoplastic flap technique in which he made a U-shaped skin incision over the dorsum of the nose. This incision looks like the dual incisions for bilateral external ethmoidectomy with their lower ends joined by a curved incision just below the junction of the nasal bones and the upper lateral nasal cartilages. Macbeth then retracted superiorly a bone flap consisting of the nasal bones. The septum was approached next and a submucous resection performed up to the anterior wall of the sphenoid sinus. The sphenoid sinus was subsequently entered.

Netzer and McCoy[14] described a lateral rhinotomy approach to the septum and thence to the sphenoid sinus. Both Macbeth's method and that of Netzer and McCoy leave an obvious scar and a possible nasal deformity.

Nonsurgical Hypophysectomy.

In addition to surgical ablation of the pituitary gland, other modalities have been used to treat pituitary adenomas and selectively destroy the anterior pituitary function to palliate metastatic disease or to control diabetic retinopathy and malignant exophthalmos. Although these techniques are considered nonsurgical procedures by their proponents, they entail some degree of dissection except the use of external radiation. The modalities to be reviewed are: Ultrasonic irradiation, cryosurgery, gold and yttrium implant, stereotaxic thermal ablation and external radiation.

Ultrasonic Irradiation. Ultrasonic irradiation was described by Arslan[25] in 1973 in his report on 41 cases of acromegaly. He approached the capsule of the pituitary through a transseptal transsphenoidal approach. The ultrasonic probe was pressed firmly against the capsule and irradiation was administered at 3 megahertz frequency with intensity from 30 to 40 W/cm^2 lasting 20 minutes or more. He maintained that this approach eliminated the surgical risk. However, this was not entirely correct because a transseptal transsphenoidal opening of the sella was required. As ultrasound at frequencies suitable for pituitary cell destruction is not transmitted by air and is very rapidly absorbed by bone, it becomes necessary to expose the capsule surgically. Furthermore, the course of ultrasonic destruction lacked precision. Arslan[25] reported the results of 31 patients in which 20 patients improved from a subjective standpoint. Complications or lack of complications of this procedure were not discussed in his presentation.

Cryohypophysectomy. Cross, et al.,[26] described the stereotaxic transsphenoidal cryosurgical treatment of acromegaly. A hollow metal probe was inserted under fluoroscopic guidance through the nasal cavity and sphenoid sinus into the pituitary fossa. An aspiration biopsy was taken followed by freezing the fossa to between $-100°$ C and $-180°$ C for 10 to 15 minutes continuously or for 4 separate cycles of 2 to 3 minutes each. Individual freezing sessions were terminated by controlled return to normal body temperature at the probe tip. Core muscle plugs were used to seal the surgical defect in the pituitary floor. Of the 13 cases reported, one patient developed a CSF leak which lasted three days and had a transient upper quadrantanopia. Two cases developed bacterial meningitis, one case had transient III nerve palsy, and one case developed permanent diabetes insipidus.

Richards, et al.,[27] found it difficult to control the destructive action of cryosurgery. Complications such as meningitis and ocular nerve palsies were high. DiTullio and Rand,[28] advocates of stereotaxic cryohypophysectomy, reported a 13% morbidity. Angell James[9] reported an incidence of 15% ocular palsies with cryohypophysectomy. He further explained that complete ablation of the gland was not easy to achieve by cryosurgery because of the rapidly flowing blood in the intercommunicating sinuses which warms the surrounding tissues.

Gold and Yttrium Implants. Bateman[21] reported in 1962 a series of 18 patients with diffuse metastasis from breast carcinoma in whom he implanted radioactive gold grain into the pituitary by the transnasal route. Only 7 patients demonstrated the effects of hypophysectomy and in these

7 patients, 2 had visual defects. He therefore abandoned the implantation of radioactive gold grains for implantation of irradiated yttrium pellets with the help of an image intensifier. Bateman later abandoned this technique altogether in favor of surgical hypophysectomy. He concluded that to use radioactive material successfully it was necessary to know 1) the volume and shape of the tissue to be irradiated, 2) the dose necessary to produce the required biological effect, and 3) the limit of the dose necessary to avoid undesirable effects. Radiographic studies can measure the size of the pituitary fossa but not all of the fossa is filled with the pituitary gland. Since distance between the gland and the optic chiasm is variable, implant irradiation becomes hazardous. Macbeth[21] agreed that the implantation of radioactive material poses problems such as a hazard to surrounding vital tissues, bone necrosis, and the risks of an incomplete functional ablation.

Ray, et al.,[29] implanted yttrium 90 to treat 22 patients with diabetic retinopathy. General anesthesia was used and a sheathed trochar was inserted through each nostril guided by fluoroscopy. Complications related to this procedure developed in about half of the patients. Five patients died as a direct result of these complications, and two died of vascular complications of diabetes. One patient lost useful vision in one eye, one died of massive epistaxis 11 months after the procedure. An autopsy on the latter case revealed erosion of the cavernous portion of the internal carotid artery due to radiation necrosis. One patient died of hemorrhage during an attempt to remove one of the metal screws which had caused meningitis. Persistent pneumocephalus developed in one patient whose diaphragma sellae was found to be perforated secondary to radiation necrosis.

Riskaer, et al.,[30] and Hartog, et al.,[31] reported similar complication rates with radioactive implants.

Gold gives off gamma rays with more tissue penetration than yttrium 90 and thus is more hazardous to surrounding tissues. The latter gives off beta radiation which causes less surrounding tissue necrosis. However, from the above reports, even the yttrium 90 implant is hazardous. Angell James[3] felt that interstitial irradiation with yttrium 90 was a definite risk to the ocular nerves and gave rise to secondary infection in the necrotic radiated gland thus making CSF rhinorrhea and meningitis more likely.

Stereotaxic Thermal Ablation. Zervas and Hamlin[32] reported 312 cases of stereotaxic radiofrequency thermal hypophysectomy. The probe was placed in the sphenoid sinus through a transnasal sphenoidectomy approach. Through a 2 mm puncture of the posterior wall of the sphenoid sinus the electrode was introduced into the sella turcica. Destruction was achieved by radiofrequency conducted through the soft malleable electrode. Through a small stylet at the tip of the electrode, 10 to 20 small lesions were made to achieve total hypophysectomy. Each lesion was created by applying the tip temperature of 80° C for 40-60 seconds. Zervas and Hamlin[32] pointed out that the advantage of using heat is that the destruction does not extend beyond the confines of the pituitary since heat is easily carried away by the circulating blood in the cavernous sinus or carotid artery as well as by the CSF above the diaphragma sellae. This protective mechanism is not available in radiation and less effective in cryohypophysectomy. However, the authors did report two visual impairments, one temporary and one permanent, as well as two deaths secondary to meningitis. There were 15 cases of CSF rhinorrhea. Two contraindications to stereotaxic radiofrequency thermal hypophysectomy became apparent in this series: 1) increased intracranial pressure, 2) erosion of the sellar floor. These two conditions increased the incidence of CSF rhinorrhea.

External Radiation. It is generally agreed that postoperative radiation has improved the long-term results in patients with pituitary adenoma. German and Flanigan[19] reviewed Cushing's series and found 42% control for five years or more with surgery alone, while 75% of the patients were controlled for five years or more when postoperative radiation was given. Hayes, et al.,[23] reported comparable percentages of 45% without postoperative radiation and 79% with postoperative radiation. Ray and Patterson's[24] statistics were 78% and 92% respectively. However, Svien and Colby's[25] series showed 92% control with surgery alone and, with only a slight improvement of their statistics, 95.25% control if combined with postoperative radiation. Stern and Batzdorf[26] reported a 94% control with total hypophysectomy alone.

Furstenberg and Blatt[27] advocated treating small pituitary adenomas with 3,000 rads in three weeks through two lateral fields. They recommended surgery only for the following categories: *1.* The imminent possibility of blindness or rapidly decreasing visual fields. *2.* Severe intractable headache not relieved by radiation therapy. *3.* Large lesions. *4.* Radiation failures. *5.* When the diagnosis is in doubt.

Sheline, et al.,[28] recommended 4,500 to 5,000 rads over a four and a half week period. They pointed out that cystic lesions do not respond well to radiation. Williams[29] believed that external radiation as a primary therapy was not very effective. Improvement, if present, takes some months to become apparent. Complications such as brain necrosis have been reported. DiTullio and Rand[28] reported optic vasculitis, memory loss, central scotomata, empty sella syndrome, and brain necrosis as some of the complications seen. They also felt that external radiation used as the only form of therapy was not very effective in the control of pituitary tumors. However, when used as a postoperative mode of therapy, it has proved useful in controlling recurrences of pituitary adenoma.

In order to obtain tissue diagnosis of a pituitary tumor, open biopsy is needed either transcranially or transsphenoidally. A closed needle biopsy is both hazardous and unreliable. Once the sella has been approached surgically, the tumor might well be removed. Hence, when external radiation is used as the only mode of therapy, no histological diagnosis is made.

Since normal pituitary cells do not respond to a safe dosage of radiation, external radiation alone is unable to suppress endocrine function sufficiently to palliate breast and prostate metastases.

HISTOLOGY AND PHYSIOLOGY OF THE PITUITARY GLAND.

The pituitary derives its name from pituita meaning mucus.[11] According to Galen, as reported by Hirsch,[12] the mucus was formed in the brain and discharged through the nose. The other name, hypophysis (hypo = under, physis = growth), was given by von Soemmering[12] in 1798.

The pituitary gland is made up of two lobes, the anterior and posterior lobes or the adenohypophysis and the neurohypophysis. The adenohypophysis (anterior lobe) is made up of pars distalis, pars tuberalis and pars

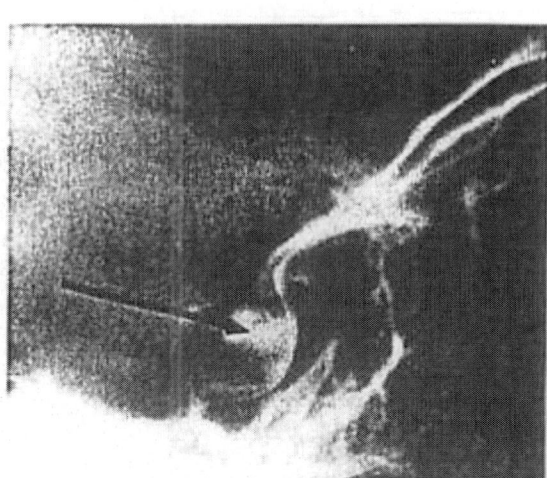

Fig. 1. Calcification within the sella in craniopharyngioma.

intermedia. The pars distalis is also known as pars anterior or pars glandularis. The neurohypophysis (posterior lobe) is made up of the neural lobe (pars nervosa) and the neural stalk. The pars intermedia separates the two lobes. However, in terms of structure and function the pars intermedia is part of the anterior lobe. The adenohypophysis is derived from stratified squamous epithelium of the primitive buccal cavity by the evagination of Rathke's pouch (craniopharyngeal duct). Thus it has the same anlage as tooth enamel.

The neurohypophysis is derived from the floor of the third ventricle of developing neuroectoderm. Hence, the pituitary is attached to the third ventricle by a stalk known as the infundibulum which is about 1 cm in length. The pars distalis and pars tuberalis are made up of three cell types named according to their staining characteristics: eosinophile, basophile, and chromophobe cells. The latter are not stainable by either eosin or hematoxylin. The eosinophiles are small, granular and stain red with acid eosin dyes. The basophiles are large cells containing coarse cytoplasmic granules and stain with basic dyes such as blue hematoxylin. The fourth cell type, not always present, is the squamous epithelial cell which is a remnant of the embryonal development from the oral cavity. Occasionally, these cells give rise to hypophyseal duct tumors or craniopharyngiomas. Histologically they are identical to the odontogenic ameloblastomas. Calcification in these tumors is frequently seen (Fig. 1).

Although the chromophobe cells are least numerous, the incidence of chromophobe tumors is greatest.[12,23] Next in frequency are the eosinophilic tumors. Eosinophilic tumors usually grow toward the sphenoid sinus and do not usually interfere with the optic nerve or chiasma. They cause acromegaly and severe headaches. Chromophobe tumors usually grow in all directions. They can give rise to visual symptoms as well as to endocrine dysfunction, e.g., amenorrhea. Basophilic adenomas are extremely rare and are an occasional cause of Cushing's disease characterized by hypertension, hirsutism, protein depletion, increased fragility of blood vessels, "buffalo hump," "moon facies," and osteopenia.

The anterior lobe produces the following hormones:

1. Somatotrophic hormone (STH) or growth hormone which regulates the growth of the body. Its target organ is protein tissue and it is secreted by the eosinophilic cells.

2. Gonadotrophic hormone (the follicle stimulating hormone and the luteinizing hormone). The absence of gonadotrophic hormone will lead to delayed appearance or disappearance of the secondary sexual characteristics and amenorrhea in women.

3. Prolactin or lactogenic hormone.

4. Thyrotrophic hormone (Thyroid Stimulating Hormone — TSH).

5. Adrenocorticotrophic hormone (ACTH) stimulates the adrenal cortex. Its absence can lead to hypoglycemia, postural hypotension, decreased strength and stamina.

6. Beta lipotropin.

The pars intermedia secretes a melanocytic hormone which is part of beta lipotropin.

The posterior lobe or neurohypophysis is made up of:

1. Neuroglia which are the supporting protoplasmic network of this nervous tissue. They are fusiform cells called pituicytes with several processes and brown pigment in their cytoplasm.

2. Nerve fibers

3. Hyaline bodies.

4. Some basophiles.

The neurohypophysis secretes antidiuretic hormone (ADH or vasopressin) and oxytocin. These hormones are actually formed in the hypothalamus and transported to the neurohypophysis for storage and release. ADH maintains the water balance in the body by controlling re-absorption of water by the kidney tubules. Oxytocin promotes uterine contraction and assists in the expulsion of milk from the mammary glands.

The release of pituitary hormones is controlled by the hypothalamus. In the adenohypophysis, this is probably initiated by chemical activators or releasing factor carried in the portal blood. For the neurohypophysis, the messages are carried by nerve fibers within the stalk.

The anterior lobe is supplied by a series of superior hypophyseal arteries arising from the supraclinoid portion of each internal carotid artery as well as the anterior and posterior cerebral arteries. The posterior lobe is supplied by the inferior hypophyseal artery which is a branch of the internal carotid artery within the cavernous sinus.

APPLICATION OF TRANSSPHENOIDAL APPROACH.

Pituitary surgery is performed for the removal of pituitary tumors, to palliate metastases from breast carcinoma, prostate carcinoma and melanoma, as well as for the control of diabetic retinopathy and malignant exophthalmos. The transsphenoidal route can be used to drain, remove or biopsy lesions of the sphenoid sinus and parasellar region. At the 1977 American Otological Society Meeting, Montgomery[40] described the trans-ethmoidosphenoidal route for draining cystic lesions of the petrous apex.

Pituitary Tumors.

Chromophobe adenoma is the most common type of pituitary adenoma and constitutes 10% of all intracranial tumors.[35] Chromophobe adenoma does not secrete hormones but compresses the eosinophilic and basophilic cells which secrete hormones thus causing endocrine dysfunction such as amenorrhea, decreased libido, hypoadrenalism and hypothyroidism. Eosinophilic adenoma leads to acromegaly in adults or gigantism in children in addition to causing decreased libido. Severe headache occurs frequently with pituitary tumors.

Acromegaly is a progressive, disfiguring and a potentially fatal disease.[38] Evans, et al.,[41] reported a 50% death rate in acromegalics before middle age and 90% mortality before the sixth decade. The cause of death varied from intracerebral tumor extension to diabetic coma. According to Wright, et al.,[42] cardiovascular disease secondary to strain on the heart was the most frequent cause of death in acromegalics.

Encroachment by any pituitary tumor on the optic chiasm or optic nerves most commonly causes bitemporal hemianopsia. Chamlin, et al.,[43] reported that 86% of 156 cases of pituitary adenoma had bitemporal hemianopsia. Limitation of extraocular eye movements is observed when the III, IV, or VI nerves are involved. A sudden loss of vision associated with hemorrhage within the pituitary tumor is occasionally seen. This is called pituitary apoplexy. Summers[44] reported a case of nasal obstruction caused by a recurrent chromophobe adenoma which eroded the anterior clinoids, posterior clinoids, pituitary fossa, sphenoid sinus, bilateral greater and lesser wings of the sphenoid. White and Warren[45] in 1945 reviewed 338 pituitary adenomas and reported only 8 cases where the tumors were large enough to obstruct the nasopharynx. Kay, et al.,[46] reported 3 lesions of such size among 192 patients. In the series reported here, the pituitary adenoma in one case had eroded into the nasopharynx (refer to case reports).

Breast Carcinoma.

Angell James[8,9] indicated that estrogen, progesterone, prolactin and growth hormone seem to enhance the growth or the spread of metastases of breast carcinoma. Hypophysectomy eliminates prolactin, growth hormone, adrenocorticotrophic hormone, follicle stimulation hormone and luteinizing hormone while suppressing estrogen and progesterone levels. In general, patients who responded to bilateral oophorectomy and androgen therapy also responded to hypophysectomy.

Hamberger, et al.,[16] indicated that 80% of young women who had undergone successful oophorectomy can expect good results from hypophysectomy. In older women hypophysectomy as a primary procedure produced remission in about 30% of the cases.

The criteria of objective evaluation of breast carcinoma metastases remission are: *1*. Healing of skin lesions. *2*. Recalcification of bone metastases. *3*. Reduction in size of lung metastases. *4*. Relief of pain.

Hypophysectomy to palliate breast carcinoma metastases has met with varying degrees of success.[24] McGuire, et al.,[41] mentioned that in random series, regardless of the type of endocrine therapy employed, objective tumor regression occurred in only 20-40% of breast cancer patients.

The basis for endocrine manipulation with sex hormones or surgical deprivation of hormones (oophorectomy or hypophysectomy) for the treatment of breast carcinoma, prostate carcinoma, and melanoma metastases is still subject to controversy and needs further investigation. Recently an upsurge of interest in endocrine therapy has resulted from the development of assays that can determine with considerable confidence those breast cancer patients who will or will not respond to endocrine therapy.[47] It has been found that normal target tissues including mammary glands contain specific receptors for hormones. When malignant transformation occurs the cell may retain or shed the receptor sites. If the cell retains the receptor sites, its growth and function like that of the normal cell can potentially be regulated by its hormonal environment. If the cell loses these receptors following malignant transformation, it is no longer recognized as a target cell by circulating hormones and hence its growth is not dependent on endocrine influence. This leads to the implication that malignant tumor with hormonal receptor sites (e.g., estrogen receptor sites) is under the influence of the hormones and its growth can therefore be hampered by endocrine deprivation. Methods for assay of these receptor sites are described in an article by McGuire, et al.[47] Hence, in many centers, a specimen of the primary breast carcinoma tissue is analyzed for estrogen receptor sites. In the event of metastases or advanced disease, endocrine manipulation such as hypophysectomy is recommended only for those tumors with high estrogen binding receptor sites. McGuire, et al.,[47] reported a 55% success rate with surgical endocrine ablation in 107 patients with positive estrogen receptor site values, while only 8% responded in the 94 patients with negative estrogen receptor site values. However, it should be emphasized that endocrine manipulation only palliates the metastases and eases the bone pain temporarily, even in the so-called successful group.

Diabetic Retinopathy.

Houssay and Biasotti[18] demonstrated a marked improvement in the diabetes of pancreatectomized animals after hypophysectomy. Poulson[10] reported in 1953 that a patient who had a selective necrosis of the anterior lobe of the hypophysis had a permanent cure of his diabetic retinopathy. Hence, it would seem that the most physiologic approach to the treatment of progressive diabetic retinopathy would be a selective but complete anterior hypophysectomy. Of the anterior pituitary hormones with an influence on carbohydrate metabolism, the growth hormone has the most potent anti-insulin property.

Angell James[5] established the following criteria for anterior hypophysectomy for diabetic retinopathy:

1. There should be a predominantly hemorrhagic retinopathy which is obviously threatening vision.

2. That neither retinitis proliferans nor extensive retinal degeneration should affect both eyes severely.

3. That renal failure is absent.

4. That the patient is intelligent enough to comprehend the operation and follow a replacement therapy regimen.

Hardy and Ciric[56] reported on 17 patients with progressive diabetic retinopathy who underwent hypophysectomy (11 selective anterior hypophysectomies and 6 total hypophysectomies). Ten patients with 8-19 months follow-up had lasting improvement of their retinopathy. Five patients with 3-7 months follow-up showed rapid amelioration in the pathological findings of the fundi. In contrast, it is fairly well agreed that the progression of diabetic neuropathy as well as of peripheral vascular disease has not been demonstrably altered by hypophysectomy.[51] Hamberger, et al.,[19] reported that, in addition to improvement of the retinopathy, all of their 26 cases became insulin-sensitive and the tendency to acidosis disappeared.

Prostatic Carcinoma.

Gonadotrophic and growth hormones are suspected of proliferating prostatic carcinoma. A hypophysectomy eliminates these hormones. Angell James[5] reported on 14 patients with advanced prostatic carcinoma who underwent hypophysectomy. At 6 months postoperatively, he calculated a 14% remission rate and 7% at 12 months.

Murphy, et al.,[52] reported on 24 patients with disseminated prostatic carcinoma. They demonstrated good correlation between the rates of remission and the degree of growth hormone suppression. Among the cases with evident growth hormone suppression, 42.9% had a satisfactory remission while those cases with no evidence of growth hormone suppression had 0% remission. The major urinary androgenic fractions (androsterone, etiocholanolone, dehydroisoandrosterone) showed an immediate and sustained decrease in those patients manifesting clinical remission.

Melanoma and Malignant Exophthalmos.

Angell James[8,9] pointed out that the spread of melanoma may be enhanced by estrogen, progesterone, growth hormone, and melanocytic hormone. Hypophysectomy would eliminate the growth hormone, melanocytic hormone, and ACTH while suppressing the levels of estrogen and progesterone. He discussed 7 cases of malignant melanoma treated with hypophysectomy. The remission rate was 14% six months postoperatively. He also expressed the theory that eliminating thyrotrophic stimulating hormone and suppressing thyroxine may help malignant exophthalmos.

Sphenoid Lesions.

Sphenoid lesions usually give rise to vertex headache, retro-orbital pain, or throbbing head pain on leaning forward. The more advanced cases additionally cause nasal congestion, visual disturbance such as diplopia, and facial numbness over the distribution of the ophthalmic nerve. Bitemporal hemianopsia and endocrine malfunction are rarely noted in sphenoid lesions. Wyllie, et al.,[53] who reviewed 45 cases of sphenoid lesions gave the following distribution: 21 cases of chronic sphenoid sinusitis, 8 cysts or mucoceles, 5 pyoceles, 6 primary tumors of the sphenoid, 2 fibrous dysplasia, 2 rhinoliths, and 1 polyp. In Watson's[54] series of 127 cases of primary carcinoma of the paranasal sinuses, only one originated in the sphenoid sinus. Wyllie, et al.,[53] reported two cases of sphenoid sinus squamous

TABLE 1.
Differential Diagnosis of Sellar and Parasellar Lesion.

Chromophobe adenoma (80% of pituitary adenomas)
Eosinophilic adenoma (15% of pituitary adenomas)
Basophilic adenoma (5% of pituitary adenomas)
Craniopharyngioma
Aneurysm of the internal carotid artery
Empty sella syndrome
Metastatic tumors
Optic and/or hypothalamus glioma
Hamartoma of the hypothalamus
Ectopic pinealoma, teratoma, dermoid
Meningioma
Prepontine lesions — chordoma
Mucocele of the sphenoid sinus
Sellar abscess secondary to sphenoiditis
Fibrous dysplasia
Granulomatous disease
Bony tumors of the sphenoid

cell carcinoma, two of lymphoepithelioma, one undifferentiated carcinoma, and one adenocarcinoma. Hallberg and Begley[55] found no sphenoid sinus involvement in their review of 51 cases of osteoma of the paranasal sinuses. Brunner[56] pointed out that fibrous dysplasia rarely involves the sphenoid bone because it arises from precartilaginous bone rather than membranous bone. Townsend and DeSanto[57] diagnosed a fibrous dysplasia with sarcomatous degeneration through a transseptal biopsy. DeBartolo and Vrabec[58] treated 4 encephaloceles through a transnasal and transethmoidal approach. Henry, et al.,[59] employed this approach for lesions of the clivus such as chordomas and meningiomas. In the author's series, a case of chondrosarcoma of the sphenoid bone in a 14-year-old boy was encountered in which the sublabial transseptal transsphenoidal approach was used to biopsy and partially remove the lesion (see case reports).

PREOPERATIVE CARE.

It is important that these patients be seen and evaluated by a team consisting of an endocrinologist, neurosurgeon, ophthalmologist, otolaryngologist, and an oncologist in the case of metastatic disease.

Preoperative work-up of these patients includes:

1. Complete blood count, prothrombin time, partial thromboplastin time, platelet count, liver function tests (including alkaline phosphatase), and serum electrolytes, serum calcium and phosphorus determination in cases of metastatic disease.

2. Control of diabetes mellitus.

3. Routine chest X-ray and EKG. The EKG gives a baseline of myocardial activity regarding both rhythm and voltage. Changes in the "T" wave may indicate a variation in circulating blood cortisol or thyroid hormone

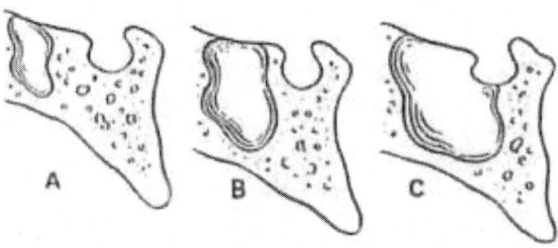

Fig. 2A. Diagrammatic representation of sellar presentation. (A) Conchal. (B) Presellar. (C) Sellar.

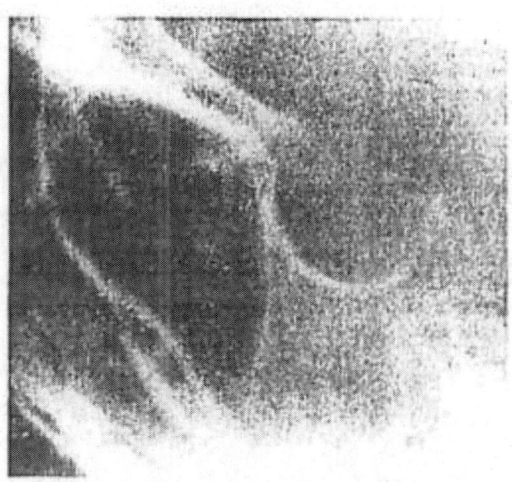

Fig. 2B. Presellar type of presentation.

problem. A postoperative depression of the "T" wave may indicate insufficient circulating cortisone.

4. Endocrine work-up to include:

(a) Morning and afternoon serum cortisol levels.

(b) Serum cortisol levels, growth homone levels, prolactin levels following insulin hypoglycemia.

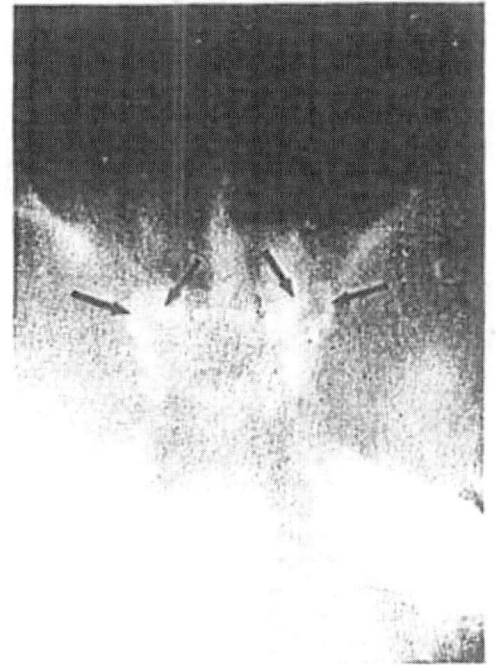

Fig. 3. Submentovertical laminogram showing carotid calcification.

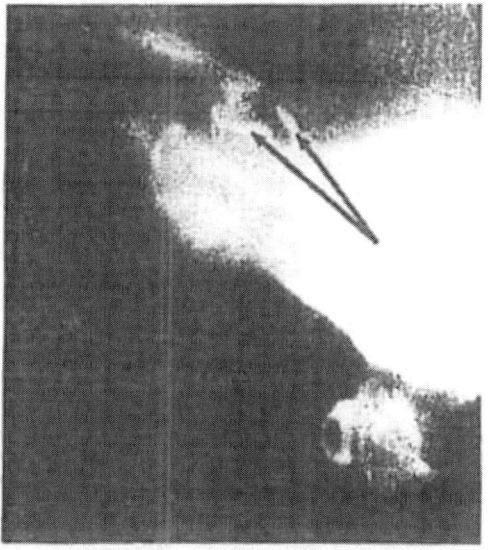

Fig. 4. Lateral laminogram showing carotid calcification.

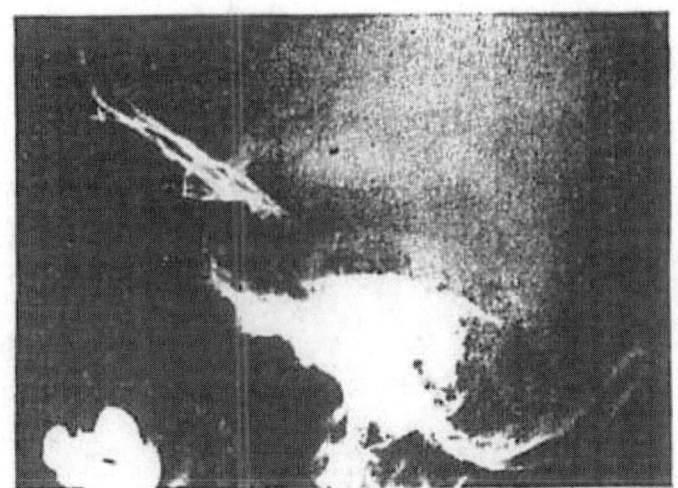

Fig. 5. Lateral X-ray showing double floor of sella secondary to pituitary adenoma.

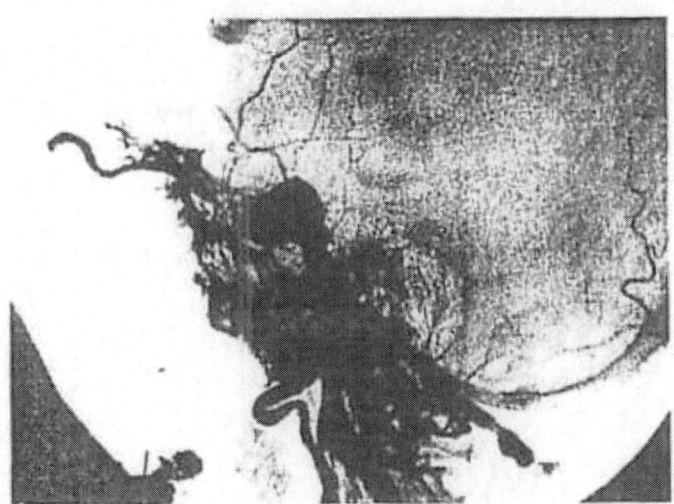

Fig. 6. Carotid aneurysm eroding into the sella.

(c) T_3, T_4, T_7, Thyrotropin Releasing Factor (TRF).
(d) Metapyrone test.
(e) Urine 17-OH steroids and 17-OH keto steroids.
(f) LH, FSH, estrodiol and testosterone levels.
(g) Urine and serum osmolalities after overnight water deprivation.
(h) Arginine infusion test.

5. Radioisotope scans of liver, spleen, bone and brain, in cases of metastatic disease.

6. Determination of the Estrogen Receptor Sites of the primary breast carcinoma tissue, where possible.

7. A-P, lateral and submentovertical laminograms of the sphenoid sinus and sella turcica. It is important to locate the position of the intersphenoidal septum which may not be in the midline and may lead to the internal carotid artery (Figs. 29-A and B). This septum is best seen in the submentovertical view. The sellar presentation into the sphenoid sinus is important when planning a transsphenoidal hypophysectomy. This is best seen in the lateral view. Hamberger, et al.,[16] estimated that 86% of the pituitary fossa presents as a bulge into the sphenoid sinus. Eleven percent are of the presellar type in which the pneumatization is anterior to the sella and 3% are of the conchal type in which there is a thick bony partition between the sphenoid sinus and the sella turcica (Figs. 2-A and B). It is important to differentiate calcification of the carotid siphon from calcification within the sella as in craniopharyngioma (Figs. 1, 3 and 4). At times, a calcified carotid artery can give rise to the so-called "double floor" appearance to falsely suggest a pituitary adenoma. The "double floor" appearance in the true lateral view in the case of a pituitary adenoma is due to partial erosion of the sellar floor (Fig. 5).

8. Arteriography (bilateral carotid and vertebrobasilar, if indicated) is useful for ascertaining the position of the cavernous portion of the internal carotid arteries and all segments of the anterior cerebral arteries. It helps to rule out a carotid aneurysm eroding into the sella (Fig. 6). Arteriography helps delineate the vascular pattern of a pituitary adenoma and may outline the extent of its suprasellar extension.

9. Pneumoencephalogram is used to determine the status of the floor of the third ventricle and the chiasmatic cistern. It provides the most accurate delineation of a suprasellar extension of pituitary tumors both in the lateral and frontal projections. It also rules out an "empty sella syndrome" in which the subarachnoid recess herniates into the sella mimicking a mass lesion.

10. Computerized tomography is used to ascertain the status of the lateral ventricles and the degree of parasellar and suprasellar extensions of a pituitary tumor.

11. Isotope scanning is rarely helpful in pituitary lesions until they have become so large as to be detectable by other means. Hence, isotope scanning is not indicated in the evaluation of these patients.

12. Visual fields.

13. Nose and throat cultures taken 48 hours before surgery to determine the flora and its sensitivity to antibiotics.

14. Ampicillin or oxacillin is usually given 24 hours preoperatively and maintained for 5 to 7 days after surgery.

15. 50 mg cortisone acetate is administered every 6 hours the day before surgery. On the day of surgery, 100 mg of hydrocortisone is given intramuscularly. This is repeated intraoperatively.[23]

POSTOPERATIVE CARE.

The patient's anterior nasal packing is removed five to seven days postoperatively. A urinary Foley catheter monitors hourly output. Urine osmolality, electrolytes and specific gravity are measured. In most instances, postoperative diabetes insipidus is transient and relatively mild, lasting 12 to 48 hours. In these cases, only replacement fluid therapy is required. A diagnosis of diabetes insipidus is made if the urine output is greater than 250 cc per hour with a specific gravity of 1.005 or less. When diabetes insipidus occurs, pitressin (usually the oil suspension preparation) is required. In our series, three cases of permanent diabetes insipidus required the use of pitressin nasal spray. Postoperative replacement therapy with steroids and thyroxin is indicated if hypophysectomy is performed.

SURGICAL ANATOMY.

The skull dissections and the whole head sections with radiographic correlations were prepared for this dissertation to illustrate the surgical anatomy for the sublabial transseptal transsphenoidal hypophysectomy.

The adult male pituitary gland weighs between 350 and 800 mg while an adult female pituitary gland weighs between 450 and 900 mg. In the female, the weight of the pituitary gland changes with pregnancy. The gland measures about 12 mm horizontally, 8 mm vertically and 8 mm anteroposteriorly. It lies in a depression on the roof of the sphenoid sinus called the sella turcica. On lateral view, the sella should not be more than 1.7 cm in A-P diameter and not more than 1.4 cm in depth. Zervas[80] and Bergland, et al.,[81] pointed out that, although preoperative radiographic studies can demonstrate the dimensions of the sella turcica, they cannot define the limits of the hypophysis in all cases. In the majority of cases the hypophysis conforms to the dimensions of the sella turcica, particularly along the anterior, inferior and posterior contours. The lateral borders of the hypophysis are bound by soft tissues and by the cavernous sinuses making the exact determination of the width of the gland impossible from preoperative radiographs. The superior margin is similarly difficult to estimate. Anterior to the sella turcica lies the tubercle of sella (tuberculum sellae or olivary eminence); posterior to it lies the dorsum sellae. Antero-laterally on each side are the anterior clinoid processes (Fig. 7, page 28). Posterolaterally on each side are the posterior clinoid processes. It is of interest to note that the surface identifications of the sella turcica are one inch anterior to and one inch above the external auditory meatus.

The chiasmatic sulcus is a transverse groove located between the optic foramina. It lies between the tuberculum sellae and limbus sphenoidalis.

Forming a roof to the sella is a part of the dura mater called diaphragma sellae. This is pierced by a stalk called the infundibulum which in turn connects the pituitary gland to the floor of the third ventricle of the brain.

The cavernous sinuses form the lateral walls and contain the III, IV, the first division of the V, VI nerves and the internal carotid artery. The two cavernous sinuses intercommunicate by a network of venous channels some of which span the anterior capsule of the hypophysis. This network is known as the circular sinus or intercavernous sinus. The usual location of the carotid artery is within the cavernous sinus lateral to the sella (Figs. 8-A and B). However, the carotid artery may be more medial and traverses the sella or may be exposed within the sphenoid sinus. Care

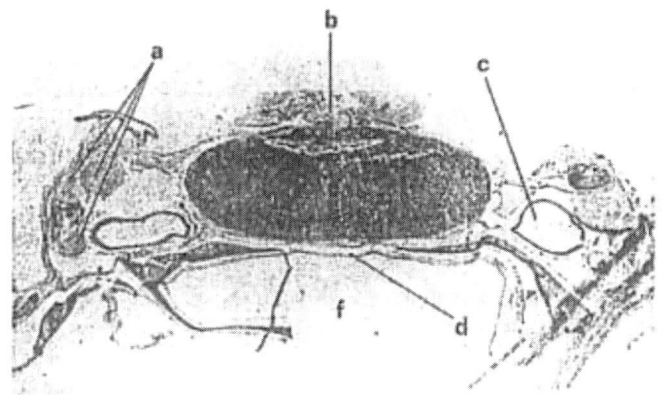

Fig. 8A. Histological slide of the sellar area. (a) Cranial nerves III, IV, V, VI. (b) Pituitary stalk. (c) Carotid artery. (d) Circular sinus (intercavernous sinus). (e) Pituitary gland. (f) Sphenoid sinus.

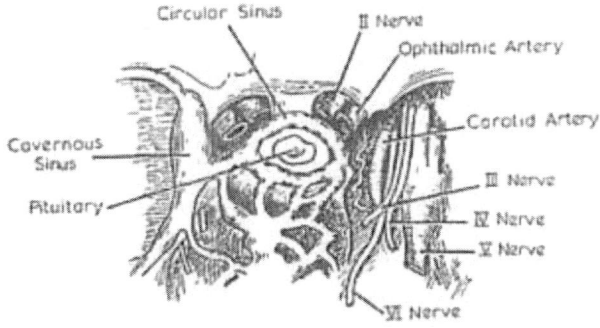

Fig. 8B. Vital structures in the parasellar area.

should be taken in the preoperative work-up to identify a carotid aneurysm or a tortuous carotid (Fig. 6). The carotid sulcus is noticeable on the sphenoid bone lateral to the sella (Fig. 7, page 28). Although the width of the hypophysis corresponds to the distance between the carotid grooves, in some cases the arteries are tortuous and compress into the gland medially as well as inferiorly.

The gland is covered by dura only. The pia arachnoid covers the stalk of the pituitary but does not reach beyond the diaphragma sellae. Unless the arachnoid is violated, no CSF leak ensues. Hence at surgery, unless the diaphragma sellae is penetrated, there should be no cerebrospinal fluid leak. Therefore, tumors of the anterior lobe are actually extradural thus, perhaps, explaining the respectable mortality rate of surgical removal, even prior to the antibiotic era. The level of the diaphragma sellae should span from the anterior aspect of the dorsum sellae to the tuberculum sellae, but it is important to know that such is not always the case. There may be pockets of arachnoid encroaching on the gland. A pocket that could lead to a CSF fistula after surgery was found in 17% of Zervas'[65] specimens and in 20% of Bergland's[61] material.

Bergland, et al.,[61] studied fresh autopsy materials and made the following observations:

1. In 80% of the specimens, the optic chiasm lies over the diaphragma sellae and pituitary. In 9%, it is prefixed, i.e., it is anteriorly displaced and lies over the tuberculum sellae. In 11% it is postfixed, i.e., it lies over the dorsum sellae.

2. In 20% of his specimens, pockets of arachnoid protrude into the sella increasing the chances of a CSF leak after transsphenoidal hypophysectomy. In 39% of the series, the opening for the stalk was greater than 5 mm. In 10%, the diaphragma sellae was considered too thin to prevent CSF rhinorrhea after surgical manipulation. However, in the opinion of the author, with the use of fascia plug over the sella and fatty connective tissue obliteration of the sphenoid sinus, CSF rhinorrhea can be avoided even in these unfavorable situations.

3. The average distance between the two carotid siphons was 14 mm. However, the spread was from 4 mm to 23 mm. In 22% of his specimens, the carotid was close enough to the gland to distort it.

4. The thickness of the anterior bony floor of the sella measures 1 mm in 72% of the specimens. The posterior bony floor is thicker and consists of spongiosum bone. In children, before pneumatization of the sphenoid bone has taken place, the anterior floor can be as thick as 20 mm.

Renn and Rhoton[62] studied 50 adult sellae. They noted anatomical variants of interest to the transsphenoidal hypophysectomy surgeon as well as to the transcranial hypophysectomy surgeon.

Of interest to the transsphenoidal hypophysectomy surgeon:

1. A thin diaphragm — 62%.

2. A large opening in the diaphragma sellae through which passes the stalk — 56%.

3. An intersphenoidal septum that is off the midline — 47%.

4. The absence of intersphenoidal septum — 28%.

5. A presellar presentation with no "pituitary bulge" into the sphenoid sinus — 20%.

6. Thick sellar floor — 18%.

7. A carotid artery that approaches within 4 mm of the midline — 10%.

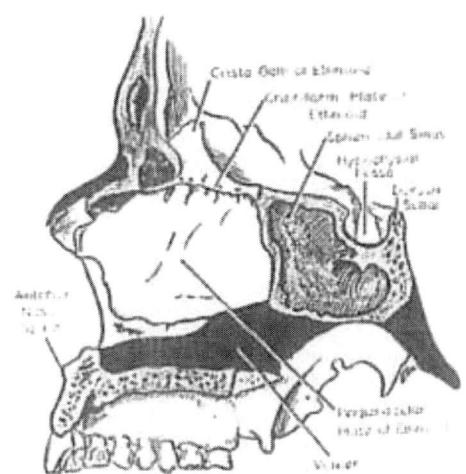

Fig. 9. Midline sagittal section.

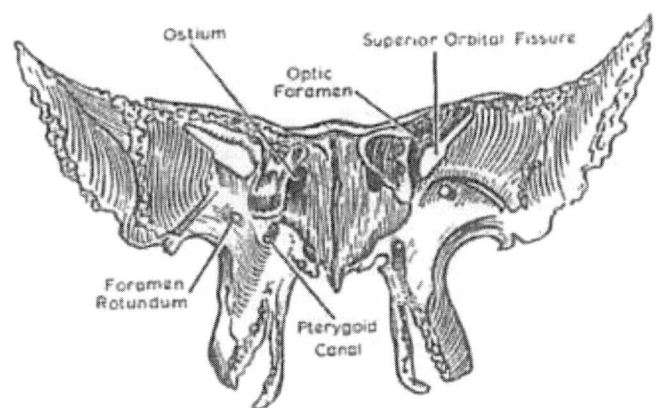

Fig. 10. Anterior view of the sphenoid bone.

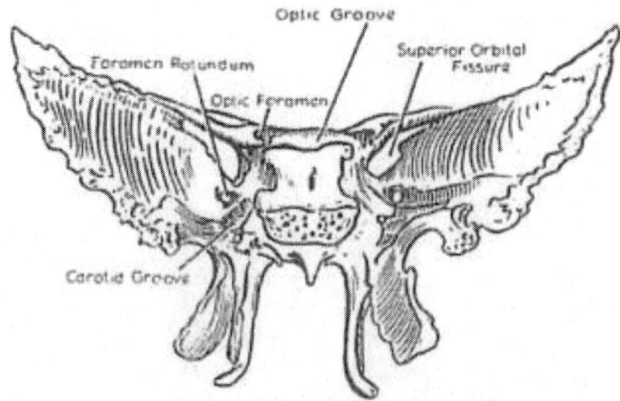

Fig. 11. Posterior view of the sphenoid bone.

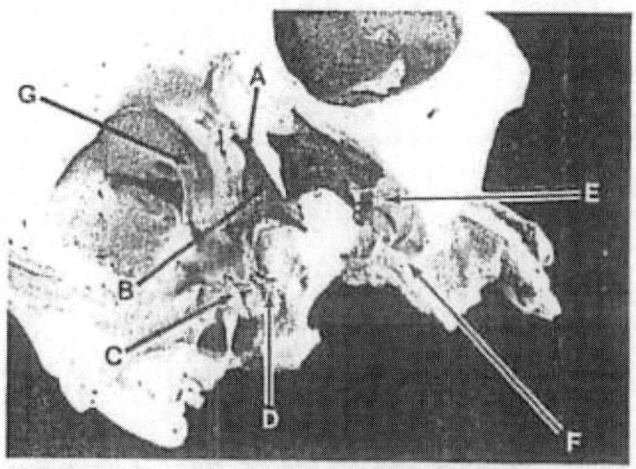

Fig. 12. Skull dissection. (A) Sphenoid sinus. (B) Sphenoid rostrum. (C) Lateral pterygoid plate. (D) Medial pterygoid plate. (E) Medial wall of maxillary sinus. (F) Anterior nasal spine. (G) Medial wall of orbit.

8. Large anterior intercavernous sinus — 10%.

9. A bare carotid artery without bony protection in the sphenoid sinus — 4%.

10. Bony defect within the optic canal exposing the optic nerves in the sphenoid sinus — 4%.

Of interest to the transcranial hypophysectomy surgeon:

1. Prominent protruding tuberculum sella — 44%.

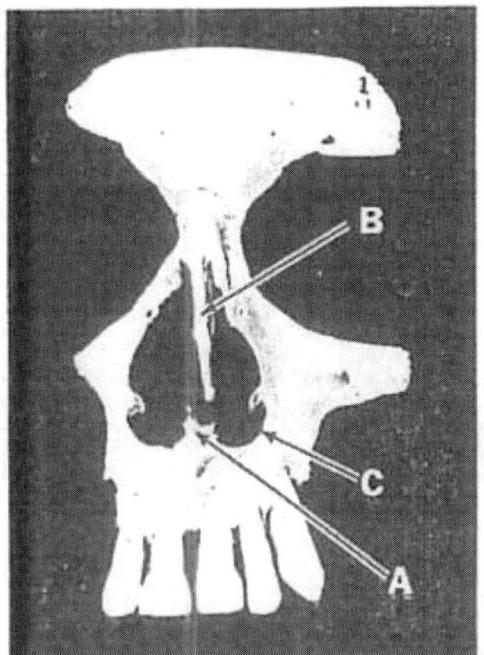

Fig. 13. (A) Anterior nasal spine. (B) Septal bone. (C) Pyriform aperture.

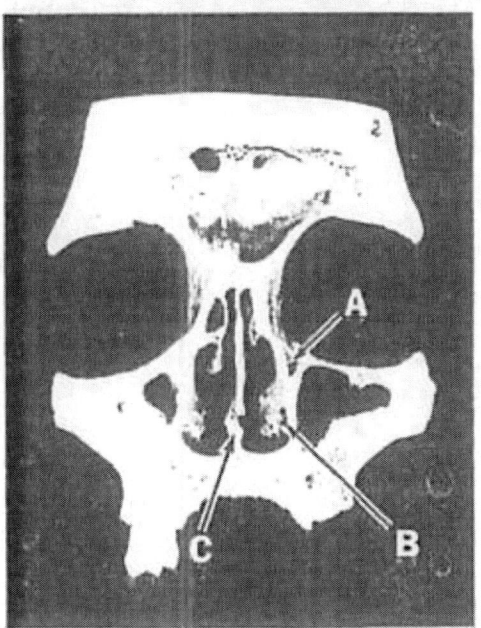

Fig. 14. (A) Nasolacrimal fossa. (B) Nasolacrimal opening. (C) Vomer.

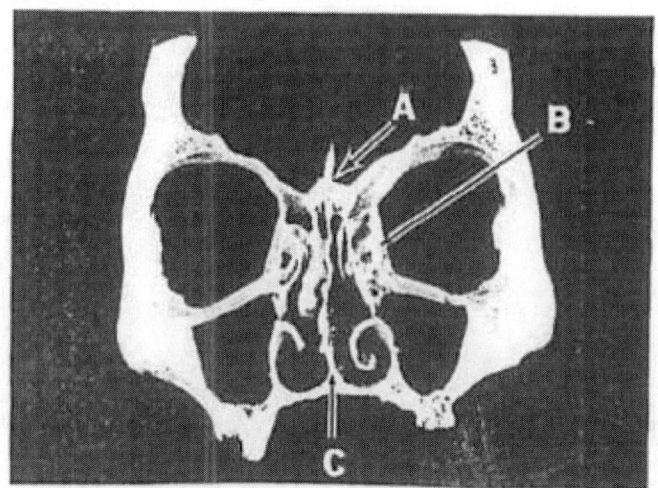

Fig. 15. (A) Crista Galli. (B) Lamina papyracea. (C) Vomer.

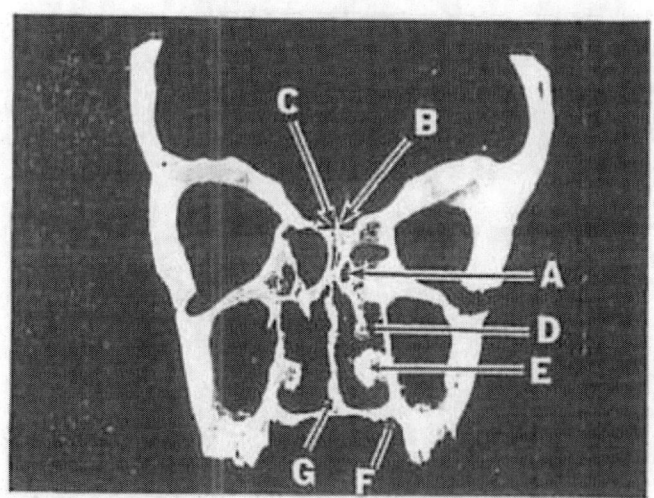

Fig. 16A. (A) Anterior ethmoid cell. (B) Crista Galli. (C) Cribriform plate. (D) Middle turbinate. (E) Inferior turbinate. (F) Palatine groove. (G) Vomer.

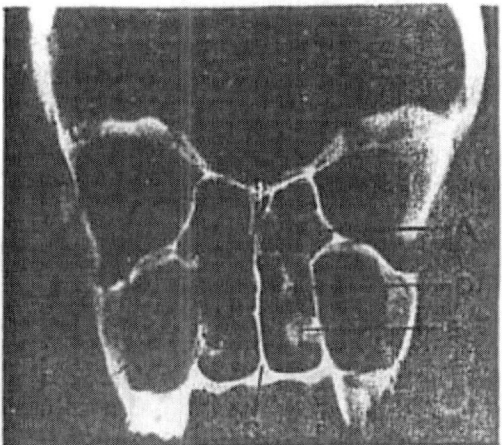

Fig. 16B. (A) Anterior ethmoid cell. (B) Crista Galli. (C) Cribriform plate. (D) Middle turbinate. (E) Inferior turbinate. (F) Palatine groove. (G) Vomer.

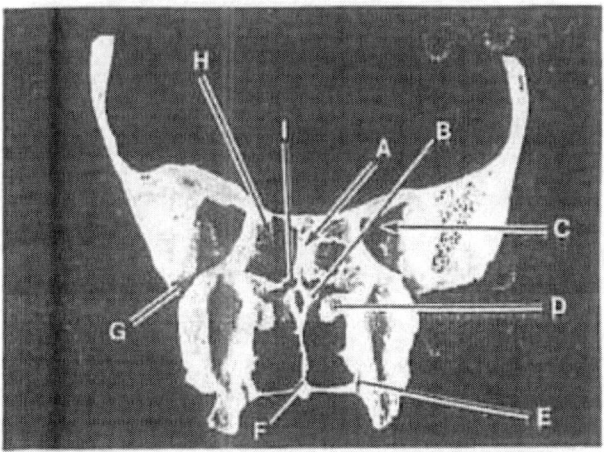

Fig. 17A. A) Sphenoid crest. (B) Sphenoid rostrum. (C) Superior orbital fissure. (D) Middle turbinate. (E) Greater palatine canal. (F) Vomer. (G) Inferior orbital fissure. (H) Posterior ethmoid cell. (I) Sphenoid ostium.

2. Prefixed chiasm — 10%.

3. The carotid artery within 4 mm of the midline — 10%.

Figures 9, 10, and 11 are a diagrammatic representation of the midline sagittal section, an anterior view of the sphenoid bone and a posterior view of the sphenoid bone respectively. Figure 12 is of a skull dissection in which the right maxilla has been removed together with the infraorbital rim and orbital floor to reveal the sphenoid sinus as well as the lateral and medial pterygoid plates. Figures 13 to 20 show the A-P cuts of a dry skull

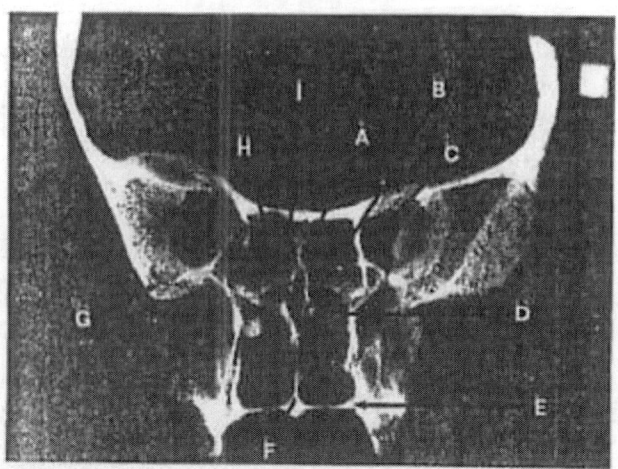

Fig. 17B. (A) Sphenoid crest. (B) Sphenoid rostrum. (C) Superior orbital fissure. (D) Middle turbinate. (E) Greater palatine canal. (F) Vomer. (G) Inferior orbital fissure. (H) Posterior ethmoid cell. (I) Sphenoid ostium.

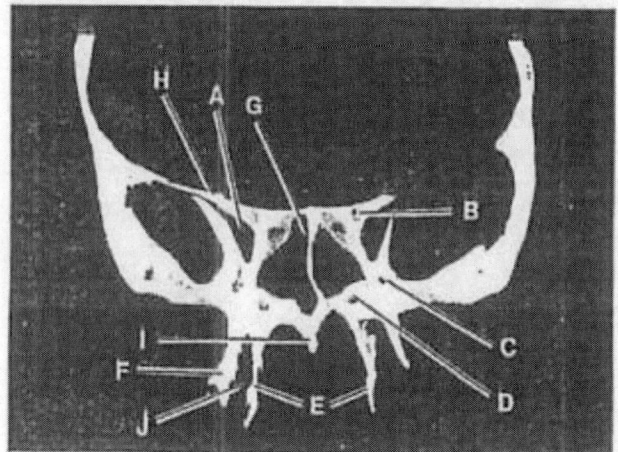

Fig. 18A. (A) Superior orbital fissure. (B) Optic canal. (C) Foramen rotundum. (D) Pterygoid canal. (E) Medial pterygoid plate. (F) Lateral pterygoid plate. (G) Intersphenoidal septum. (H) Lesser wing of sphenoid. (I) Sphenoid rostrum. (J) Pterygoid fossa.

illustrating the tomographic anatomy in this region from anterior to posterior. Figures 7, 21, and 22 are skull sections painted to help identify the vital structures that are to be avoided or identified during surgery.

Figures 23 to 31 are submentovertical sections (inferior to superior) of a whole preserved human head to illustrate the pertinent anatomy. These specimens are now cast in lucite for use as a 3-dimensional teaching aid for resident training or postgraduate education. It is of interest to note that this particular specimen has a deviated intersphenoidal septum lead-

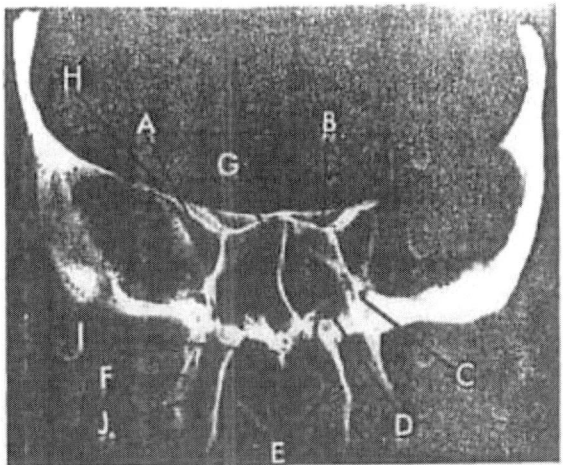

Fig. 18B. (A) Superior orbital fissure. (B) Optic canal. (C) Foramen rotundum. (D) Pterygoid canal. (E) Medial pterygoid plates. (F) Lateral pterygoid plate. (G) Intersphenoidal septum. (H) Lesser wing of sphenoid. (I) Sphenoid rostrum. (J) Pterygoid fossa.

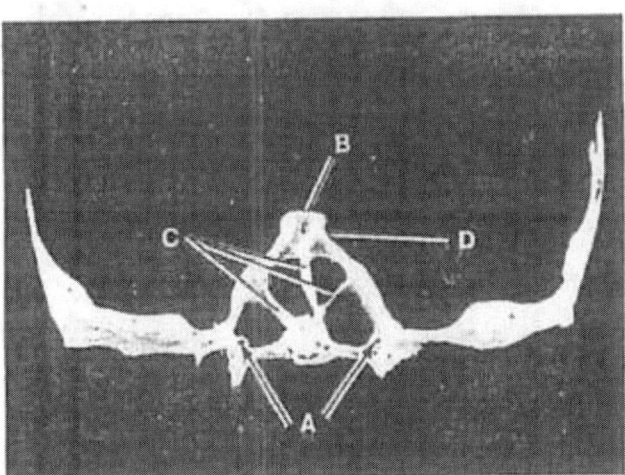

Fig. 19A. (A) Pterygoid canals. (B) Tuberculum sellae. (C) Intersphenoidal septi. (D) Depression of carotid sulcus.

ing towards the carotid artery as shown in Figure 29. As pointed out previously, preoperative submentovertical laminography is essential to determine the direction of the intersphenoidal septum. In reviewing 100 consecutive routine sinus X-rays, the author found that 34% of patients have a deviated intersphenoidal septum. Hence, unless guided by preoperative laminography, the intersphenoidal septum is a misleading "midline" structure. The vomer and the center of the sphenoid rostrum are more reliable landmarks.

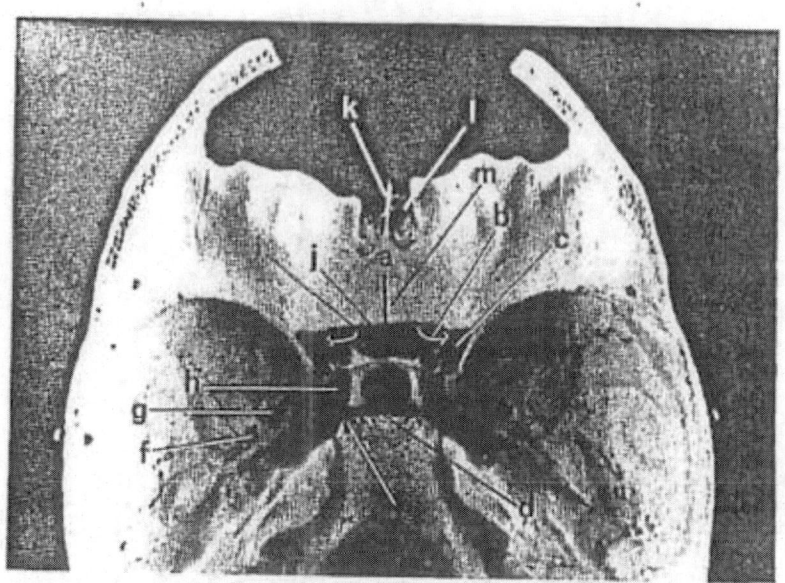

Fig. 7. (a) Tuberculum sellae. (b) Optic canal. (c) Anterior clinoid process. (d) Dorsum sellae. (e) Posterior clinoid process. (f) Foramen spinosum. (g) Foramen ovale. (h) Carotid canal. (i) Chiasmatic sulcus. (j) Limbus sphenoidalis. (k) Crista galli. (l) Cribriform plate. (m) Planum sphenoidale.

Appendix 2. Articles by Doctor Lee

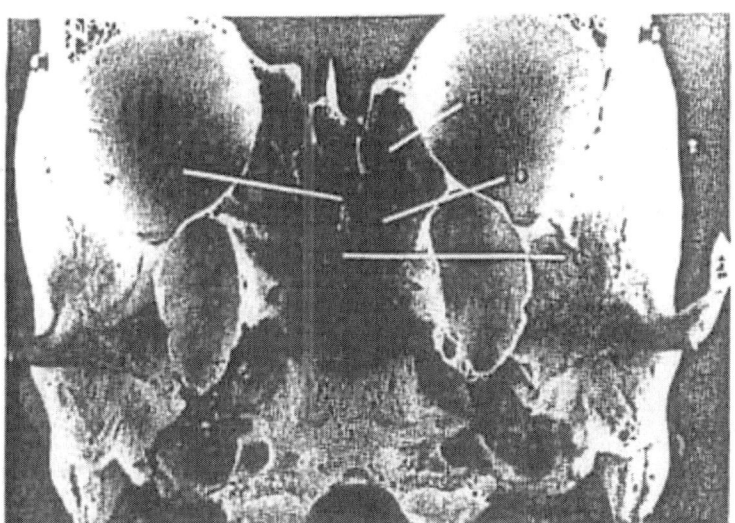

Fig. 21. (a) Ethmoid cells. (b) Sphenoid ostium. (c) Sphenoid rostrum. (d) Perpendicular plate of the ethmoid.

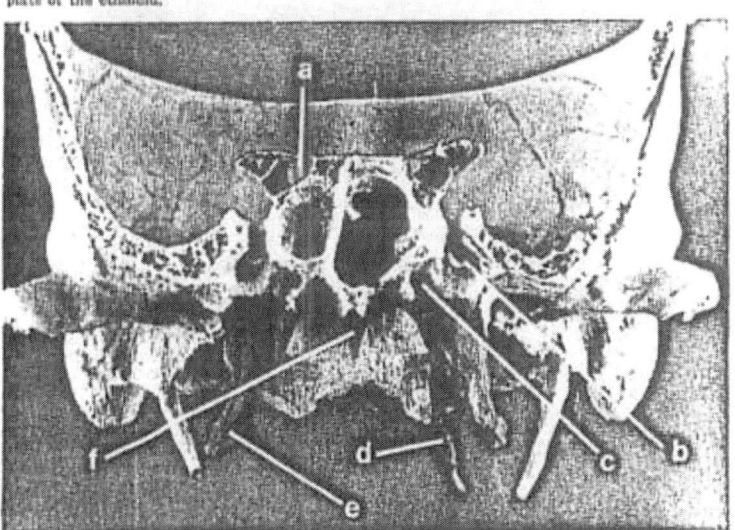

Fig. 22. (a) Optic canal. (b) Foramen rotundum. (c) Pterygoid canal. (d) Medial pterygoid plate. (e) Lateral pterygoid plate. (f) Sphenoid rostrum.

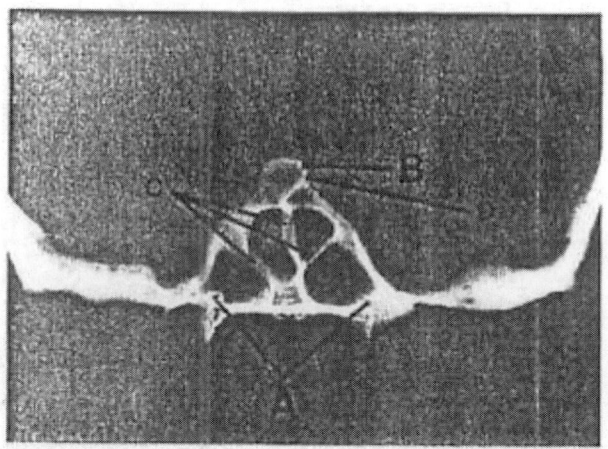

Fig. 19B. (A) Pterygoid canals. (B) Tuberculum sellae. (C) Intersphenoidal septi. (D) Depression of carotid sulcus.

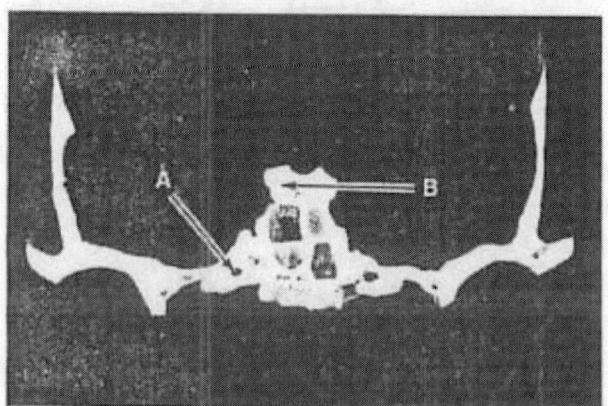

Fig. 20A. (A) Pterygoid canal. (B) Dorsum sellae.

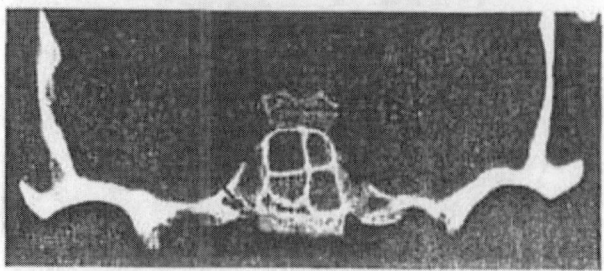

Fig. 20B. (A) Pterygoid canal. (B) Dorsum sellae.

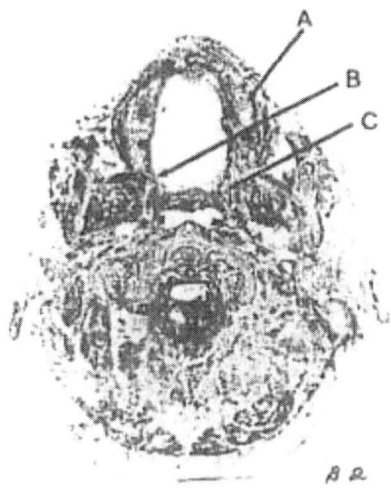

Fig. 23. (A) Maxillary antrum. (B) Hamulus. (C) Medial pterygoid plate.

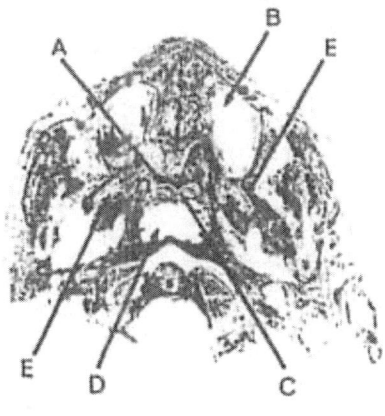

Fig. 24. (A) Hard palate. (B) Maxillary antrum. (C) Posterior nasal spine. (D) Nasopharynx. (E) Lateral pterygoid plate.

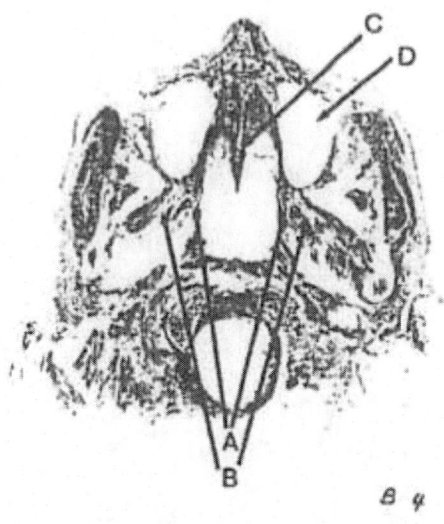

Fig. 25A. (A) Medial pterygoid plates. (B) Lateral pterygoid plates. (C) Vomer. (D) Maxillary sinus.

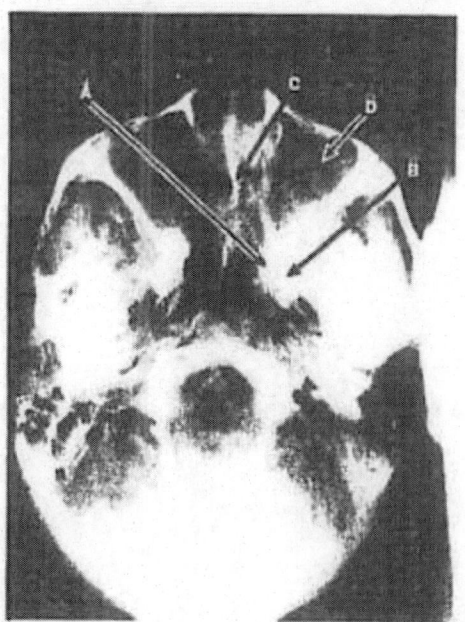

Fig. 25B. (A) Medial pterygoid plates. (B) Lateral pterygoid plates. (C) Vomer. (D) Maxillary sinus.

Appendix 2. Articles by Doctor Lee

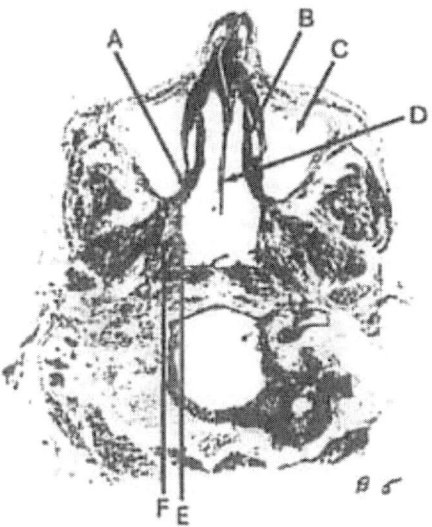

Fig. 26. (A) Greater palatine canal. (B) Inferior turbinate. (C) Maxillary sinus. (D) Vomer. (E) Medial pterygoid plate. (F) Lateral pterygoid plate.

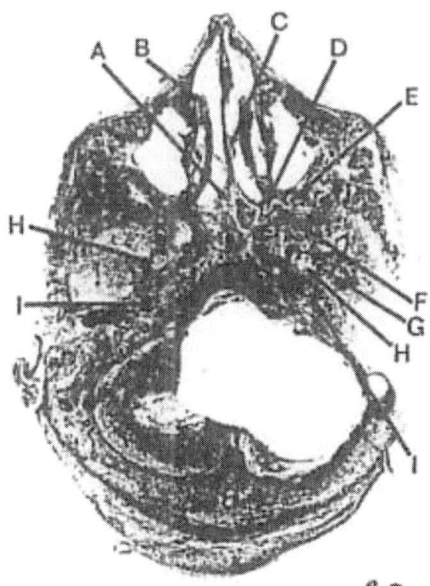

Fig. 27A. (A) Sphenoid rostrum. (B) Inferior turbinate. (C) Vomer. (D) Medial pterygoid plate. (E) Lateral pterygoid plate. (F) Pterygoid fossa. (G) Foramen spinosum. (H) Foramen ovale. (I) Carotid canal.

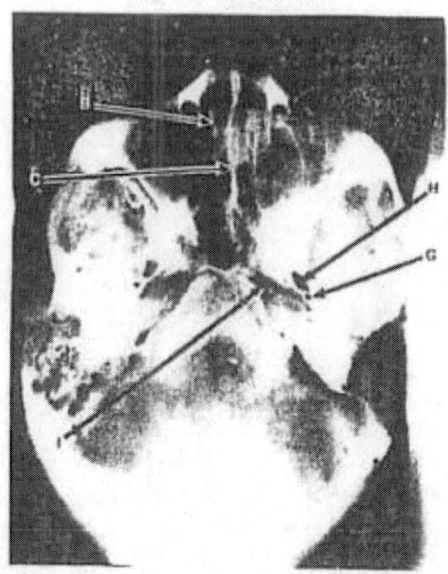

Fig. 27B. (B) Inferior turbinate. (C) Vomer. (G) Foramen spinosum. (H) Foramen ovale. (I) Carotid canal.

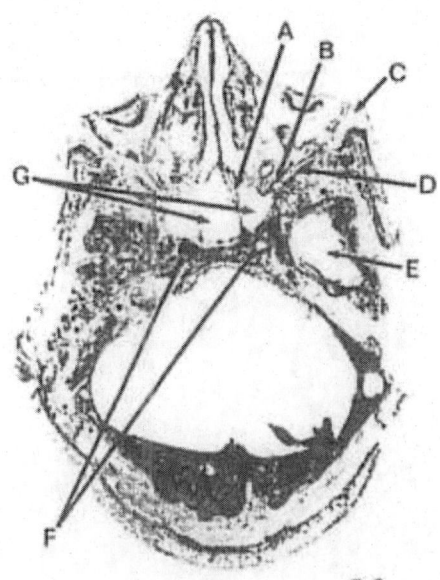

Fig. 28. (A) Intersphenoidal septum. (B) Foramen rotundum. (C) Zygoma. (D) Greater wing of the sphenoid. (E) Middle cranial fossa. (F) Carotid canals. (G) Sphenoid sinus.

Appendix 2. Articles by Doctor Lee

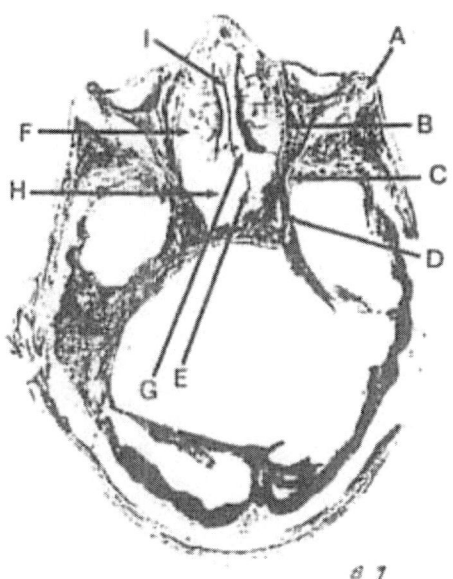

Fig. 29A. (A) Zygoma. (B) Lamina papyracea. (C) Superior orbital fissure. (D) Carotid artery. (E) Intersphenoidal septum. (F) Posterior ethmoid cells. (G) Sphenoid ostium. (H) Sphenoid sinus. (I) Perpendicular plate of the ethmoid.

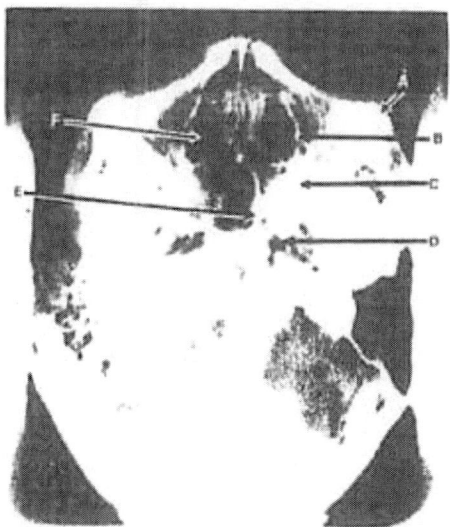

Fig. 29B. (A) Zygoma. (B) Lamina papyracea. (C) Superior orbital fissure. (D) Carotid artery. (E) Intersphenoidal septum. (F) Posterior ethmoid cells.

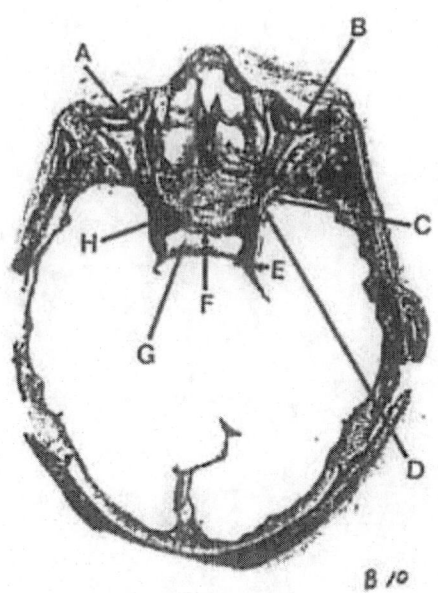

Fig. 36. (A) Planum sphenoidale. (B) Floor of optic canal. (C) Superior orbital fissure. (D) Anterior clinoid process. (E) Posterior clinoid process. (F) Tuberculum sellae. (G) Sella turcica. (H) Carotid artery.

SURGICAL TECHNIQUE.

The following technique is similar to that of Hardy[7] with modifications by the author.

The patient is placed in the position shown in Figure 32-A, with the operative field slightly elevated above the heart for better hemostasis. Slight hyperextension of the neck allows a better line of vision. Elevation of the lower extremities prevents pooling of blood to avoid hypotension and flexion of the knee is for the patient's comfort. The author prefers to operate from the right side of the patient. The dissection is done without magnification until the sphenoid sinus is encountered. An operating microscope with a 400 mm objective lens and angled eyepiece is placed as in an otologic case for the right ear. This arrangement allows a comfortable working posture for the surgeon (Fig. 32-B).

After induction of general anesthesia, the operative field is injected with 9 cc of 1% lidocaine with epinephrine 1:100,000 concentration.[63] Cotton applicators dusted with 300 mg of cocaine flakes are introduced into the nose to decongest the nasal mucosa as in routine rhinoplasty. Excellent hemostasis is very important in the transseptal route. Special attention is given to draping so as to avoid placing metallic towel clips in the path of a lateral or A-P X-ray to be taken intraoperatively. The sublabial incision is made with a cutting bovie current (Figs. 33-A and B). This incision

Appendix 2. Articles by Doctor Lee

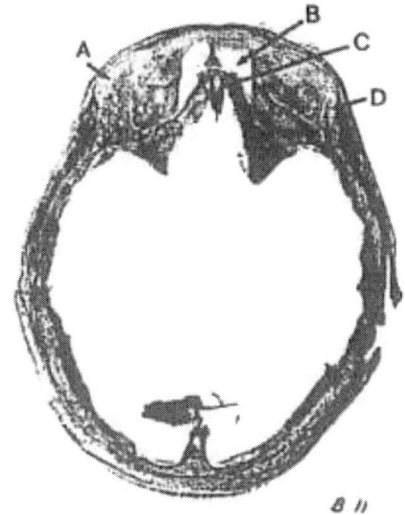

Fig. 31. (A) Zygoma. (B) Frontal sinus. (C) Crista Galli. (D) Greater wing of the sphenoid.

Fig. 32A. Diagrammatic representation to show positioning of operating table.

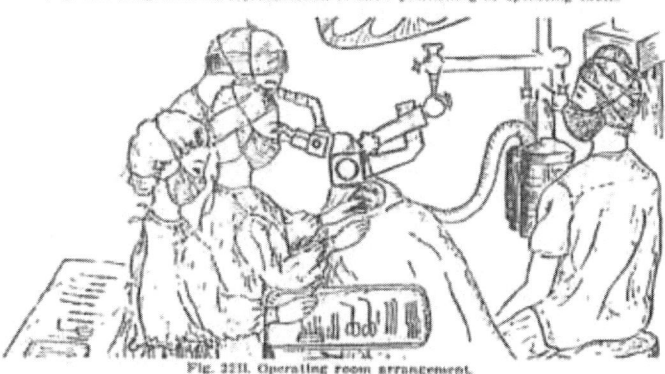

Fig. 32B. Operating room arrangement.

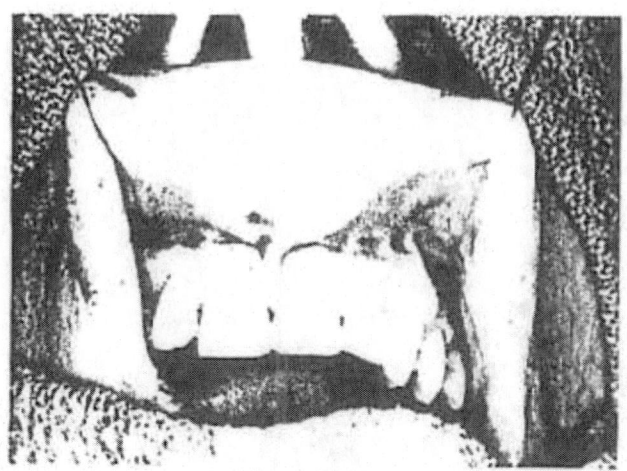

Fig. 33A. Incision.

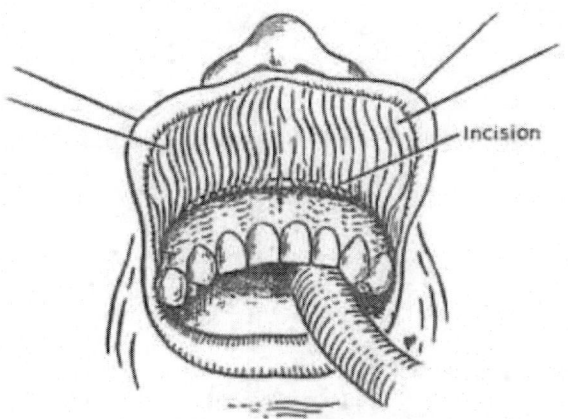

Fig. 33B. Incision.

transects the nerve endings of the superior labial branch of the infraorbital nerve causing temporary anesthesia of the upper lip.

The right pyriform aperture is identified and the mucous membrane is elevated, creating an "inferior tunnel" (Figs. 34-A and B). The caudal aspect of the septum is identified and the mucoperichondrium elevated on the ipsilateral side as in routine septoplasty. The elevation is carried past the perpendicular plate of the ethmoid (Figs. 35-A and B). The left "inferior tunnel" is made (Figs. 36-A and B). This dissection is carried posteriorly to the level of the perpendicular plate. However, the mucoperichondrium of the cartilaginous septum on this side is left intact for two

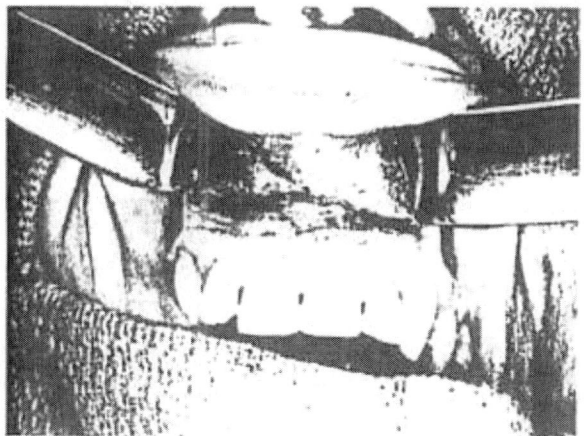

Fig. 34A. Elevating right floor of nose.

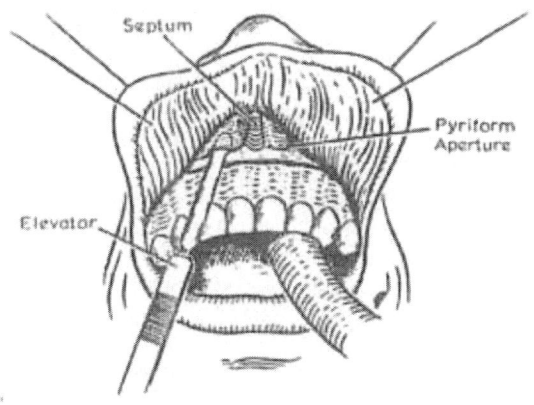

Fig. 34B. Elevating right floor of nose.

reasons: 1) It is not necessary to elevate it, 2) Should one need to return for recurrence of pituitary adenoma, this side will afford a fresh operative field. The anterior nasal spine is removed with a rongeur (Figs. 37-A and B).

Figure 38 illustrates the air drill removing part of the floor of the pyriform aperture to allow better seating and proper angulation of the blades of the self-retaining speculum to point towards the sella turcica. Excessive bone removal in this region will damage the branches of the anterior-superior dental nerve innervating the incisors and canines. Good hemostasis of the bone should be achieved with cautery or the use of a diamond

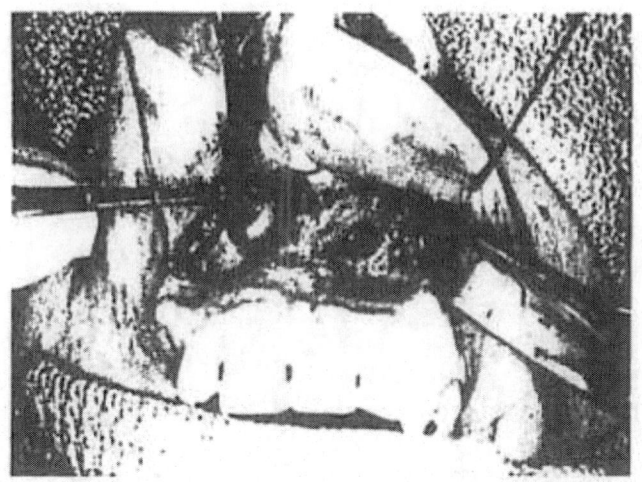

Fig. 35A. Elevating right mucoperichondrium of septum.

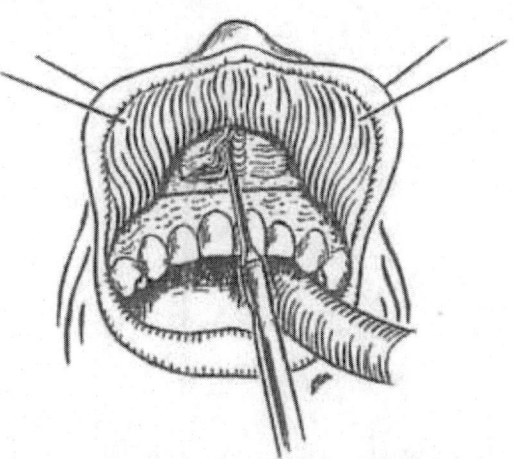

Fig. 35B. Elevating right mucoperichondrium of septum.

bur. The cartilaginous septum is then carefully dislocated to the left carrying with it the intact left mucoperichondrium. It is important at this step to elevate the mucoperiosteum of the perpendicular plate of the ethmoid on the left side as well as on the right to avoid a septal perforation. Part of the perpendicular plate of the ethmoid is then removed to visualize the sphenoid rostrum. It is important to stay in the midline and this is done by "keeping an eye" on the vomer since the intersphenoidal septum is an unreliable landmark as pointed out previously. The self-retaining speculum is then inserted and opened. Figure 39 shows the speculum blades in relation to the septum, mucoperichondrium and nasal mucosa.

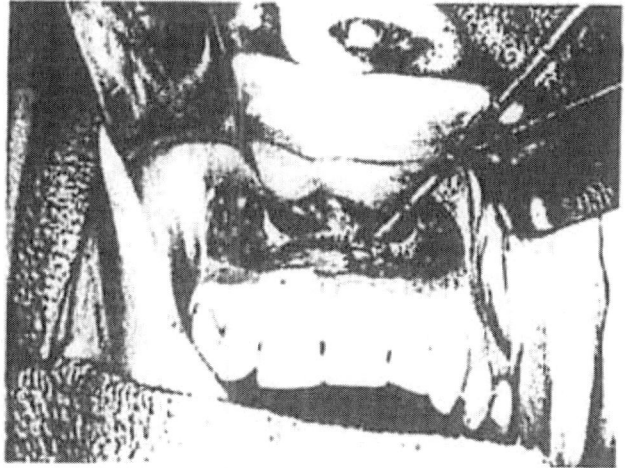

Fig. 36A. Elevating left floor of nose.

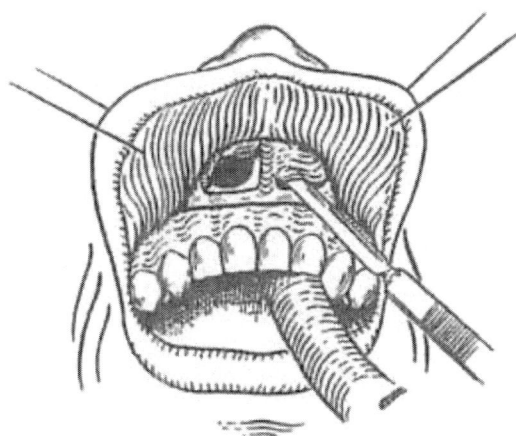

Fig. 36B. Elevating left floor of nose.

The lateral movement of the speculum blades is limited by the width of the pyriform apertures anteriorly and by the mid-portion of the medial pterygoid plates posteriorly. It is important not to fracture the pyriform apertures, the medial pterygoid plates, the medial walls of the orbits and the medial walls of the maxillary sinuses. Once past the pyriform apertures, the distance between the mid-portion of the two medial pterygoid plates is the narrowest width in the path of the speculum. The depth of introduction of the blades of the speculum depends on the pneumatization and presentation of the sphenoid sinus. The contour of the blades of the self-retaining speculum is designed to gain maximum working space for

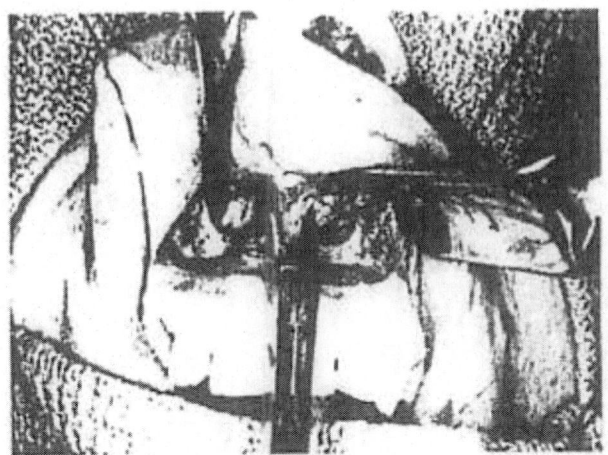

Fig. 27A. Removing anterior nasal spine.

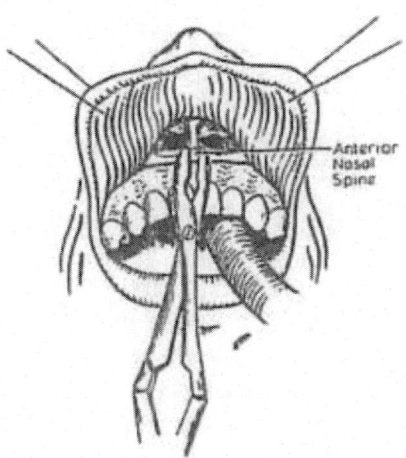

Fig. 27B. Removing anterior nasal spine.

bimanual manipulation and the effective use of the operating microscope. (See Section on Development of New Instruments.)

Figures 40-A and B illustrate the introduction of the self-retaining speculum. The anterior wall of the sphenoid is removed with the sphenoid punch and Kerrison rongeurs, care being taken to avoid the vital structures discussed previously. A good landmark to identify at this point is the ostia of the sphenoid sinus with the mucosa displaced laterally. A

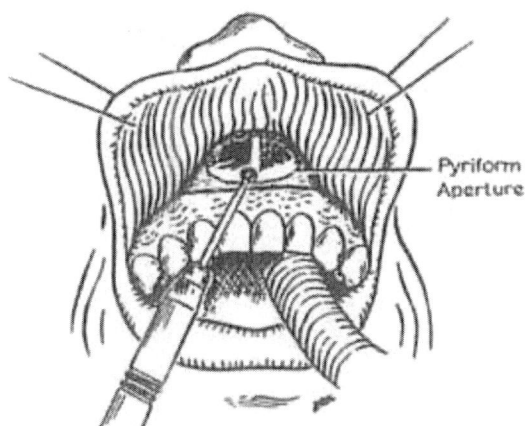

Fig. 38. Removing anterior bony floor of nose.

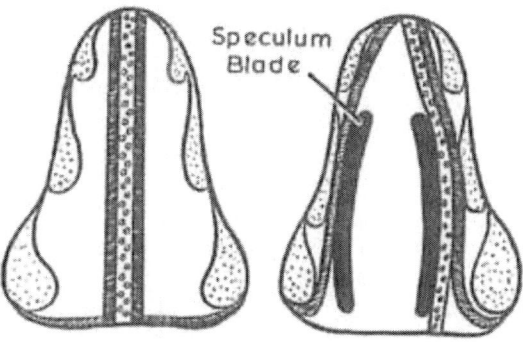

Fig. 39. Positioning of speculum blades in relation to septal cartilage and mucoperichondrium.

branch of the sphenopalatine artery usually lies inferior to the ostium. A sphenoid septum deviating extremely to one side may erroneously lead the unsuspecting surgeon to the carotid artery or cavernous sinus. In approximately 86% of the sphenoid bones,[10] the pneumatization is such that the sella presents itself into the sphenoid sinus (sellar type, Fig. 2). In this case, the anterior wall of the sella is thin and can be removed with the sphenoid curettes. However, even in these circumstances, the use of a diamond bur achieves complete hemostasis and prevents untoward injury to the circular sinuses (Figs. 8-A and B).

In cases where the presellar arrangement is encountered, the use of a diamond bur is very helpful. Usually a window about 1.5 x 1.5 cm is made

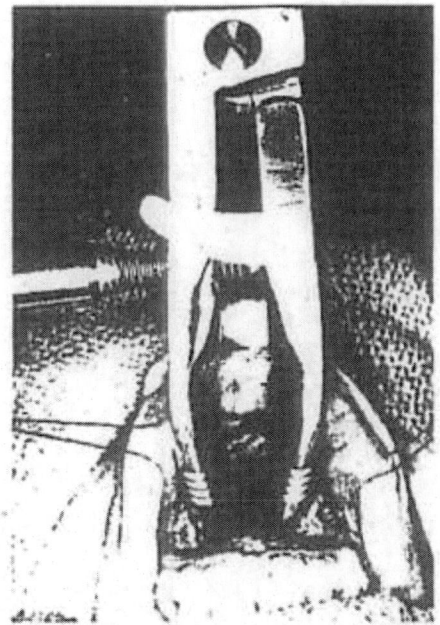

Fig. 40A. Introducing the self-retaining speculum.

through the posterior wall of the sphenoid sinus. A cruxiate incision is made in the dura, care being taken to avoid the venous lakes. Careful bimanual dissection is carried out with pituitary dissectors and curettes. Under magnification the two lobes of the pituitary appear different in color. The anterior lobe appears yellowish with a glistening capsule and becomes whitish when gentle pressure is applied. The posterior lobe appears gelatinous and greyish red in color. It is important to work between the dura and the hypophyseal capsule. Working in the extracapsular cleavage plane allows easier separation of the anterior lobe from the posterior lobe and helps to identify the stalk. Hardy[7] suggested using a cotton pledget to hold back the stalk and the posterior lobe while gently teasing out the anterior lobe in selective anterior hypophysectomy. During resection of a pituitary adenoma, the adenoma usually appears gelatinous and purplish-grey in color. Unlike the normal pituitary, the adenoma does not have a capsule. In fact, the dura is the "capsule" of the tumor. As previously pointed out, unless the diaphragma sellae is violated, there should be no CSF leak. When a CSF leak does occur it is controlled with a fascia graft placed against the opening.

Unlike the pituitary adenoma which has no capsule, a craniopharyngioma has a thick membrane. It usually contains a brownish fluid with cholesterol crystals. The normal pituitary with its own capsule lies outside the capsule surrounding the craniopharyngioma. Hence, with careful dissection under microscopic magnification, it is possible to avoid damage to the normal gland. Since the craniopharyngioma is quite adherent to the dia-

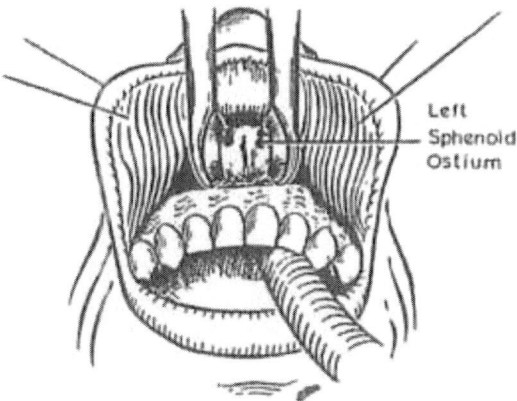

Fig. 40B. Introducing the self-retaining speculum.

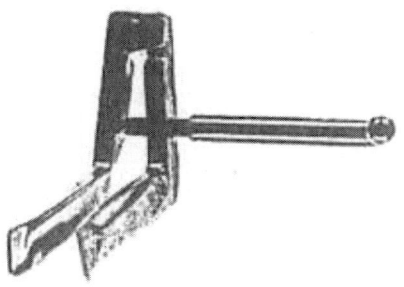

Fig. 41. Self-retaining speculum.

phragma sellae, a small CSF leak is not uncommon during removal of these tumors.

At the conclusion of the surgery, the dura defect is closed with fascia obtained from the right thigh. All mucosa is removed from the sphenoid sinus and the cavity is obliterated with fatty connective tissue. The sublabial incision is closed with interrupted 3-0 chromic catgut. The nasal cavities are packed with vaseline gauze impregnated with bacitracin ointment as for septoplasty.

DEVELOPMENT OF NEW INSTRUMENTS.

At the time we started performing this procedure, the most commonly used self-retaining speculum was the Hardy's Modified Cushing Bi-Valve Speculum. It fulfilled the purpose, but many surgeons, including our team, felt that the mechanical leverage was poor, requiring "sheer force" to open the self-retaining speculum. In addition, the tips of the speculum did

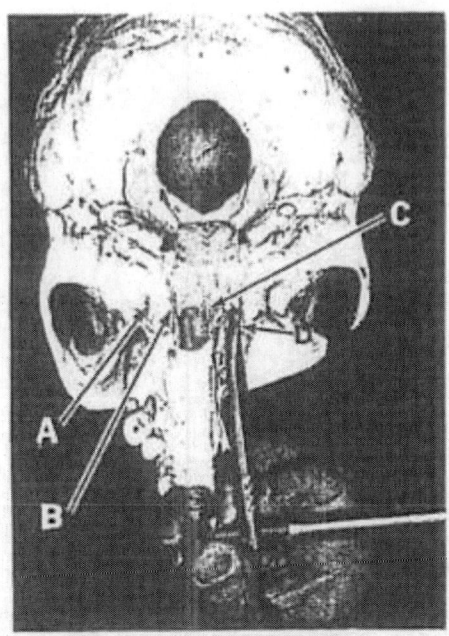

Fig. 42. Submentovertical view of the self-retaining speculum in a dissected skull. (A) Lateral pterygoid plate. (B) Medial pterygoid plate. (C) Sphenoid rostrum. (D) Flared tip of speculum.

not retract the mucosa laterally. Working with a toolmaker, the self-retaining speculum, as shown in Figures 40-A and 41, was devised by the author and is currently commercially available. Its mechanical advantage permits opening the blades with smooth and easy finger-tip motion. The speculum blades are flared at the tips to better hold the mucosa laterally, providing a wider operative field (Fig. 42).

Due to limitations imposed laterally by the medial wall of the orbit (Fig. 12), the self-retaining speculum blades cannot rest on an axis between the anterior nasal spine and the sella but need to rest inferior to the sella as illustrated in Figures 43-A and B. Furthermore, the blades should not rest parallel to the palate. Lowering the bony ridges lateral to the anterior nasal spine (Fig. 38) permits the tips of the speculum to be directed slightly upwards.

The distal portions of the speculum blades rest on the medial wall of the maxilla or on the mid-portion of the medial pterygoid plates (Fig. 42). The space between the two medial pterygoid plates being the narrowest width in the path of the speculum, it is helpful to determine a measurement of this distance preoperatively from A-P laminograms. The zygomatic-temporal suture line lies approximately in the same plane as the medial pterygoid plates in an A-P laminogram. Placing surface metallic markers at the zygomatic-temporal suture line on the patient when the X-ray is taken will aid in calculating the actual distance between the medial pterygoid plates. Figures 44 and 45 show markers placed on the

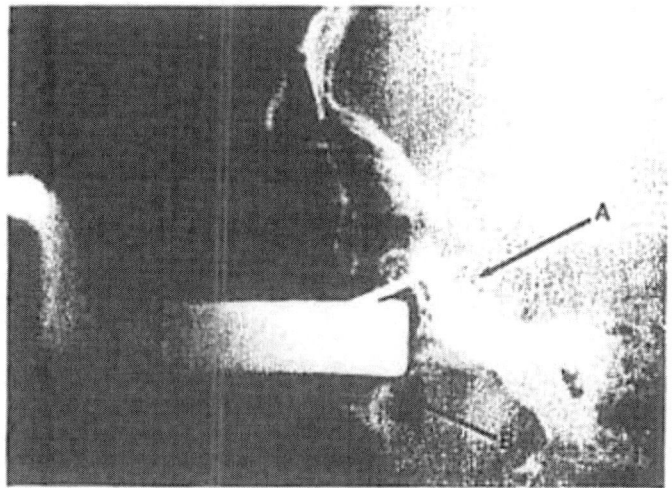

Fig. 43A. (A) Sella. (B) Medial pterygoid plates.

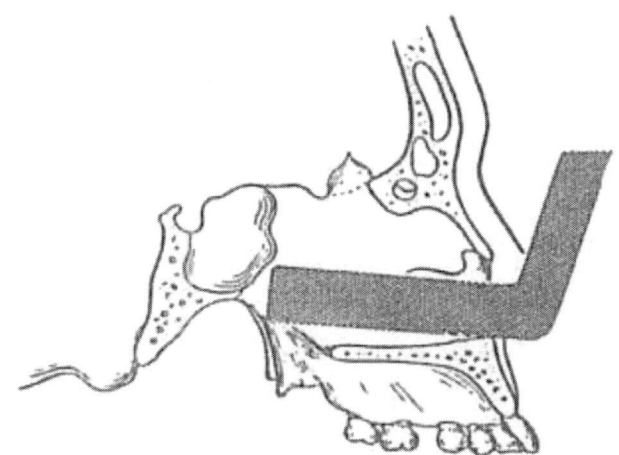

Fig. 43B. Diagrammatic representation of self-retaining speculum in position.

zygomatic-temporal suture line as well as on the medial pterygoid plates in a skull. The actual distance between the zygomatic markers can be measured on the skull or on the patient (x'y'). The radiographic distances xy and ab can be measured on the X-ray. Hence, the "unknown" distance between the medial pterygoid plates (a'b') in the case of a patient can be derived from the following formula:

$$a'b' = \frac{x'y'}{xy} \times ab$$

The formula applied to the skull shown in Figure 44 is:

$$a'b' = \frac{11.5}{15.5} \times 3.5 = 2.6 \text{ cm}$$

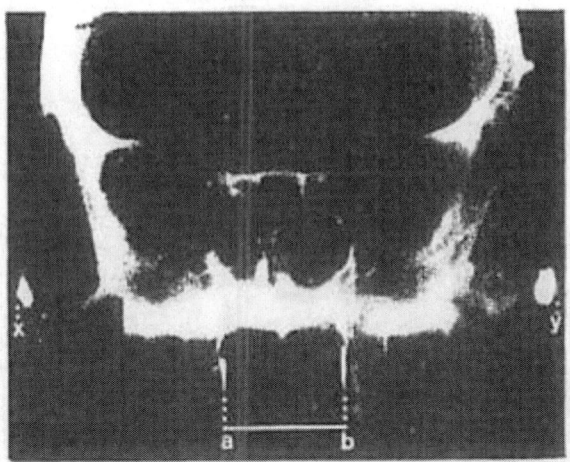

Fig. 44. A-P Laminogram of skull. (x,y) Markers on the temporo-zygomatic suture line. (a,b) Markers on the mid-portions of the medial pterygoid plates.

TABLE II.
Distance Between the Mid-Portions of the Medial Pterygoid Plates in 25 Adult Specimens.

Specimen	Measurement	Specimen	Measurement	Specimen	Measurement
1	2.8 cm	10	2.8 cm	18	2.9 cm
2	2.7 cm	11	2.7 cm	19	2.7 cm
3	2.4 cm	12	2.8 cm	20	2.6 cm
4	2.6 cm	13	2.6 cm	21	2.7 cm
5	2.5 cm	14	2.8 cm	22	2.8 cm
6	2.4 cm	15	2.6 cm	23	2.6 cm
7	2.7 cm	16	2.6 cm	24	2.5 cm
8	2.6 cm	17	2.8 cm	25	2.7 cm
9	2.8 cm				

Similarly, the distance between the two medial walls of the posterior maxillary sinuses can be predetermined.

The distance between the right and left medial pterygoid plates was measured in 25 adult specimens and found to be between 2.4 and 2.9 cm.

A gauge placed on the front of the instrument is calibrated to measure the opening of the tips of the blades (Fig. 40-A). Use of the gauge and the knowledge of preoperative measurements eliminate guesswork in achieving a safe and yet maximal operating aperture. This is particularly important in a patient with a small skull or with congenital anomaly (Fig. 46).

The proximal ends of the speculum blades are flat externally to reduce the width of the opened blades to accommodate the narrow pyriform aperture. The rest of the blades are convex externally to conform to the contour of the nasal cavity and concave internally to provide a wide operative

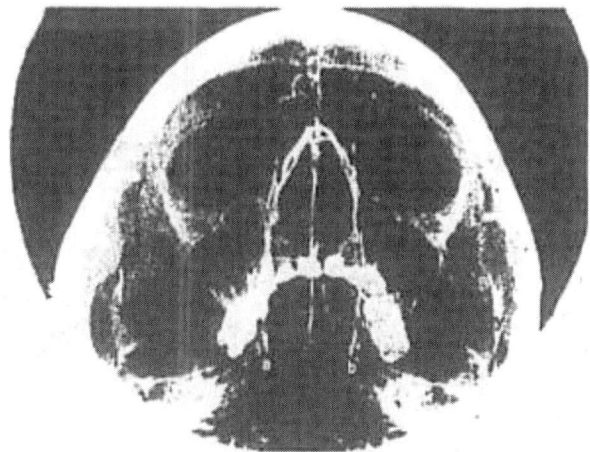

Fig. 45. Waters' view showing the same markers.

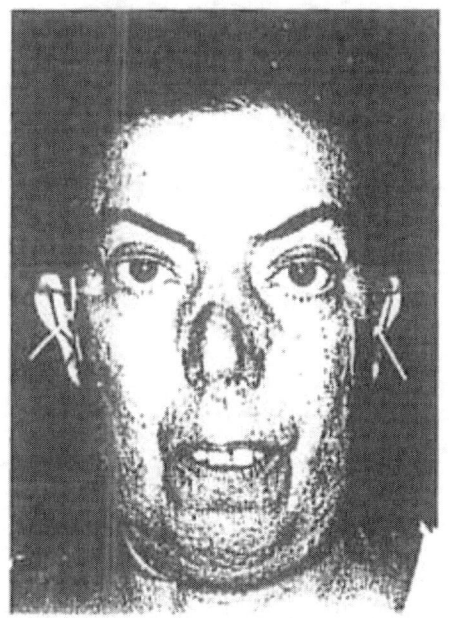

Fig. 46. Arrows point to lead markers on a patient with severe high arched palate and other anomalies.

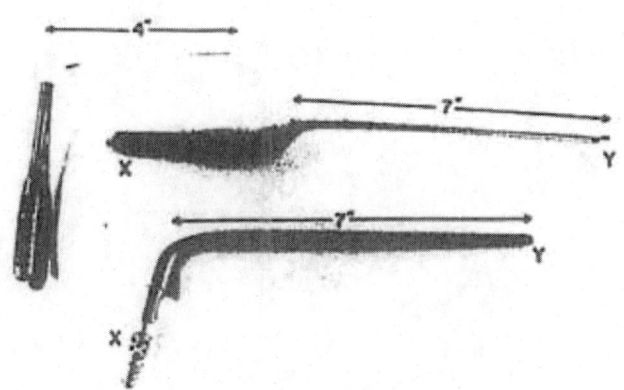

Fig. 47. Nasal speculum, Bayonet forcep, Nasal suction.

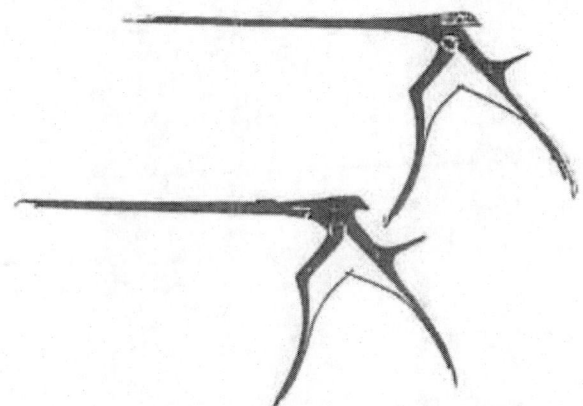

Fig. 48. Sphenoid punches.

field. From an engineering standpoint, the strength of the blade is greatly enhanced by this curved construction. The amount of force required to open the speculum to achieve an adequate operative field is surprisingly great.

To complement this self-retaining speculum, currently available instruments were modified to make them more suitable to our needs. A 4" insulated nasal speculum, a 7" insulated bayonet forceps, and a 7" insulated nasal suction were made (Fig. 47). The insulation in the suction tube and the bayonet forceps was omitted at both the proximal end and the distal tip to allow the use of cautery for hemostasis. One millimeter up-biting

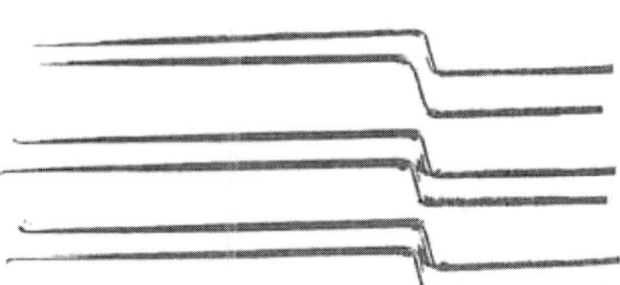

Fig. 49. Sphenoid curettes.

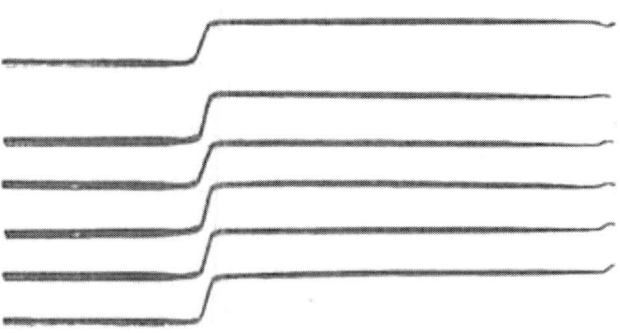

Fig. 50. Pituitary dissectors.

and down-biting sphenoid punches 7½" long were made (Fig. 48). Sphenoid curettes (cup sizes 3/16", 1/8", 3/32", each up and down), pituitary dissectors, ring curettes and pituitary knives were mounted on a bayonet handle with a working arm of 7¼" (Figs. 49, 50 and 51).

A 30° air drill, hand balanced to provide a firm grip, using small diamond burs and a working arm of 7", was designed with an air drill company (Figs. 52-A, B and C). The 30° angle was selected as the one offering the least interference with vision during manipulation. A well balanced air drill with the proper angle adds to the safety and ease of removing the posterior wall of the sphenoid sinus as contrasted to chiselling.

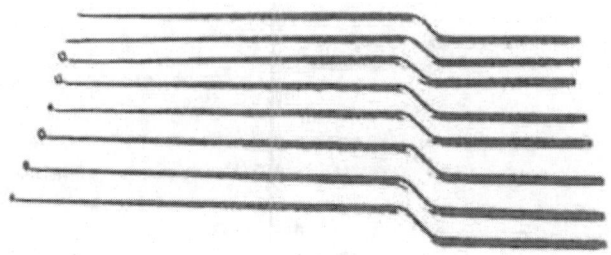

Fig. 51. Pituitary knives and ring curettes.

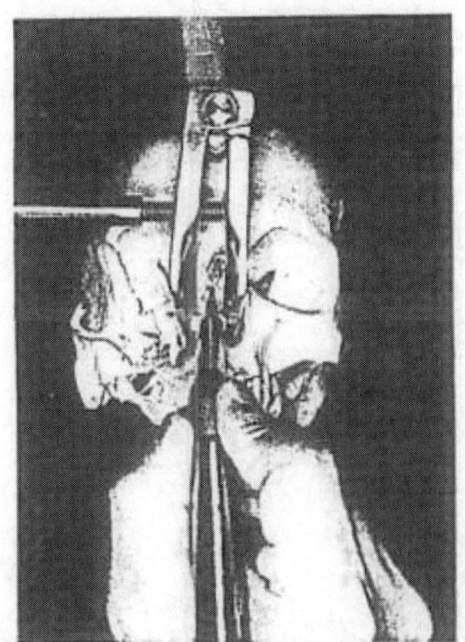

Fig. 52A. One way of holding the 30° Air drill. Note unobstructed view of bur tip.

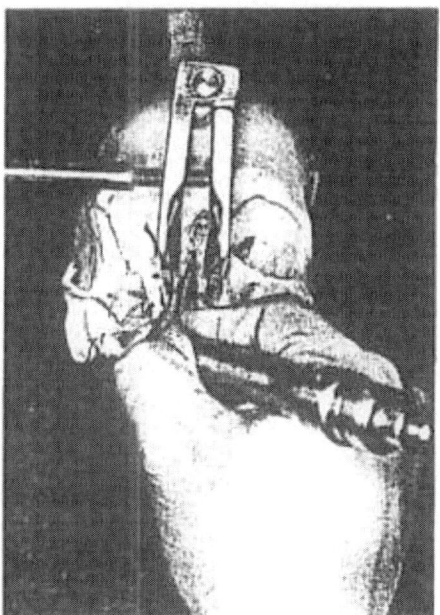

Fig. 5211. Another way of holding the 30° Air drill.

Since diamond burs are used, the drilling achieves hemostasis while removing bone. When used with care, it can uncover the circular sinus gently without damaging the sinus. The use of the drill is especially appropriate in a presellar or conchal type of sphenoid pneumatization. It is also of great help when exposing and partially removing a chondrosarcomatous lesion of the sphenoid bone for biopsy.

RESULTS AND COMPLICATIONS.

The literature on the efficacy of hypophysectomy for pituitary tumors, metastases from breast and prostate carcinoma and diabetic retinopathy has been discussed previously.

In the author's series of 30 cases of sublabial transseptal transsphenoidal approach, 13 were for palliation of breast carcinoma, 15 for pituitary adenoma, 1 for craniopharyngioma, and 1 for biopsy of a chondrosarcoma of the sphenoid bone. No operative mortality, CSF rhinorrhea, visual damage, carotid or cavernous sinus hemorrhage, fracture of medial pterygoid plate or maxilla was encountered in this series.

Table III outlines the complication rates of several reported transsphenoidal hypophysectomy series including that of the author's. Among the 51 cases of CSF rhinorrhea reported by Angell James,[a] five did not respond to conservative therapy consisting of daily lumbar puncture and bed rest in the head elevated position. Surgical repair was necessary in each of these five cases.

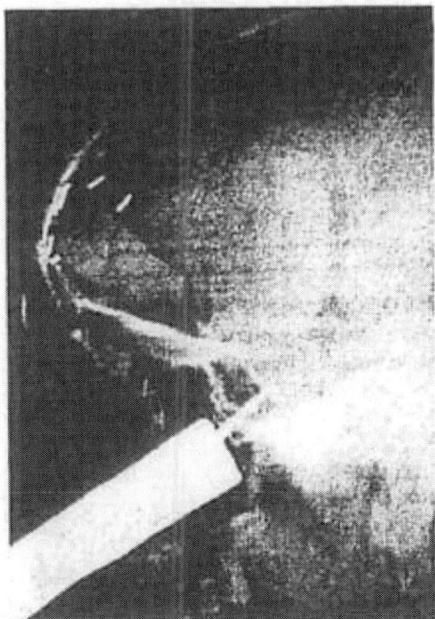

Fig. 52C. 20° Air drill in use.

Hardy[1] reported over 300 cases but did not report on complications. In another article covering 17 patients who underwent selective anterior hypophysectomy, he mentioned one case of CSF rhinorrhea.[20]

In Hudson and Kenan's[21] series, one patient died secondary to a tear in the anterior cerebral artery when a portion of the cribriform plate broke off during removal of the anterior surface of the sphenoid sinus. Bateman[21] reported one death secondary to anterior cerebral artery bleeding and one due to subarachnoid hemorrhage. In two of his cases there was sufficient bleeding from the anterior communicating sinuses to require termination of the procedure.

Postoperative anesthesia and paresthesia of the upper lip and teeth lasted no longer than six months in the author's series. Three patients reported no anesthesia or paresthesia of the upper lip and incisors. Nasal airway was normal in all cases postoperatively as evidenced by history and clinical examination. Rhinometric air flow studies were performed in the last eight cases and found to be within normal limits in each nasal passage after surgery. Two patients who had deviated nasal septums with nasal obstruction preoperatively enjoyed an improved nasal airway after surgery.

Among the 13 patients with breast carcinoma, four had no indications of any favorable response to hypophysectomy. Six of these patients had significant reduction in pain for three to six months. Four patients showed objective signs of decrease in bone metastases and one patient's supra-

TABLE III.
Complications.

	Total No.	CSF Rhinorrhea	Diabetes Insipidus (Permanent)	Meningitis	Carotid or Cavernous Hemorrhage	Ophthalmic Disturbance	Mortality
Angell James[1]	345	51	NI	11	0	2	26
Van Gilder[25]	94	2	3	3	0	0	1
Zervas and Gordy[26]	65	7	NI	5	0	0	0
Baker[13]	18	6	NI	6	2	0	1
Roth, et al.[17]	55	6	10	3	0	1	0
Kirchner and Van Gilder[21]	67	2	1	4	0	2	1
Macbeth[22]	36	NI	NI	2	1	0	2
Cross, et al.[20]	13	3	1	2	0	1	0
Hudson and Kenan[24]	38	4	1	1	0	1	1
Bateman[23]	22	NI	NI	3	0	0	2
Author's	30	0	3	2	0	0	0

NI = No Information.

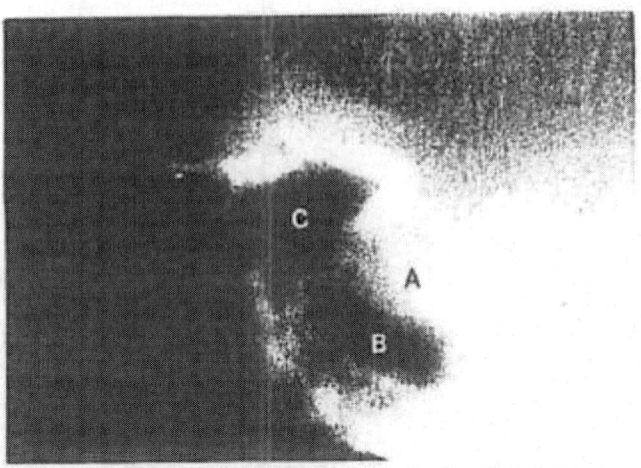

Fig. 53. Pituitary tumor eroding into the sphenoid sinus. (A) Sella turcica. (B) Pituitary adenoma in the sphenoid sinus. (C) Sphenoid sinus.

clavicular mass decreased from 5 cm x 4 cm in size to 2 cm x 1 cm within six months after surgery. Four patients are living and relatively well at this writing. These results are comparable to cases reported in the literature. It should be emphasized again that hypophysectomy for metastatic disease is only a palliative measure.

A long follow-up is necessary for pituitary adenomas to evaluate the results properly. Hence it would not be proper to actually give a meaningful report at this writing on the 15 cases of pituitary adenomas. However, five patients with disturbance in menstrual cycle or libido preoperatively enjoy normal sexual activities postoperatively. Two patients with hypothyroidism preoperatively are now euthyroid. Four patients are maintained on cortisone and synthroid postoperatively — one patient on synthroid alone. Two patients are on testosterone. Those patients with preoperative headache improved considerably after surgery.

CASE PRESENTATION.

Six diverse cases are presented here.

Case 1. A 52-year-old white male presented to the otolaryngologist's office for evaluation of a unilateral 60 db sensorineural hearing loss. Routine work-up confirmed the diagnosis of probable Ménière's disease with minimal vestibular disturbance.

A submentovertical X-ray demonstrated a questionable density in the sphenoid sinus. Further radiographic studies showed erosion of the sella with a large soft tissue mass in the sphenoid sinus (Fig. 53). Computerized tomography outlined the lesion (Fig. 54). Neurological examination was normal. Endocrinological studies, arteriography and pneumoencephalography were also normal. The patient was explored through the sublabial transseptal transsphenoidal approach and a chromophobe adenoma was encountered. Total gross tumor removal was accomplished except for possible remnants along the walls of the cavernous sinus. The patient had an uneventful postoperative course without developing diabetes insipidus. Postoperative radiation therapy was administered. No endocrine replacement therapy was needed and the patient returned to normal daily activity.

Case 2. A 58-year-old white male was hospitalized for evaluation of dyspepsia and acromegaly. Laboratory studies showed elevated growth hormone levels. Skull films showed marked erosion of the base of the skull, including involvement of the left ethmoid sinus, left anterior clinoid,

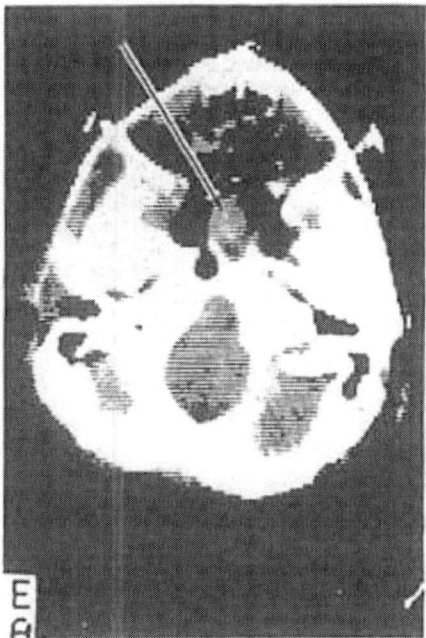

Fig. 54. Computerized tomography of patient in Case 1. Arrow points to the pituitary adenoma.

medial part of the left sphenoid wing, entire sphenoid sinus, sella turcica, and the rostral half of the clivus. The tumor mass was visible in the nasopharynx as outlined by the Pantopaque (Fig. 55). Angiography confirmed a massive tumor extending from the posterior nasal region to the foramen magnum with relatively mild suprasellar intracranial extension.

The day following angiography, progressive left orbital pain, marked left visual loss, ophthalmoplegia and lethargy evolved. An emergency repeat angiography revealed an increased mass effect, felt to be secondary to pituitary apoplexy. An emergency procedure utilizing the sublabial transseptal transsphenoidal technique, combined with nasopharyngeal dissection decompressed the bulk of the tumor mass, which on histological section proved to be a chromophobe adenoma. No evidence of recent hemorrhage or cyst formation was found. Two hours postoperatively, eye signs did not improve and the patient became more lethargic. Re-exploration of his transsphenoidal surgical site showed no compression from a hematoma. Bifrontal craniotomy was subsequently performed for further decompression of the optic nerves. The tumor was very dense and adherent to the suprasellar region, including the optic nerves. Total tumor removal was not feasible. Enterococcal meningitis developed postoperatively which responded to antibiotic therapy. The patient gradually improved and was discharged after completion of a course of radiotherapy. The patient remained blind in the left eye. A postcraniotomy left hemiparesis resolved in three months. He is currently maintained on cortisone acetate and thyroid extract.

Case 3. A 57-year-old white female was admitted to the hospital following a syncopal episode. Eighteen years prior to admission, she received radiotherapy (4,000 rads) for an enlarged sella turcica, presumed to be secondary to pituitary adenoma since no tissue diagnosis was made. At that time the patient was asymptomatic with normal endocrine and visual fields. The patient did well until ten years prior to admission when she developed a bitemporal hemianopsia with decreased visual acuity. Endocrine studies were again normal. Skull films revealed complete erosion of the sella turcica, including the dorsum sellae. Pneumoencephalography revealed a large sellar mass with extension close to the foramen of Monro and retro-displacement of the rostral brain stem. Significant hydrocephalus was not present. She was again treated with radiotherapy and received 3,000 rads. The patient did well until one and a half years prior to admission when she developed a slow, progressive decrease in higher cognitive function and visual acuity.

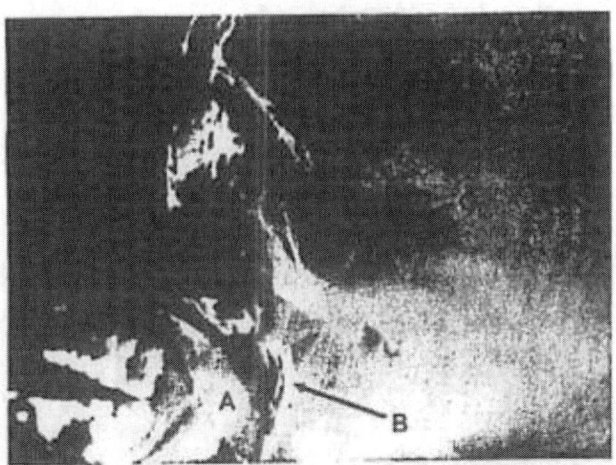

Fig. 55. Pituitary adenoma eroding into the nasopharynx. (A) Edematous soft palate. (B) Pantopaque outlining irregular nasopharyngeal mass. (C) Sella turcica.

On the day of the present admission the patient was found semiresponsive at home. After admission she rapidly returned to a normal level of sensorium following large doses of steroids and antibiotics. Work-up for pituitary apoplexy and/or meningitis was negative. Endocrine studies revealed low normal function. Bilateral optic pallor with bitemporal hemianopsia, the left being greater than the right, was present. Visual acuity was 20/50 on the left and 20/30 on the right. Skull films and tomography revealed complete erosion of the sella with disruption of its floor. The brain scan was within normal limits and an EEG revealed diffuse slowing. A computerized tomography scan revealed a large sellar mass with extension to the level of the foramen of Monro with indentation of the floor of the third ventricle, moderate hydrocephalus, and retro-displacement of the rostral brain stem (Fig. 56-A). Angiography confirmed the computerized tomography scan results.

The patient refused to consider transcranial approach surgery. A sublabial transseptal transsphenoidal approach to the tumor was performed. Approximately two thirds of the tumor mass was removed at surgery. Permanent histological sections revealed a chromophobe pituitary adenoma. The patient's postoperative course was benign except for transient diabetes insipidus. She was discharged on the ninth postoperative day on endocrine replacement therapy (cortisone acetate 37.5 mg q.i.d. and dessicated thyroid 2 grains q.d.). Postoperatively, her visual field testing revealed definite improvement bilaterally, the left greater than the right. Visual acuity was 20/30 bilaterally. She is currently being followed closely. She has resumed her normal daily activities. A postoperative computerized tomogram showed decreased density of the tumor site (Fig. 56-B).

Case 4. M. M. is a 48-year-old right-handed white male who was admitted for evaluation of a recurrent pituitary adenoma. In 1968, he developed bitemporal hemianopsia. His symptoms progressed and, in 1970, he underwent craniotomy to remove the pituitary chromophobe adenoma. No postoperative radiotherapy was given and he was not placed on replacement therapy. In 1971, he was re-evaluated because of a decrease in libido and generalized malaise. He was then placed on cortisone, testosterone and thyroid extract. Two months prior to his admission in February 1976, he developed increasing visual symptoms, especially in the left eye. On examination he was noted to have bitemporal hemianopsia. Brain scan revealed evidence of increased uptake in the suprasellar region. Three vessel angiography revealed displacement of one segment of the carotid artery bilaterally suggesting widening of the carotid siphon areas. Pneumoencephalography revealed extension of the tumor near the level of the foramen of Monro. Computerized tomography outlined the recurrent tumor with its suprasellar extension. Polytomography showed erosion of the sellar floor into the sphenoid sinus. Insulin tolerance test was abnormal and serum cortisol levels were low.

In spite of a confirmed suprasellar extension, it was decided to approach this tumor through the sublabial transseptal transsphenoidal route because of previous transcranial surgery and the morbidity associated with the previous transcranial approach. At the time of the surgery, a large portion of the tumor was removed. Dissection was carried 4 to 5 mm above the level of the

Appendix 2. Articles by Doctor Lee

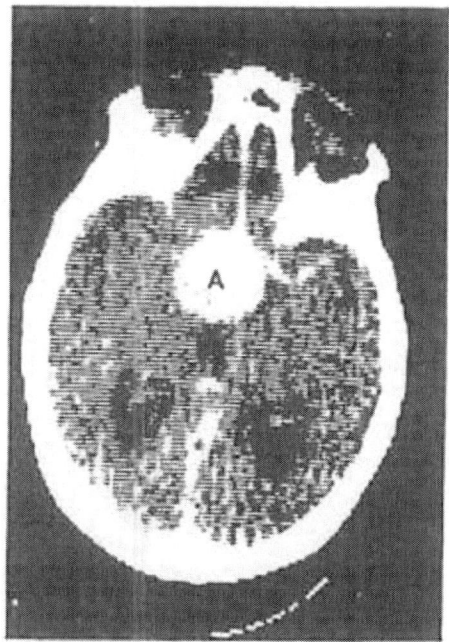

Fig. 56A. Preoperative CT scan of patient in Case 3 showing pituitary adenoma (A).

diaphragma sellae until the capsule of the tumor was identified. The dura defect was closed with a fascia plug and the sphenoid sinus filled with fatty connective tissue after its mucosa was completely stripped. The patient had an uneventful postoperative course. No CSF leak developed. Transient diabetes insipidus was present during the immediate postoperative course. The patient was put on a course of postoperative radiation. He is currently over one and a half years postoperative. He has shown improvement in his visual acuity and fields. He is still maintained on cortisone, testosterone and thyroid extract.

Case 5. J. K. is a 62-year-old white male who presented with left retro-orbital pain. Past medical history was noncontributory other than a pituitary tumor diagnosed in 1961 for which the patient received a full course of radiation therapy. At that time he was asymptomatic and the enlarged sella was an incidental finding in a routine skull film taken for evaluation of head trauma. No tissue diagnosis was obtained. He did well until two weeks prior to admission in 1977 when he had severe left retro-orbital pain. Visual fields were normal. Repeat skull films showed further destruction of the dorsum sellae as compared to previous films. At this time, the only positive findings were bilateral optic disc pallor and a decrease in vascularity of the small arterioles crossing the disc edges. Visual fields were intact. Laboratory investigation showed him to be hypothyroid. Prolactin and growth hormone levels were normal. CT scan showed an extremely expanded sella turcica. Polytomography and a pneumoencephalogram showed no suprasellar extension although the floor of the sella was eroded. Neuro-ophthalmological studies disclosed a visual acuity of 20/20 on the left and 20/30 on the right with an enlarged blind spot on the right secondary to old macula disease. He was on cortisone acetate 25 mg and thyroid extract 1 grain per day.

A sublabial transseptal transsphenoidal removal of pituitary adenoma was performed uneventfully. However, the pathological specimen showed pleomorphism with mitosis, suggestive of malignant degeneration of the chromophobe adenoma. Radiation consultation was obtained and the patient is currently undergoing postoperative radiation therapy.

Case 6. A 14-year-old white school boy was admitted to a hospital on December 14, 1975 because of diplopia and headache. The past medical history revealed the patient to have no evidence of injury to the eyes or head.

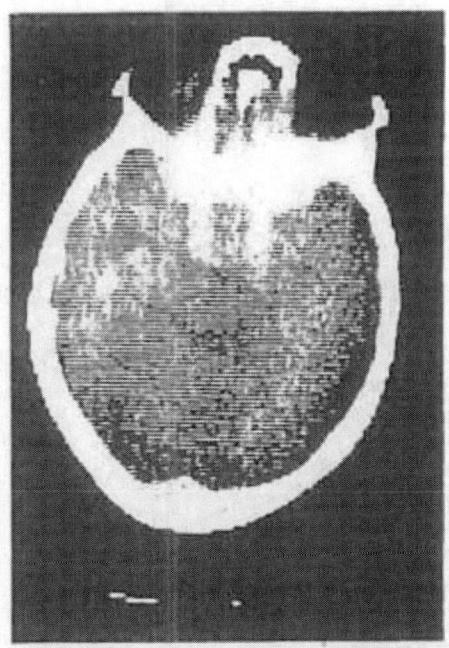

Fig. 56B. Postoperative CT scan of patient in Case 3 showing resolution of tumor.

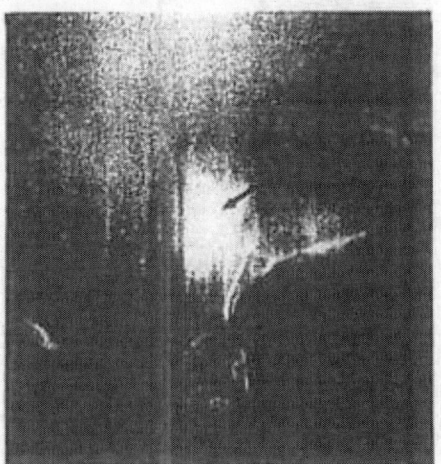

Fig. 57A. Arrow points to increased density in sphenoid bone chondrosarcoma in laminogram.

Appendix 2. Articles by Doctor Lee

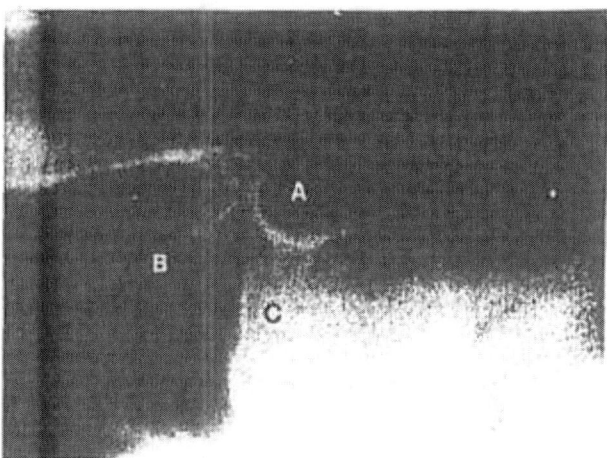

Fig. 57B. Lateral laminogram of lesion. (A) Sella turcica. (B) Sphenoid sinus. (C) Chondrosarcoma.

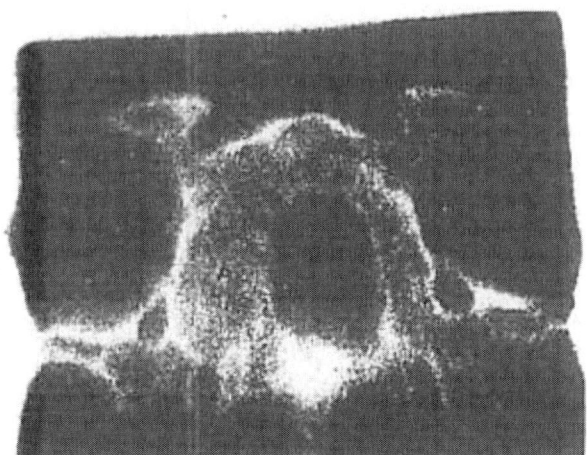

Fig. 57C. A-P Laminogram. (A) Chondrosarcoma. (B) Sphenoid sinus.

Physical examination was completely within normal limits except for a slight gaze palsy of the right lateral rectus and diplopia on right lateral gaze. There were no other focal or other cranial nerve signs and no evidence of papilledema. The remainder of the neurological examination with respect to motor reflex and sensory system as well as cerebellar systems were completely within normal limits. Endocrine studies were also normal.

Radiographic studies demonstrated a cartilaginous mass with foci of calcification in the base of the sphenoid on the right with extension into the parasellar region and involvement of the cavernous sinus (Figs. 57-A, B and C). There was also evidence of tumor within the dorsum sellae with extension superiorly on the right with erosion of the right posterior clinoid process and parasellar calcification. Angiography demonstrated lateral displacement of the right internal carotid artery as it approaches the cavernous sinus.

Following investigative work-up the tumor of the right sphenoid was biopsied and partially removed with the air drill through a sublabial transseptal transsphenoidal approach.

Using intraoperative radiographic control with fluoroscopy, multiple biopsies of vital areas of this bony and cartilaginous tumor were performed. During surgery it was determined that the tumor was within the body of the sphenoid bone, extending to the floor of the sella turcica and posteriorly to the right of the sella well beyond the posterior clinoid and into the right parasellar region.

Postoperative packing and dressing was similar to that used for transseptal transsphenoidal hypophysectomy. No CSF rhinorrhea was noted and the patient had an uncomplicated postoperative course except for a transient right III nerve weakness. He was discharged nine days after surgery.

Pathological diagnosis revealed this to be a low-grade osteochondrosarcoma and the patient was treated postoperatively with radiation therapy. At the time of this report, the patient is asymptomatic with no evidence of diplopia or headache.

CONCLUSIONS.

The sublabial transseptal transsphenoidal approach to the hypophysis and parasellar region is a safe and simple procedure; however, the surgeon must be thoroughly familiar with the surgical anatomy, position the patient properly and have access to appropriate instrumentation. Vital structures to identify or avoid during surgery include the optic canals, carotid arteries, circular sinuses, cavernous sinuses, III, IV, V, VI cranial nerves, foramen rotundum, medial walls of the orbits and maxillary sinuses, medial pterygoid plates and pterygoid canals.

The intersphenoidal septum which is deviated in 34 to 47% of patients is an unreliable midline landmark. The vomer and center of the sphenoid rostrum are more consistent structures for locating the midline. These and other structures have been illustrated with the aid of specially prepared whole head specimens and skull dissections. Preoperative laminography and measurements of key distances within the skull help avoid damage to vital structures including the medial pterygoid plates and medial walls of the maxillary sinuses.

The surgical technique, including positioning of the patient, has been described. The advantages of the self-retaining speculum and other instruments have been discussed. The use of the gauge on the self-retaining speculum prevents excessive opening of the speculum blades.

A series of 30 cases has been reported. No operative mortality, CSF rhinorrhea, visual damage, carotid or cavernous sinus hemorrhage, fracture of the medial pterygoid plate or maxilla was encountered in this series. Three patients developed diabetes insipidus and two patients had meningitis which responded to antibiotic therapy.

ACKNOWLEDGMENT.

My special thanks go to Drs. I. Goodrich, A. Greenberg, and F. Robinson who performed the neurosurgical part of the operation as well as cared for these patients from the neurological standpoint. Dr. Goodrich was consulted for the design of the pituitary dissectors, knives and ring curettes.

I am indebted to Dr. Daniel Miller and Dr. Howard Smith for generously giving of their time to review this manuscript.

I am grateful to my wife, Linda, for her editorial assistance, medical illustrations, typing and proofreading.

BIBLIOGRAPHY.

1. CHIARI, O.: Uber eine Modification der Schloffer'schen Operation von Tumoren der Hypophyse. Wien Klin Wchnschr., 25:5, 1912.

2. Cushing, H.: Partial Hypophysectomy for Acromegaly. *Am. Surg.*, 50:1002, 1909.

3. Cushing, H.: The Pituitary Body and Its Disorders. J. B. Lippincott Company, Philadelphia, Pa., 1912.

4. Hirsch, O.: Uber Methoden der Operativen Behandlung von Hypophysistumoren auf endonasalem Wege. *Arch. Laryngol. Rhinol.*, 24:129-177, 1910.

5. Burian, K.: Transsphenoidal Operation for Tumors of the Pituitary Gland. *Arch. Otolaryngol.*, 86:449-452, 1967.

6. Montgomery, W. W.: Transethmoidosphenoidal Hypophysectomy with Septal Mucosal Flap. *Arch. Otolaryngol.*, 78:68-77, 1963.

7. Hardy, J.: Transsphenoidal Hypophysectomy. *J. Neurosurg.*, 34:582-594, 1971.

8. James, J. A.: The Hypophysis. *J. Laryngol. Otol.*, 81:1283-1307, 1967.

9. James, J. A.: Transethmosphenoidal Hypophysectomy. *Arch. Otolaryngol.*, 86:256-264, 1967.

10. Hamberger, C. A., et al.: Transantrosphenoidal Hypophysectomy. *Arch. Otolaryngol.*, 74:22-28, 1961.

11. Baker, D. C. and Bridges, T. J.: Transantrosphenoidal Hypophysectomy. *Trans. Am. Acad. Ophthalmol.*, 68(1):60-64, 1964.

12. Hirsch, O.: Symptoms and Treatment of Pituitary Tumors. *Arch. Otolaryngol.*, 55:268-306, 1952.

13. Horsley, V.: Address in Surgery: On the Technic of Operations on the Central Nervous System. *Br. Med. J.*, 2:411, 1906.

14. Proust, R.: Chirurgie de l'Hypophyse. *J. Chir.*, 1:668, 1908.

15. Kanavel, A. B.: Removal of Tumors of the Pituitary Body by an Infranasal Route. *J.A.M.A.*, 53:1704, 1909.

16. Kanavel, A. B. and Grinker, J.: Removal of Tumors of the Pituitary Body. *Surg. Gynecol. Obstet.*, 10:414, 1910.

17. Halstead, A. E.: Remarks on the Operative Treatment of Tumors of the Hypophysis: Report of Two Cases Operated on by an Oro-Nasal Method. *Surg. Gynecol. Obstet.*, 10:494, 1910.

18. Bakay, L.: Results of 300 Pituitary Adenoma Operations (Prof. Herbert Olivecrona's Series). *J. Neurosurg.*, 7:240, 1950.

19. German, W. J. and Flanigan, S.: Pituitary Adenomas: A Follow-Up Study of the Cushing Series. *Clin. Neurosurg.*, 10:72-81, 1962.

20. Kirchner, J. A. and Van Gilder, J. C.: Transethmoidal Hypophysectomy. *Trans. Am. Acad. Ophthalmol. Otolaryngol.*, 80:391-396, 1975.

21. Bateman, G. H.: Transsphenoidal Hypophysectomy. A Review of 70 Cases Treated in the Past Two Years. *Trans. Am. Acad. Ophthalmol. Otolaryngol.*, 63:103-110, 1962.

22. Trible, W. M. and Morse, A. E.: Transpalatal Hypophysectomy. *The Laryngoscope*, 75:1116-1122, 1965.

23. Macbeth, R. and Hall, M.: Hypophysectomy as a Rhinological Procedure. *Arch. Otolaryngol.*, 75:440-450, 1962.

24. Netzer, H. R. and McCoy, E. G.: Transseptal Transsphenoidal Hypophysectomy. *Arch. Otolaryngol.*, 86:252-255, 1967.

25. Arslan, M.: Ultrasonic Hypophysectomy in Acromegaly. Report of 41 Cases. *Otol. Rhinol. Laryngol.*, 35:134-140, 1973.

26. Cross, J. N., et al.: Treatment of Acromegaly by Cryosurgery. *Lancet*, 1:215-216, 1972.

27. Richards, S. H., Thomas, J. P. and Kilby, D.: Transethmoidal Hypophysectomy for Pituitary Tumours. *Proc. R. Soc. Med.*, 67:889-892, 1974.

28. Di Tullio, M. V., Jr. and Rand, R. W.: Efficacy of Cryohypophysectomy in the Treatment of Acromegaly. *J. Neurosurg.*, 46(1):1-11, 1977.

29. Ray, B. S., et al.: Pituitary Ablation for Diabetic Retinopathy. II. Results of Yttrium 90 Implantation in the Pituitary Gland. *J.A.M.A.*, 203:107-109, 1968.

30. Riskaer, N., Foc, C. V. M. and Hommelgaard, T.: Transsphenoidal Hypophysectomy in Metastatic Cancer of the Breast. *Arch. Otolaryngol.*, 74:483-493, 1961.

31. Hartog, M., et al.: Partial Pituitary Ablation with Implants of Gold-198 and Yttrium 90 for Acromegaly. *Br. Med. J.*, 2:396-398, 1965.
32. Zervas, N. T. and Hamlin, H.: Stereotaxic Thermal Pituitary Ablation. *Acta Neurochir.*, Suppl. 21:165-168, 1974.
33. Hayes, T. P., Davis, R. A. and Raventos, A.: The Treatment of Pituitary Chromophobe Adenomas. *Radiology*, 98:149-153, 1971.
34. Ray, B. S. and Patterson, R. H., Jr.: Surgical Experience with Chromophobe Adenomas of the Pituitary Gland. *J. Neurosurg.*, 34:726-729, 1971.
35. Svien, H. J. and Colby, M. Y.: Pituitary Chromophobe Adenomas: Comparative Results of Surgical and Roentgen Treatment. *Behav. Neuropsychiatry*, 1:35-39, 1969.
36. Stern, W. E. and Batzdorf, U.: Intracranial Removal of Pituitary Adenomas. An Evaluation of Varying Degrees of Excision from Partial to Total. *J. Neurosurg.*, 33:564-573, 1970.
37. Furstenberg, A. C. and Blatt, I. M.: Transsphenoidal Approach to the Pituitary Gland. *The Laryngoscope*, 65:420-430, 1955.
38. Sheline, G. E., Boldrey, E. B. and Phillips, T. L.: Chromophobe Adenomas of the Pituitary Gland. *Am. J. Roentgenol.*, 92:160-173, 1964.
39. Williams, R. A.: Hypophysectomy for Pituitary Tumours. *Proc. R. Soc. Med.*, 67:881-885, 1974.
40. Montgomery, W. W.: Transsphenoid Approach to Cystic Lesions of the Petrous Apex. Presented at the American Otology Society, Boston, Mass., May 1977.
41. Evans, H. M., Griggs, J. H. and Dixon, J. S.: The Pituitary Gland: The Physiology and Chemistry of Growth Hormone. Edited by G. W. Harris and B. T. Donovan, University of California Press, Berkeley/Los Angeles, pp. 439-491, 1966.
42. Wright, A. D., Hill, D. M. and Lowy, C.: Mortality in Acromegaly. *Q. J. Med.*, 39:1-16, 1970.
43. Chamlin, M., Davidoff, L. M. and Feiring, E. H.: Ophthalmologic Changes Produced by Pituitary Tumors. *Am. J. Ophthalmol.*, 40:353-368, 1955.
44. Summers, G. W.: Nasal Obstruction Caused by a Pituitary Chromophobe Adenoma. *The Laryngoscope*, 86:1718-1721, 1976.
45. White, J. C. and Warren, S.: Unusual Size and Extension of a Pituitary Adenoma. *J. Neurosurg.*, 2:126-139, 1945.
46. Kay, S., Lees, J. K. and Stout, A. P.: Pituitary Chromophobe Tumors of the Nasal Cavity. *Cancer*, 3:695-704, 1950.
47. McGuire, W. L., et al.: Current Status of Estrogen and Progesterone Receptors in Breast Cancer. *Cancer*, 39:2934-2947, 1977.
48. Houssay, B. A. and Biasotti, A. A.: Diabetes Pancreática de los Perros Hipofisoprivos. *Rev. Soc. Argent. Biol.*, 6:251-269, 1930.
49. Poulson, J. E.: Houssay Phenomenon in Man: Recovery from Retinopathy in Case of Diabetes with Simmond's Disease. *Diabetes*, 2:7-12, 1953.
50. Hardy, J. and Ciric, I. S.: Selective Anterior Hypophysectomy in the Treatment of Diabetic Retinopathy. *J.A.M.A.*, 203:95-100, 1968.
51. Ray, B. S., et al.: Pituitary Ablation for Diabetic Retinopathy. *J.A.M.A.*, 203:78-84, 1968.
52. Murphy, G. P., et al.: Hypophysectomy and Adrenalectomy for Disseminated Prostatic Carcinoma. *J. Urol.*, 105:817-825, 1971.
53. Wyllie, J. W., III, Kern, E. B. and Djalilian, M.: Isolated Sphenoid Sinus Lesions. *The Laryngoscope*, 83:1252-1265, 1973.
54. Watson, W. L.: Cancer of Paranasal Sinuses. *The Laryngoscope*, 52:22-42, 1942.
55. Hallberg, O. E. and Begley, J. W., Jr.: Origin and Treatment of Osteomas of the Paranasal Sinuses. *Arch. Otolaryngol.*, 51:750-760, 1950.
56. Brunner, H.: Fibrous Dysplasia of Facial Bones and Paranasal Sinuses. *Arch. Otolaryngol.*, 55:43-54, 1952.
57. Townsend, G. L. and DeSanto, L. W.: Malignant Change in Sphenoid Sinus Fibrous Dysplasia. *Arch. Otolaryngol.*, 92:267-271, 1970.
58. DeBartolo, H. M. and Vrabec, D.: Sphenoid Encephalocele. *Arch. Otolaryngol.*, 103:172-174, 1977.

Appendix 2. Articles by Doctor Lee

59. HENRY, H. M., HARDY, J. and MOODY, R.: Transsphenoidal Hypophysectomy: A Laboratory Approach and Commentary. *J. Surg. Oncol.*, 8(6):513-522, 1976.

60. ZERVAS, N. T.: Stereotaxic Radiofrequency Surgery of the Normal and the Abnormal Pituitary Gland. *N. Engl. J. Med.*, 280:429-437, 1969.

61. BERGLAND, R. M., RAY, B. S. and TORACK, R. M.: Anatomical Variations in the Pituitary Gland and Adjacent Structures in 225 Human Autopsy Cases. *J. Neurosurg.*, 28:93-99, 1968.

62. RENN, W. H. and RHOTON, A. L., JR.: Microsurgical Anatomy of the Sellar Region. *J. Neurosurg.*, 43:288-298, 1975.

63. SEAH, C. H. and LEE, K. J.: Local Anesthesia. Chapter 20, The Otolaryngology Boards. Edited by K. J. Lee, The Medical Examination Publishing Co., Inc., New York, 1973.

64. HUDSON, W. R. and KENAN, P. D.: Transsphenoidal Management of Pituitary Adenomas and Other Selected Lesions of the Sella Turcica. THE LARYNGOSCOPE, 84:1159-1169, 1974.

65. VAN GILDER, J. C.: The Place of Hypophysectomy in the Management of Metastatic Breast Cancer. *Conn. Med.*, 39:3-4, 1975.

66. ZERVAS, N. T. and CORDY, P. D.: Radiofrequency Hypophysectomy for Metastatic Breast and Prostatic Carcinoma. *Surg. Clin. North Am.*, 47:1279-1285, 1967.

67. ROTH, J. A., ET AL.: Transnasal Transsphenoidal Approach to the Sella. THE LARYNGOSCOPE, 87:47-57, 1977.

APPENDIX 3. PATIENT HANDOUTS

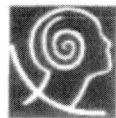

K. J. LEE, M.D., F.A.C.S., P.C.
SOUTHERN NEW ENGLAND EAR, NOSE, THROAT & FACIAL PLASTIC
SURGERY GROUP, LLP

University Towers, 98 York Street, New Haven, CT 06511 - (203) 777-4005

HOME CARE FOLLOWING DIRECT LARYNGOSCOPY

1. Complete voice rest for 24 hours following surgery. After this time remember to talk normally but do not whisper. Whispering is more harmful than talking.

2. Talking for the next 3 to 4 days should be kept to a minimum; avoid raising your voice at any time. DO NOT WHISPER.

3. After recovering from the anesthetic effects, use your own judgment regarding diet.

4. A sore throat may be present. Take Tylenol or pain medication as prescribed.

5. Please call the office to make an appointment for 10 to 14 days after surgery.

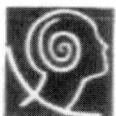

K. J. LEE, M.D., F.A.C.S., P.C.
SOUTHERN NEW ENGLAND EAR, NOSE, THROAT & FACIAL PLASTIC
SURGERY GROUP, LLP

University Towers, 98 York Street, New Haven, CT 06511 - (203) 777-4005

HOME CARE FOLLOWING LASER SURGERY FOR HEMANGIOMA

1. Use your own judgment regarding diet.

2. During hospitalization, you will learn to apply bacitracin ointment to the laser site. This is to be started as soon as you arrive home and continued three times a day until you return to the office for your postoperative visit.

3. You must keep the laser site completely dry for three days. After the third day, you may wash the area gently with Dove soap and warm water. Pat completely dry and apply bacitracin ointment as directed.

4. You can expect some pain. Take Tylenol or pain medication as prescribed.

5. Office follow-up is necessary. Please call the office to make an appointment five to seven days after surgery.

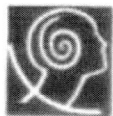

K. J. LEE, M.D., F.A.C.S., P.C.
SOUTHERN NEW ENGLAND EAR, NOSE, THROAT & FACIAL PLASTIC
SURGERY GROUP, LLP

University Towers, 98 York Street, New Haven, CT 06511 - (203) 777-4005

HOME CARE FOLLOWING NASAL POLYPECTOMY/ETHMOIDECTOMY

1. Rest quietly for the first 48 hours after leaving the hospital. Continue to rest at least 2 hours per day for the remainder of the week. Plan to remain home from school or work for 7-10 days. Please consult Dr. Lee for any specifics.

2. Sleep in a position in which the patient's head is elevated 30° to 45° or higher. No bending, lifting or any physical exertion.

3. Use your own judgment regarding diet.

4. During hospitalization, the patient will learn to change the "drip pad." Please ask the nurse to teach you. This involves applying a gauze pad under the nose with a piece of tape. This is to be continued and changed periodically at home as necessary. A moderate amount of pinkish drainage or light bleeding is to be expected. This "drip pad" is nothing more than a bib. It is "nonmedical." If there is no drainage, you may not need to use the "drip pad." In addition, you will have a nasal packing which will stay in your nose for 4-7 days after surgery. Please do not remove the packing.

5. Expect some fever. If the temperature is over 101.5° F, please call Dr. Lee's office.

6. Take Tylenol or pain medication as prescribed.

7. If excessive sneezing should occur, please take Actifed which can be purchased at the pharmacy without a prescription. Also, remember to sneeze with your mouth open.

8. Following surgery, swelling and bruising may be seen around the eyes and nose.

9. If significant bleeding is seen, please call the office at 777-4005. If for some reason you cannot reach someone at this number, please go to St. Raphael's Emergency Room.

10. Office follow-up is necessary. Please call the office to make an appointment for 4-7 days after surgery. At this time, the packing will be removed from your nose.

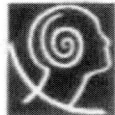

K. J. LEE, M.D., F.A.C.S., P.C.
SOUTHERN NEW ENGLAND EAR, NOSE, THROAT & FACIAL PLASTIC SURGERY GROUP, LLP

University Towers, 98 York Street, New Haven, CT 06511 (203) 777-4005

HOME CARE FOLLOWING SEPTOPLASTY/RHINOPLASTY

1. Rest quietly for the first 48 hours after leaving the hospital. Continue to rest at least 2 hours per day for the remainder of the week. Plan to remain home from school or work for 7-10 days. Please consult Dr. Lee.

2. Sleep in a position in which the patient's head is elevated 30° to 40° or higher. No bending, lifting or any physical exertion.

3. Use your own judgment regarding diet.

4. During hospitalization, the patient will learn to change the "drip pad." Please ask the nurse to teach you. This involves applying a gauze pad under the nose with a piece of tape. This is to be continued and changed periodically at home as necessary. A moderate amount of pinkish drainage or light bleeding is to be expected. This "drip pad" is nothing more than a bib. It is "nonmedical." If there is no drainage, you may not need to use the "drip pad."

5. Expect some fever. If the temperature is over 101.5° F, please call Dr. Lee's office.

6. Take Tylenol or pain medication as prescribed.

7. If excessive sneezing should occur, please take Actifed, which can be purchased at the pharmacy without a prescription. Also, remember to sneeze with your mouth open.

8. Following surgery, swelling and bruising may be seen around the eyes and nose, more commonly with a rhinoplasty and seldom seen with septoplasty alone. A light ice pack may be applied over the eyes for the first 48 hours.

9. If significant bleeding is seen, please call the office at 777-4005. If for some reason you cannot reach someone at this number, please to go to St. Raphael's Emergency Room.

10. Office follow-up is necessary. Please call the office to make an appointment for 5-7 days after surgery.

11. If you have rhinoplasty performed, avoid a suntan or sunburn for 3 months and avoid contact sports for 1 month.

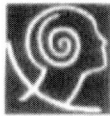

K. J. LEE, M.D., F.A.C.S., P.C.
SOUTHERN NEW ENGLAND EAR, NOSE, THROAT & FACIAL PLASTIC SURGERY GROUP, LLP

University Towers, 98 York Street, New Haven, CT 06511 · (203) 777-4005

HOME CARE FOLLOWING TONSILLECTOMY AND ADENOIDECTOMY

1. If significant bleeding is seen, please call the office (777-4005) at once. If, for some reason you cannot reach the office, go at once to the Hospital of St. Raphael's Emergency Room.

2. Rest quietly for 48 hours, after leaving the hospital, and then rest at least 2 hours a day for the remainder of the week.

3. Children who have had tonsil and adenoid surgery should not go back to school for at least one week. The recovery time is less if only the adenoids are removed.

4. For the first few days, food should be soft and nourishing such as milk, soups, ice cream, soft boiled eggs, etc. It is important to drink plenty of liquids. Avoid acid foods and drinks such as citrus juices. Popsicles are a good source of fluid.

5. Expect some fever. If over 101.5° F please call the office.

6. Expect earache after removal of the tonsils.

7. Take liquid Tylenol or prescribed pain medication as directed.

8. A white or gray membrane may form where tonsils are removed. This is normal healing, do not try to remove it.

Office follow-up is necessary. Please call the office and make an appointment for 7 to 10 days after discharge from the hospital.

HOME CARE FOLLOWING DRAINAGE OF FLUID OR INSERTION OF PLASTIC DRAIN TUBES IN THE EARS

1. Do not wash your hair or allow water near the ears before follow-up visit.

2. After follow-up visit, when washing your hair, use a large piece of lambs wool or cotton coated with Vaseline as a plug for the ears.

3. Swimming is not allowed while drain tubes are in the ears unless special custom fitted ear molds are used.

4. Drain tubes are painless. If pain or visible drainage develops, please call the office.

5. It is important that you keep return appointments so that the drain tubes can be periodically inspected.

K. J. LEE, M.D., F.A.C.S., P.C.
SOUTHERN NEW ENGLAND EAR, NOSE, THROAT & FACIAL PLASTIC
SURGERY GROUP, LLP

University Towers, 98 York Street, New Haven, CT 06511 - (203) 777-4005

POSTOPERATIVE EXPECTATIONS IN CANALPLASTY-MEATOPLASTY

1. There will be a turban-type dressing for the first 48 hours after surgery. In 2 days after surgery the dressing will be changed to band-aids.
   a. Do not get the ear wet under any circumstances.
   b. Do not wash your hair until the inner packing is removed and you have obtained your doctor's permission and instructions.
   c. Do not expect to swim for the first 6 weeks after surgery. Thereafter, get your doctor's permission before swimming.

2. The outer packing and the sutures will be removed in the office one week after surgery. The inner packing will be removed 2 weeks after surgery. Thereafter, you would need follow-up visits about once in 10 days until the inside wound is healed which takes approximately 4 to 6 weeks after the surgery. The first checkup should be one week after the surgery, so please call the office (777-4005) for an appointment.

3. Due to the skin incision behind the ear, the skin of the outer ear will be numb for several months. After the first 48 hours, you may experience some pain that is easily controlled by Darvon or similar strength medication. Should you have severe pain, severe dizziness or a temperature of over 101° F, please call 777-4005.

4. There may be a slight pinkish discharge. Change the outer cotton and band-aids. Should you experience heavy discharge, please call 777-4005.

5. You can be on the diet that you are accustomed to before the surgery.

6. Please discuss your type of occupation with your doctor so that he can advise you on the length of your disability period.

7. Your hearing may be muffled until all packings are removed and swelling has subsided.

Appendix 3. Patient Handouts

**Southern New England Ear, Nose, Throat
and Facial Plastic Surgery Group, LLP**
(Head and Neck Surgery)

POSTOPERATIVE EXPECTATIONS IN STAPEDECTOMY

1. Under most circumstances, you can expect to be discharged 2 days after surgery. Of course, should you feel "weak" or for any medical reason you would like to stay an extra day or two, this can be arranged.

2. Due to the packing in the ear and to the operative swelling, your hearing may not seem to have improved right after surgery. To allow time for healing a valid hearing test is not obtained sooner than 4 weeks after surgery.

3. You may be somewhat dizzy, nauseated and even vomit the day of surgery. We advise you to lie flat in bed with the operated ear up. You can get up to use the bathroom provided you obtain the nurse's help. You can have liquids after the surgery.

4. You may get up and have a regular diet the next day. Please do not move fast, turn quickly or stoop over. Be generally careful.

5. Your dressing consists of an inner packing, an outer piece of cotton and 2 band-aids. If the dressing is dry, do not change it. Should you have slightly pinkish discharge, replace the outer cotton and the band-aids. Do not clean the ear canal (hole) at all. Should you have heavy discharge, please call 777-4005.

6. After you have been discharged, please call us should you experience severe dizziness, nausea and vomiting, or severe earache not controlled with Darvon or similar strength medications. Please call us if your temperature is over 100.6° F.

7. For the first 2 weeks after surgery,
    a. Do not blow your nose hard.
    b. If you have to sneeze, do so with your mouth open.
    c. Do not fly unless you have discussed this with your doctor.
    d. For the first 10 days, do not get the ear wet under any circumstances. You can expect to wash your hair and go swimming 10 days after surgery with your doctor's permission. Driving is PROHIBITED until you have discussed it with your doctor.

8. Please call 777-4005 for an appointment to be seen one week after surgery. The packing and sutures will be removed.

9. Please discuss your occupation with your doctor so that he can advise you regarding the length of your disability period.

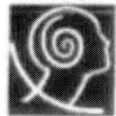

K. J. LEE, M.D., F.A.C.S., P.C.
SOUTHERN NEW ENGLAND EAR, NOSE, THROAT & FACIAL PLASTIC
SURGERY GROUP, LLP

University Towers, 98 York Street, New Haven, CT 06511 - (203) 777-4005

POSTOPERATIVE EXPECTATIONS IN TYMPANOPLASTY-MASTOIDECTOMY

1. There will be a turban-type of dressing for the first 48 hours after surgery. In 2 days after surgery the dressing will be changed to band-aids.

2. For the first two weeks after surgery,
   a. Do not blow your nose hard.
   b. If you have to sneeze, do so with your mouth open.
   c. Do not get the ear wet under any circumstances.
   d. Do not wash your hair until the inner packing is removed and you have obtained your doctor's permission and instructions.
   e. Do not expect to swim for the first 6 weeks after surgery. Thereafter, get your doctor's permission before swimming.

3. If you have to fly, consult your doctor first.

4. The outer packing and sutures will be removed in the office 1 week after surgery. The inner packing will be removed 2 weeks after surgery. Thereafter, you would need follow-up office visits about once in 10 days until the inside wound is healed which takes approximately 4 to 6 weeks after the surgery. The first checkup should be 1 week after the surgery, so please call 777-4005 for an appointment.

5. Due to the skin incision behind the ear, the skin of the outer ear will be numb for several months. After the first 48 hours, you may experience some pain that is easily controlled by Darvon or similar strength medication. Should you have severe pain, severe dizziness or a temperature over 100.6° F, please call 777-4005.

6. There may be slight pinkish discharge. Change the outer cotton and band-aids. Should you experience heavy discharge, please call 777-4005.

7. You can be on the diet that you are accustomed to before the surgery.

8. Please discuss your type of occupation with your doctor so that he can advise you on the length of your disability period.

9. We expect hearing improvement in some patients undergoing mastoidectomy-tympanoplasty and not in others. Due to the fact that the new eardrum has to "thin out" and epithelize, the hearing improvement may not be noticeable until 6 weeks after surgery.

Appendix 3. Patient Handouts

Risks and Complications of Surgery

The following is a list of possible complications in your proposed surgery though some complications are rarer than others, they could happen. In any human endeavor, there are many unknowns. Hence, it is impossible to have a complete list of possible complications. If you are not satisfied with any explanation, please feel free to ask your Doctor. In the event of non-urgent surgery, feel free to postpone the surgery until you believe that the potential benefit of the surgery outweighs the risks. If you would like, we encourage you to obtain a second opinion. Please discuss possible anesthesia complications with the anesthesiologist as he/she is responsible for the delivery of anesthesia. In cases where there is a specimen sent to the Pathologist for interpretation, it is the responsibility of the Pathologist to render the diagnosis. If you have doubt or wish, please communicate directly with the Pathologist.

Cancer Surgery

1. Pain
2. Infection
3. Bleeding
4. Numbness
5. Scarring
6. Failure of the surgery
7. Allergic reaction to medicine or materials
8. It would be to your advantage to obtain the consultation of an oncologist and radiotherapist even if you believe that their services are not necessary. The doctor may not force you to obtain such consultation in some cases, but he/she would highly recommend it. In other cases, it is mandatory to obtain such consultations.
9. Swallowing and breathing difficulty
10. Taste and smell abnormalities
11. Loss of vital organ or major blood vessel and nerves and the inherent suffering when such structures are removed.

I have read the above and am willing to accept the risks of surgery and believe that the potential benefits outweigh the potential risks.

_____   Chart # _____
Name of Patient

_____   _____
Date   Signature of patient or guardian

_____   _____
Name of Doctor   Signature of Doctor

Risks and Complications of Surgery

The following is a list of possible complications in your proposed surgery though some complications are rarer than others, they could happen. In any human endeavor, there are many unknowns. Hence, it is impossible to have a complete list of possible complications. If you are not satisfied with any explanation, please feel free to ask your Doctor. In the event of non-urgent surgery, feel free to postpone the surgery until you believe that the potential benefit of the surgery outweighs the risks. If you would like, we encourage you to obtain a second opinion. Please discuss possible anesthesia complications with the anesthesiologist as he/she is responsible for the delivery of anesthesia. In cases where there is a specimen sent to the Pathologist for interpretation, it is the responsibility of the Pathologist to render the diagnosis. If you have doubt or wish, please communicate directly with the Pathologist.

Face Lift/Blepharoplasty

1. Pain
2. Infection
3. Bleeding
4. Numbness
5. Scarring
6. Failure of the surgery
7. Allergic reaction to medicine or materials
8. Eye injury, possible blindness in Blepharoplasty
9. Miscellaneous

I have read the above and am willing to accept the risks of surgery and believe that the potential benefits outweigh the potential risks.

_____   Chart # _____
Name of Patient

_____   _____
Date   Signature of patient or guardian

_____   _____
Name of Doctor   Signature of Doctor

Risks and Complications of Surgery

The following is a list of possible complications in your proposed surgery though some complications are rarer than others, they could happen. In any human endeavor, there are many unknowns. Hence, it is impossible to have a complete list of possible complications. If you are not satisfied with any explanation, please feel free to ask your Doctor. In the event of non-urgent surgery, feel free to postpone the surgery until you believe that the potential benefit of the surgery outweighs the risks. If you would like, we encourage you to obtain a second opinion. Please discuss possible anesthesia complications with the anesthesiologist as he/she is responsible for the delivery of anesthesia. In cases where there is a specimen sent to the Pathologist for interpretation, it is the responsibility of the Pathologist to render the diagnosis. If you have doubt or wish, please communicate directly with the Pathologist.

Laryngoscopy

1. Pain
2. Infection
3. Bleeding
4. Numbness
5. Scarring
6. Failure of the surgery
7. Allergic reaction to medicine or materials
8. Voice abnormalities
9. Aspiration
10. Airway problem
11. Dental problem
12. Lip, gum, teeth, neck injury
13. Miscellaneous

I have read the above and am willing to accept the risks of surgery and believe that the potential benefits outweigh the potential risks.

_____   Chart # _____
Name of Patient

_____   _____
Date   Signature of patient or guardian

_____   _____
Name of Doctor   Signature of Doctor

Risks and Complications of Surgery

The following is a list of possible complications in your proposed surgery though some complications are rarer than others, they could happen. In any human endeavor, there are many unknowns. Hence, it is impossible to have a complete list of possible complications. If you are not satisfied with any explanation, please feel free to ask your Doctor. In the event of non-urgent surgery, feel free to postpone the surgery until you believe that the potential benefit of the surgery outweighs the risks. If you would like, we encourage you to obtain a second opinion. Please discuss possible anesthesia complications with the anesthesiologist as he/she is responsible for the delivery of anesthesia. In cases where there is a specimen sent to the Pathologist for interpretation, it is the responsibility of the Pathologist to render the diagnosis. If you have doubt or wish, please communicate directly with the Pathologist.

Middle Ear Surgery

(Canalplasty, Stapedectomy, Tympanoplasty, Mastoidectomy)

1. Pain
2. Infection
3. Bleeding
4. Numbness
5. Scarring
6. Failure of the surgery
7. Allergic reaction to medicine or materials
8. Stenosis of ear canal
9. Hearing loss
10. Dizziness
11. Tinnitus (noise in the ear)
12. Graft failure
13. Facial Paralysis
14. CSF (brain fluid) leak
15. Meningitis
16. Brain abscess
17. Jaw joint problem
18. Miscellaneous

I have read the above and am willing to accept the risks of surgery and believe that the potential benefits outweigh the potential risks.

_____   Chart # _____
Name of Patient

_____   _____
Date   Signature of patient or guardian

_____   _____
Name of Doctor   Signature of Doctor

Appendix 3. Patient Handouts

Risks and Complications of Surgery

The following is a list of possible complications in your proposed surgery though some complications are rarer than others, they could happen. In any human endeavor, there are many unknowns. Hence, it is impossible to have a complete list of possible complications. If you are not satisfied with any explanation, please feel free to ask your Doctor. In the event of non-urgent surgery, feel free to postpone the surgery until you believe that the potential benefit of the surgery outweighs the risks. If you would like, we encourage you to obtain a second opinion. Please discuss possible anesthesia complications with the anesthesiologist as he/she is responsible for the delivery of anesthesia. In cases where there is a specimen sent to the Pathologist for interpretation, it is the responsibility of the Pathologist to render the diagnosis. If you have doubt or wish, please communicate directly with the Pathologist.

Myringotomy with Tube Implantation

1. Pain
2. Infection
3. Bleeding
4. Numbness
5. Scarring
6. Failure of the surgery
7. Allergic reaction to medicine or materials
8. Blocked tube
9. Tube extrusion
10. Hole in the eardrum
11. Hearing loss
12. Dizziness
13. Tinnitus (noise in the ear)
14. Facial Paralysis
15. Tube falls into middle ear
16. Inconvenience of keeping the ear dry
17. Miscellaneous

I have read the above and am willing to accept the risks of surgery and believe that the potential benefits outweigh the potential risks.

_____   Chart # _____
Name of Patient

_____   _____
Date   Signature of Patient or Guardian

_____   _____
Name of Doctor   Signature of Doctor

Risks and Complications of Surgery

The following is a list of possible complications in your proposed surgery though some complications are rarer than others, they could happen. In any human endeavor, there are many unknowns. Hence, it is impossible to have a complete list of possible complications. If you are not satisfied with any explanation, please feel free to ask your Doctor. In the event of non-urgent surgery, feel free to postpone the surgery until you believe that the potential benefit of the surgery outweighs the risks. If you would like, we encourage you to obtain a second opinion. Please discuss possible anesthesia complications with the anesthesiologist as he/she is responsible for the delivery of anesthesia. In cases where there is a specimen sent to the Pathologist for interpretation, it is the responsibility of the Pathologist to render the diagnosis. If you have doubt or wish, please communicate directly with the Pathologist.

Removal of Lesion

1. Pain
2. Infection
3. Bleeding
4. Numbness
5. Scarring
6. Failure of the surgery
7. Allergic reaction to medicine or materials
8. Need for further surgery
9. Miscellaneous

I have read the above and am willing to accept the risks of surgery and believe that the potential benefits outweigh the potential risks.

_____   Chart # _____
Name of Patient

_____   _____
Date   Signature of patient or guardian

_____   _____
Name of Doctor   Signature of Doctor

Appendix 3. Patient Handouts

Risks and Complications of Surgery

The following is a list of possible complications in your proposed surgery though some complications are rarer than others, they could happen. In any human endeavor, there are many unknowns. Hence, it is impossible to have a complete list of possible complications. If you are not satisfied with any explanation, please feel free to ask your Doctor. In the event of non-urgent surgery, feel free to postpone the surgery until you believe that the potential benefit of the surgery outweighs the risks. If you would like, we encourage you to obtain a second opinion. Please discuss possible anesthesia complications with the anesthesiologist as he/she is responsible for the delivery of anesthesia. In cases where there is a specimen sent to the Pathologist for interpretation, it is the responsibility of the Pathologist to render the diagnosis. If you have doubt or wish, please communicate directly with the Pathologist.

Salivary Gland Surgery

1. Pain
2. Infection
3. Bleeding
4. Numbness
5. Scarring
6. Failure of the surgery
7. Allergic reaction to medicine or materials
8. Facial paralysis
9. Gustatory sweating (sweating while eating or thought of eating)
10. "Crocodile" tears
11. Miscellaneous

I have read the above and am willing to accept the risks of surgery and believe that the potential benefits outweigh the potential risks.

_____   Chart # _____
Name of Patient

Risks and Complications of Surgery

The following is a list of possible complications in your proposed surgery though some complications are rarer than others, they could happen. In any human endeavor, there are many unknowns. Hence, it is impossible to have a complete list of possible complications. If you are not satisfied with any explanation, please feel free to ask your Doctor. In the event of non-urgent surgery, feel free to postpone the surgery until you believe that the potential benefit of the surgery outweighs the risks. If you would like, we encourage you to obtain a second opinion. Please discuss possible anesthesia complications with the anesthesiologist as he/she is responsible for the delivery of anesthesia. In cases where there is a specimen sent to the Pathologist for interpretation, it is the responsibility of the Pathologist to render the diagnosis. If you have doubt or wish, please communicate directly with the Pathologist.

Septum Surgery

1. Pain
2. Infection
3. Bleeding
4. Numbness
5. Scarring
6. Failure of the surgery
7. Allergic reaction to medicine or materials
8. Septal perforation
9. Atrophic or allergic rhinitis
10. Voice changes
11. Sinusitis
12. Breathing difficulty
13. Miscellaneous

I have read the above and am willing to accept the risks of surgery and believe that the potential benefits outweigh the potential risks.

_____
Name of Patient

Chart # _____

_____
Date

_____
Signature of patient or guardian

_____
Name of Doctor

_____
Signature of Doctor

Appendix 3. Patient Handouts

Risks and Complications of Surgery

The following is a list of possible complications in your proposed surgery though some complications are rarer than others, they could happen. In any human endeavor, there are many unknowns. Hence, it is impossible to have a complete list of possible complications. If you are not satisfied with any explanation, please feel free to ask your Doctor. In the event of non-urgent surgery, feel free to postpone the surgery until you believe that the potential benefit of the surgery outweighs the risks. If you would like, we encourage you to obtain a second opinion. Please discuss possible anesthesia complications with the anesthesiologist as he/she is responsible for the delivery of anesthesia. In cases where there is a specimen sent to the Pathologist for interpretation, it is the responsibility of the Pathologist to render the diagnosis. If you have doubt or wish, please communicate directly with the Pathologist.

Sinus Surgery

1. Pain
2. Infection
3. Bleeding
4. Numbness
5. Scarring
6. Failure of the surgery
7. Allergic reaction to medicine or materials
8. Eye injury
9. Meningitis
10. Brain abscess
11. CSF (brain fluid) leak
12. Major blood vessel complications
13. Persistent opening between mouth and sinus
14. Miscellaneous

I have read the above and am willing to accept the risks of surgery and believe that the potential benefits outweigh the potential risks.

_____   Chart # _____
Name of Patient

_____   _____
Date   Signature of patient or guardian

_____   _____
Name of Doctor   Signature of Doctor

Risks and Complications of Surgery

The following is a list of possible complications in your proposed surgery though some complications are rarer than others, they could happen. In any human endeavor, there are many unknowns. Hence, it is impossible to have a complete list of possible complications. If you are not satisfied with any explanation, please feel free to ask your Doctor. In the event of non-urgent surgery, feel free to postpone the surgery until you believe that the potential benefit of the surgery outweighs the risks. If you would like, we encourage you to obtain a second opinion. Please discuss possible anesthesia complications with the anesthesiologist as he/she is responsible for the delivery of anesthesia. In cases where there is a specimen sent to the Pathologist for interpretation, it is the responsibility of the Pathologist to render the diagnosis. If you have doubt or wish, please communicate directly with the Pathologist.

Thyroid Surgery

1. Pain
2. Infection
3. Bleeding
4. Numbness
5. Scarring
6. Failure of the surgery
7. Allergic reaction to Medicine or materials
8. Need for further surgery
9. Hoarseness or voicelessness
10. Breathing difficulty
11. Calcium deficiency (spasm)
12. Hormone problems
13. Miscellaneous

I have read the above and am willing to accept the risks of surgery and believe that the potential benefits outweigh the potential risks.

_____
Name of Patient

Chart # _____

_____
Date

_____
Signature of patient or guardian

_____
Name of Doctor

_____
Signature of Doctor

Appendix 3. Patient Handouts

Risks and Complications of Surgery

The following is a list of possible complications in your proposed surgery though some complications are rarer than others, they could happen. In any human endeavor, there are many unknowns. Hence, it is impossible to have a complete list of possible complications. If you are not satisfied with any explanation, please feel free to ask your Doctor. In the event of non-urgent surgery, feel free to postpone the surgery until you believe that the potential benefit of the surgery outweighs the risks. If you would like, we encourage you to obtain a second opinion. Please discuss possible anesthesia complications with the anesthesiologist as he/she is responsible for the delivery of anesthesia. In cases where there is a specimen sent to the Pathologist for interpretation, it is the responsibility of the Pathologist to render the diagnosis. If you have doubt or wish, please communicate directly with the Pathologist.

Tonsillectomy and Adenoidectomy

1. Pain & Odor
2. Infection
3. Bleeding
4. Numbness
5. Scarring
6. Failure of the surgery
7. Allergic reaction to medicine or materials
8. Dehydration
9. Stiff neck
10. Neck complication
11. Loss of sense of taste and/or smell
12. Speech abnormalities
13. Major blood vessel complication
14. Headache
15. Earache
16. Stenosis of the throat and/or nasopharynx
17. Lip, gum, teeth, neck injury
18. Miscellaneous

I have read the above and am willing to accept the risks of surgery and believe that the potential benefits outweigh the potential risks.

_____   Chart # _____
Name of Patient

_____   _____
Date   Signature of patient or guardian

_____   _____
Name of Doctor   Signature of Doctor

Risks and Complications of Surgery

The following is a list of possible complications in your proposed surgery though some complications are rarer than others, they could happen. In any human endeavor, there are many unknowns. Hence, it is impossible to have a complete list of possible complications. If you are not satisfied with any explanation, please feel free to ask your Doctor. In the event of non-urgent surgery, feel free to postpone the surgery until you believe that the potential benefit of the surgery outweighs the risks. If you would like, we encourage you to obtain a second opinion. Please discuss possible anesthesia complications with the anesthesiologist as he/she is responsible for the delivery of anesthesia. In cases where there is a specimen sent to the Pathologist for interpretation, it is the responsibility of the Pathologist to render the diagnosis. If you have doubt or wish, please communicate directly with the Pathologist.

UPPP

1. Pain
2. Infection
3. Bleeding
4. Numbness
5. Scarring
6. Failure of the surgery
7. Allergic reaction to medicine or materials
8. Swallowing difficulty
9. Dehydration
10. Breathing difficulty
11. Taste and smell abnormalities
12. Lips, gum, teeth, neck injury
13. Stenosis of throat and nasopharynx
14. Nasal regurgitation
15. Voice change
16. Miscellaneous

I have read the above and am willing to accept the risks of surgery and believe that the potential benefits outweigh the potential risks.

_____ Chart # _____
Name of Patient

_____ _____
Date   Signature of patient or guardian

_____ _____
Name of Doctor   Signature of Doctor

SURGERY APPOINTMENT FORM

DATE ENTERED				PHYSICIAN					REFERRING MD & PHONE	

STS	SDA	PEDI	23 HR	HSR	YSHH	TSC	GH	MH	MMC	MDH	SURGERY PLACE BOOKED
			SICU HOLD								

SURGERY CONFIRMED WITH _____ SURGERY DATE _____

MD'S CHART # _____ INSURANCE _____ X-RAY # _____

SSN # _____ # _____

PATIENT NAME	PARENT'S NAME	BIRTH DATE	AGE
		HOME PHONE	
ADDRESS		WORK PHONE	
MEDICATIONS	ALLERGY TO MED	OTHER PHONE/FAX	

EST. TIME OF SRG: HRS. _____ MIN. _____

ANESTHESIA
○ GENERAL
○ IV SEDATION
○ LOCAL, MONITOR ONLY

Blood Units _____

DIAGNOSIS
1. _____ (ICD9# ____)
2. _____ (ICD9# ____)
3. _____ (ICD9# ____)
4. _____ (ICD9# ____)

PROCEDURE
1. _____ (CPT# ____)
2. _____ (CPT# ____)
3. _____ (CPT# ____)
4. _____ (CPT# ____)

SPECIAL EQUIPMENT

Test	Date Done	Done at	Results Y N	Test	Date Done	Done at	Results Y N	Test	Date Done	Done at	Results Y N
H&P	☐		☐ ☐	ENT X-ray	☐		☐ ☐	Glucose	☐		☐ ☐
CBC	☐		☐ ☐	Chest X-ray	☐		☐ ☐	BUN	☐		☐ ☐
PT/PLT/C	☐		☐ ☐	EKG	☐		☐ ☐	Electrolytes	☐		☐ ☐
PTT	☐		☐ ☐	Audio	☐		☐ ☐	GH	☐		☐ ☐
Mono Spot	☐		☐ ☐	Photos	☐		☐ ☐	Bleeding Time	☐		☐ ☐
BASIC METABOLIC Elec, Gluc, Bun, Cr	☐			COMP METABOLIC B Met, Prot, Glob, AST, Alk Phos, T Bili	☐		☐ ☐		☐		☐ ☐
			☐ ☐						☐		☐ ☐

PRE-OP AT: _____

PRE-CERT # _____ SPOKE TO _____ DATE _____

Hospital Consent signed	☐	Home care handout attached	☐	Insurance signed to us	☐	Patient told NPO	☐
Office Consent signed	☐	Post Op Prescription given	☐	Cosmetic Surgery Fee Paid	☐	Hosp. Arrival time discussed	☐
				D/C Aspirin etc	☐	Pre-cert done	☐

OPERATIVE PERMIT

I authorize performance upon _____ of the following operation or procedure: _____ by Dr. _____ with the assistance of such persons from the staffs of the hospital or surgicenter who may be present.

I have been informed that certain risks are associated with such procedure or operation, that medicine and surgery are not exact sciences, and that no guarantees have been made concerning the results. In fact, the condition may be made worse.

Alternatives to surgery as well as alternative surgical procedures have been discussed. After consideration, I choose to have this surgery and understand the risk factors, possible complications, and that the operation may not be successful. Should I want a second opinion, Dr. _____ thoroughly approves and recommends it.

I understand that the anesthesiologist and not the surgeon is responsible for the delivery of anesthesia, and I shall discuss fully any possible anesthetic risks and side effects with the anesthesiologist. Similarly, I understand that the pathologist(s) is responsible for the pathological report.

We/I certify that we/I have read and fully understand the above and that the explanations therein referred to were made, and that all the blanks and statements were filled in before we/I signed.

Witness: _____ Date: _____

Signature of patient: _____

Signature of parent, guardian, spouse or companion: _____

I understand that the surgeon's fee for the proposed procedure will be $ _____ and that my insurance/Medicare may or may not cover the full amount, and that I shall be responsible for the remainder of this fee. In order to facilitate processing insurance forms, I shall fill in my portion of all insurance forms and assign the insurance payments to Dr. _____. The fee will include postoperative visits for _____ months excluding tests, x-rays and possible revision surgical procedures. The fee does not cover hospital costs, anesthesia fees, etc.

	Name of Procedure	CPT Code	ICD-9-CM Code	Fee
1st				
2nd				
3rd				
4th				
5th				
6th				
			TOTAL =	

We/I certify that we/I have read and fully understand the above and that the explanations therein referred to were made, and that all the blanks and statements were filled in before we/I signed.

Witness: _____ Date: _____

Signature of patient: _____

Signature of parent, guardian, spouse or companion: _____

INDEX

A

academic success, 14
appointments, 201, 202

B

Bible, 14, 32, 33, 162, 195
Biden, Vice President Joe, 104, 105
Buffet, Warren, xxxi, 218
bureaucracy, 191, 192, 217
Bush, President George Walker, 190

C

cancer, 133, 151, 164, 165, 198
Chief of the Medical Staff, xxiii
childhood, xv, xvii, xx, 2, 4, 5, 8, 72, 73, 181, 217
children, 2, 3, 4, 5, 8, 9, 13, 22, 32, 34, 70, 138, 149, 155, 162, 163, 183, 210, 217
China, 2, 52, 53, 93, 153
chronic ear infections, xx
Clinton, Hillary, 105, 190, 191
Clinton, President Bill, xx, 213
Cold War, 28, 37
community, 21, 73, 125, 195, 211
compassion, 127, 162, 165, 173, 190, 196, 201
compensation, 125, 212, 218, 219, 220
curriculum, 135, 136, 205
customer service, 153, 201

D

doctors, xxi, xxii, xxiii, 11, 28, 67, 86, 87, 90, 126, 127, 130, 131, 139, 145, 146, 152, 153, 155, 161, 164, 168, 169, 170, 171, 172, 173, 176, 177, 194, 198, 201, 203, 205, 207, 213, 216, 220

E

ear and sinus infec, xvii
education, xiv, 4, 16, 42, 52, 57, 161
Electronic Health Records (EHR), 104, 192

F

facial paralysis, xix, 13, 164

faith, xix, 16, 32, 47, 149, 195
family, v, vi, xi, xv, xxiii, xxxi, 2, 3, 4, 5, 6, 8, 9, 10, 20, 21, 22, 23, 26, 27, 31, 32, 34, 41, 42, 48, 49, 60, 80, 81, 82, 85, 89, 95, 111, 114, 116, 117, 129, 130, 136, 137, 147, 148, 162, 163, 164, 172, 177, 182, 195, 198, 199, 203, 204, 205, 206, 210, 215, 217, 218, 223, 225
family members, 8, 20, 34, 172, 204

G

God, vi, vii, xvii, 7, 11, 14, 15, 23, 43, 78, 133, 161, 163, 164, 165, 217
Google, 146

H

Harvard, v, xv, xxi, xxvii, xxviii, 12, 15, 16, 26, 32, 33, 35, 38, 39, 40, 41, 45, 47, 48, 56, 86, 88, 100, 119, 120, 122, 124, 125, 136, 162, 181, 195, 196, 218
head and neck surgeon, xv, 16, 43, 209, 217
health information, 220
hearing loss, 123, 149, 150, 151
herbal medicine, 161
hereditary hemorrhagic telangiectasia, 126
Hippocrates, xix, 164, 199
history, 1, 2, 16, 25, 52, 80, 121, 122, 129, 152, 202
Hong Kong, 82, 89, 153

I

inner ear, 123, 149
interoperability, 213, 214, 217

J

Japan, 220

Japanese women, 59

K

Kennedy, John Fitzgerald, 135
kindness, xv, xxi, 5, 15, 181, 187

L

Lee, Dr., vi, x, xv, xix, xx, xxi, xxxiv, 126, 150, 152, 159, 165, 167, 172, 182, 183, 184, 187

M

malaria, xx, 7
Malaya, v, xv, xxv, 2, 5, 8, 9, 10, 12, 13, 16, 19, 20, 21, 22, 27, 28, 33, 34, 35, 36, 38, 42, 46, 47, 71, 72, 77, 85, 88, 90, 91, 93, 156, 157, 160, 165
Malaysia, xxvii, 2, 15, 39, 55, 65, 73, 74, 80, 82, 83, 109, 129, 153
marriage, 60, 78, 79, 83, 99
Medicaid, 220
medical care, xx, 165, 190, 201
medical history, 202
Medicare, 190, 192, 194, 213, 220
memory, 9, 10, 16, 20, 22, 74, 155, 160
memory function, 10
mentor, 14, 16, 110, 125
military, 52, 64, 65, 131, 194
mission, 55, 130, 193, 196

N

nationalism, 27, 37
Nazi Germany, 1
New Haven, xxi, xxiii, 133, 140, 151, 176
New Zealand, 153
Nobel Prize, 27, 38

Index

nurses, 67, 87, 90, 91, 162, 201, 202, 219

O

Obama, President Barak, 103, 104, 105,
otolaryngologist, xvii, 17, 121, 122, 130, 135, 147, 197

P

parents, vii, xix, 2, 3, 5, 6, 8, 12, 15, 29, 41, 42, 44, 77, 82, 109, 129, 144, 150, 162, 163, 217
patient care, xx, 125, 196, 201, 206, 210
Penang, Malaya, xxvii, xxix, 2, 7, 12, 25, 27, 29, 33, 38, 39, 72, 88, 93, 97, 109, 156, 157, 160, 165, 218
perseverance, v, xvii, 14, 36, 92
personal life, 182, 195
physicians, 153, 196, 199, 215, 216, 220
positivity, v, xvii
Proust, Marcel, 31

R

risk management, 144, 147

S

scholarship, v, xv, 16, 26, 44, 45, 52, 53, 58, 64
school, 5, 11, 12, 13, 14, 15, 16, 17, 26, 32, 33, 36, 40, 43, 45, 47, 48, 49, 52, 53, 54, 55, 56, 57, 59, 60, 63, 71, 72, 77, 82, 85, 88, 90, 91, 92, 109, 119, 120, 122, 126, 136, 154, 156, 161, 162, 177, 185, 194, 196, 199, 210, 213, 219, 221
siblings, 4, 82, 162
Singapore, 2, 111, 146, 153, 163, 190, 191

South Africa, 44, 45
South Korea, 153
Southeast Asia, 2, 16, 27, 28, 44
surgery, v, xxi, xxii, xxiii, xxiv, xxxix, 16, 22, 69, 86, 87, 89, 90, 101, 106, 119, 120, 121, 122, 124, 125, 130, 131, 133, 135, 136, 137, 139, 140, 144, 145, 146, 150, 152, 164, 165, 173, 189, 198, 199, 201, 203, 210, 213

T

The Patient Is U Foundation, Inc. (TPIU), xix, xxii, 132, 168, 195, 196, 199, 200, 201, 206, 207, 208, 212
training, xxii, 3, 85, 87, 89, 92, 122, 130, 131, 132, 136, 162, 216
Truman, Harry S., 52

U

undergraduate education, 38, 43
United States, 12, 13, 20, 34, 57, 60, 73, 88, 129, 191, 209
universities, 12, 13, 16, 54
urologist, 121
US healthcare delivery system, v, xv

V

Vietnam, 80, 89, 129, 130, 132, 137
vision, xvii, 122, 176, 193, 210, 217

W

Washington, 73, 129, 130, 169
Watson, Professor James, xxxiv, 126, 218
White House, xxxiii, 106, 191, 192